MULTIPLE RISK FACTORS IN CARDIOVASCULAR DISEASE

STRATEGIES OF PREVENTION OF CORONARY HEART DISEASE,
CARDIAC FAILURE, AND STROKE

Medical Science Symposia Series

Volume 12

The titles published in this series are listed at the end of this volume.

Multiple Risk Factors in Cardiovascular Disease

Strategies of Prevention of Coronary Heart Disease, Cardiac Failure, and Stroke

Edited by

A. M. Gotto, Jr.
Cornell University Medical College,
New York, NY, U.S.A.

C. Lenfant
National Heart, Lung, and Blood Institute,
NIH, Bethesda, MD, U.S.A.

R. Paoletti
Institute of Pharmacological Sciences,
University of Milan, Italy

A. L. Catapano
Institute of Pharmacological Sciences,
University of Milan, Italy

and

A. S. Jackson
Giovanni Lorenzini Medical Foundation,
Houston, TX, U.S.A.

KLUWER ACADEMIC PUBLISHERS
DORDRECHT / BOSTON / LONDON

Fondazione Giovanni Lorenzini, Milan, Italy
Giovanni Lorenzini Medical Foundation, Houston, U.S.A.

A C.I.P. Catalogue record for this book is available from the Library of Congress.

ISBN 0-7923-5023-5

Published by Kluwer Academic Publishers,
P.O. Box 17, 3300 AA Dordrecht, The Netherlands.

Sold and distributed in the U.S.A. and Canada
by Kluwer Academic Publishers,
101 Philip Drive, Norwell, MA 02061, U.S.A.

In all other countries, sold and distributed
by Kluwer Academic Publishers,
P.O. Box 322, 3300 AH Dordrecht, The Netherlands.

Printed on acid-free paper

Printed in the Netherlands.

CONTENTS

PREFACE

This volume is a collection of the most significant contributions to the *4th International Symposium on MULTIPLE RISK FACTORS IN CARDIOVASCULAR DISEASE: STRATEGIES OF PREVENTION OF CORONARY HEART DISEASE, CARDIAC FAILURE, AND STROKE* held in Washington, D.C. in April 1997. The meeting focused on the risk factors for cardiovascular disease and their interactions. The need for this symposium is based on the epidemiological, clinical, and biological evidence that individuals from industrialized countries often possess two or more risk factors which synergistically increase the global risk profile. This has become more evident in recent years with the increase in life expectancy of populations in the industrialized countries. The evidence that a combination of risk factors confers a very high risk of developing cardiovascular diseases, is of pivotal interest in the process of detection of patients who will benefit the most from pharmacological treatment. Many recent epidemiological data identifying the intrinsic and environmental factors contributing to the development of atherosclerosis are discussed. These results, in parallel with basic and clinical research, underline atherosclerosis as a complex and multifactorial process involving the influences of lipids, including lipoprotein subfractions, blood pressure rheologic forces, carbohydrate tolerance, and thrombogenic factors, including fibrinogen, tissue factor, PAI-1, and homocysteine. Furthermore, the risk associated with any one of these risk factors varies widely depending on the level of the associated atherogenic risk factors. Hyper-cholesterolemia and hypertriglyceridemia, for instance, are more common than would be expected by chance among hypertensive patients. Hypertension also is more prevalent in those with abnormal lipid levels than in those with normal lipid levels. The association of many of these risk factors (upper body obesity, glucose intolerance, hyperlipemia, and high blood pressure) has been defined as the plurimetabolic syndrome or syndrome X, and is discussed in depth in this volume.

It is essential to consider a reduction in all risk factors involved in the development of atherosclerosis as the real end-point in any treatment. Special care should be used in selecting the pharmacological or nonpharmacological therapy without affecting adversely the cardiovascular profile. Hence, preventive management as well as risk estimation in individuals should be multifactorial with the goal of improving the cardiovascular risk profile, thus retarding or preventing the onset of heart or vascular disease. This is accomplished ultimately by causing existing lesions to regress, become stable, or progress more slowly, and also by preventing the formation of new lesions.

The information derived from this meeting should therefore be useful to specialists and practicing physicians in determining the diagnostic and therapeutic approach to patients presenting with multiple risk factors for cardiovascular disease.

The Editors

List of contributors

Yasunori Abe
Speros P. Martel Section of Leukocyte Biology, Department of Pediatrics, Baylor College of Medicine, Texas Children's Clinical Care Center, Ste 1130, 6621 Fannin, MC 3-2372, Houston, Texas 77030-2399, USA

Marie Christine Alessi
Laboratoire d'Hematologie, CHU Timone, 27, Bld Jean Moulin, 13385 Marseille Cedex 5, France

Lorenzo Arnaboldi
Institute of Pharmacological Sciences, University of Milan, Via Balzaretti 9, 20133 Milan, Italy

Gerd Assmann
Institute of Clinical Chemistry and Laboratory Medicine, University of Münster, Albert-Schweitzer-Strasse 33, 48149 Münster, Germany

Johan Auwerx
Unité 325 INSERM, Département d'Athérosclérose, Institut Pasteur de Lille, 1 rue du Professeur Calmette, 59019 Lille, France

Christie M. Ballantyne
Baylor College of Medicine, 6565 Fannin, M.S. A-601, Houston, Texas 77030, USA

Franco Bernini
Institute of Pharmacology and Pharmacognosy, University of Parma, 43100 Parma, Italy

Manlio Bolla
Center for Cardiopulmonary Pharmacology, Institute of Pharmacological Sciences, School of Pharmacy, University of Milan, 20133 Milan, Italy

Albino Bonazzi
Center for Cardiopulmonary Pharmacology, Institute of Pharmacological Sciences, School of Pharmacy, University of Milan, 20133 Milan, Italy

H. Bryan Brewer, Jr.
Molecular Disease Branch, National Heart, Lung, and Blood Institute, National Institutes of Health, Building 10, Room 7N115, 10 Center Drive MSC 1666, Bethesda, Maryland 20892-1666, USA

Carola Buccellati
Center for Cardiopulmonary Pharmacology, Institute of Pharmacological Sciences, School of Pharmacy, University of Milan, 20133 Milan, Italy

Peter Carmeliet
Center for Transgene Technology and Gene Therapy, Campus Gasthuisberg, Herestraat 49, University of Leuven, Leuven, B-3000, Belgium

Eugene I. Chazov
Cardiology Research Centre, Russian Academy of Medical Sciences, 3rd Cherepkovskaya Street 15a, Moscow 121552, Russia

Désiré Collen
Center for Transgene Technology and Gene Therapy, Flanders Interuniversity Institute for Biotechnology, Campus Gasthuisberg, University of Leuven, Leuven, B-3000, Belgium

Alberto Corsini
Institute of Pharmacological Sciences, University of Milan, Via Balzaretti 9, 20133 Milan, Italy

Michael H. Criqui
University of California, San Diego, Department of Family and Preventive Medicine, 9500 Gilman Drive, La Jolla, California 92093-0607, USA

Paul Cullen
Institute of Arteriosclerosis Research, University of Münster, Domagkstrasse 3, 48149 Münster, Germany

Ralph B. D'Agostino
Boston University, Department of Mathematics, Cummington Street, Boston, Massachusetts, USA

Jean Dallongeville
Unité 325 INSERM, Département d'Athérosclérose, Institut Pasteur de Lille, 1 rue du Professeur Calmette, 59019 Lille, France

Bassem El-Masri
Section of Atherosclerosis, Department of Medicine, Baylor College of Medicine, 6565 Fannin, MS A-601, Houston, Texas 77030, USA

Edzard Ernst
Department of Complementary Medicine, Postgraduate Medical School, University of Exeter, 25 Victoria Park Road, Exeter EX2 4NT, United Kingdom

Nicola Ferri
Institute of Pharmacological Sciences, University of Milan, Via Balzaretti 9, 20133 Milan, Italy

Giancarlo Folco
Center for Cardiopulmonary Pharmacology, Institute of Pharmacological Sciences, University of Milan, 20133 Milan, Italy

Aaron R. Folsom
Division of Epidemiology, School of Public Health, University of Minnesota, 1300 South Second Street, Suite 300, Minneapolis, Minnesota 55454-1015, USA

Jean-Charles Fruchart
Département d'Athérosclérose et INSERM U325, Institut Pasteur, 1, rue du Prof. Calmette, 59019 Lille Cédex, France

Remo Fumagalli
Institute of Pharmacological Sciences, University of Milan, Via Balzaretti 9, 20133 Milan, Italy

Harald Funke
Institute of Clinical Chemistry and Laboratory Medicine, University of Münster, Albert-Schweitzer-Strasse 33, 48149 Münster, Germany

Valentin Fuster
Cardiovascular Institute, Mount Sinai Medical Center, Box 1030, 1 Gustave Levy Place, New York, New York 10029-6574, USA

Antonio M. Gotto, Jr.
Cornell University Medical School, 1300 York Avenue, Room F-105, New York, New York 10021, USA

Steven M. Haffner
Department of Medicine, University of Texas Health Science Center at San Antonio, 7703 Floyd Curl Drive, San Antonio, Texas 78284-7873, USA

Hermann Haller
Franz Volhard Clinic, Wiltberg Strasse 50, 13122 Berlin, Germany

J. Alan Herd
Baylor College of Medicine, 6560 Fannin Street, Suite 1150, Houston, Texas 77030, USA

Jules Hirsch
The Rockefeller University, 1230 York Avenue, New York, New York 10021-6399, USA

Paul N. Hopkins
University of Utah, Cardiovascular Genetics Research Clinic, Cardiology Division, Department of Medicine, 410 Chipeta Way, Room 161, Salt Lake City, Utah 84108, USA

Mark C. Houston
Vanderbilt University Medical School, Hypertension Institute, 4230 Harding Road, 4th Floor, St. Thomas Medical Plaza, Saint Thomas Hospital, Nashville, Tennessee 37205, USA

Steven C. Hunt
University of Utah, Cardiovascular Genetics Research Clinic, Cardiology Division, Department of Medicine, 410 Chipeta Way, Room 161, Salt Lake City, Utah 84108, USA

M. Mohsen Ibrahim
Cardiology Department, Cairo University, 1 El-Sherifein Street, Abdin, Cairo 11111, Egypt

Terry A. Jacobson
Office of Health Promotion and Disease Prevention, Department of Medicine, Emory University School of Medicine, Thomas Glenn Building, 69 Butler St. SE, Atlanta, Georgia 30303, USA

Irène Juhan-Vague
Laboratoire d'Hematologie, CHU Timone, 27, Bld Jean Moulin, 13385 Marseille Cedex 5, France

Raymond Judware
Case Western Reserve University, School of Medicine, Molecular Cardiovascular Research Center, 10900 Euclid Ave., Cleveland, Ohio 44106, USA

William B. Kannel
Boston University School of Medicine, Framingham Heart Study, 5 Thurber Street, Framingham, Massachusetts 01701, USA

Kay T. Kimball
Design and Analysis Unit, Department of Medicine, Baylor College of Medicine, 6550 Fannin, MS 1201, Houston, Texas 77030, USA

Wolfgang Koenig
Department of Internal Med II-Cardiology, University of Ulm Medical Centre, Robert-Koch-Str. 8, D-89081 Ulm, Germany

Jean-Marc Lalouel
University of Utah, Department of Human Genetics and Howard Hughes Medical Institute, 410 Chipeta Way, Room 161, Salt Lake City, Utah 84108, USA

Eduardo G. Lapetina
Case Western Reserve University, School of Medicine, Molecular Cardiovascular Research Center, 10900 Euclid Ave., Cleveland, Ohio 44106, USA

John C. LaRosa
Tulane University Medical Center, 1430 Tulane Avenue SL 76, New Orleans, Louisiana 70112, USA

Jacques Maclouf
U348 INSERM, Hôpital Lariboisière, 75475 Paris, France

M. Rene Malinow
Division of Pathology-Immunology, Oregon Regional Primate Research Center, 505 NW 185th Ave., Beaverton, Oregon 97006-3448, USA

Eduardo Marban
Johns Hopkins School of Medicine, 720 North Rutland Ave., 844 Ross Building, Baltimore, Maryland 21205, USA

Kara L. Marchman
Office of Health Promotion and Disease Prevention, Grady Health Systems, 80 Butler Street, SE, Atlanta, Georgia 30335-3801, USA

Thomas S. McCormick
Case Western Reserve University, School of Medicine, Molecular Cardiovascular Research Center, 10900 Euclid Ave., Cleveland, Ohio 44106, USA

Ira S. Ockene
Preventive Cardiology Program, Division of Cardiovascular Medicine, University of Massachusetts Medical Center, 55 Lake Avenue North, Worcester, Massachusetts 01655, USA

Judith K. Ockene
Division of Preventive and Behavioral Medicine, University of Massachusetts Medical Center, 55 Lake Avenue North, Worcester, Massachusetts 01655, USA

Karin Osmundsen
Pronova Biocare, Strandveien 50, N-1324 Lysaker, Norway

Rodolfo Paoletti
Institute of Pharmacological Sciences, University of Milan, Via Balzaretti 9, 20133 Milan, Italy

Franco Pazzucconi
Center E. Grossi Paoletti, Institute of Pharmacological Sciences, University of Milan, Via Balzaretti 9, 20133 Milan, Italy

Henry Pownall
Section of Atherosclerosis, Department of Medicine, Baylor College of Medicine, 6565 Fannin, MS A-601, Houston, Texas 77030, USA

Pierangelo Quarato
Institute of Pharmacological Sciences, University of Milan, Via Balzaretti 9, 20133 Milan, Italy

Gerald M. Reaven
Stanford University School of Medicine and Shaman Pharmaceuticals, Inc., 213 East Grand Avenue, San Francisco, California 94080-4812, USA

Michael E. Rosenfeld
Department of Pathobiology, Box 353410, University of Washington, Seattle, Washington 98195, USA

Giuseppe Rossoni
Center for Cardiopulmonary Pharmacology, Institute of Pharmacological Sciences, School of Pharmacy, University of Milan, 20133 Milan, Italy

Angelo Sala
Center for Cardiopulmonary Pharmacology, Institute of Pharmacological Sciences, School of Pharmacy, University of Milan, 20133 Milan, Italy

Helmut Schulte
Institute of Arteriosclerosis Research, University of Münster, Domagkstrasse 33, 48149 Münster, Germany

Halit Silbershatz
Boston University, Department of Mathematics, Cummington Street, Boston, Massachusetts, USA

Cesare R. Sirtori
Institute of Pharmacological Sciences, University of Milan, Via Balzaretti 9, 20133 Milan, Italy

Sidney C. Smith, Jr.
Division of Cardiology, Center for Cardiovascular Disease, University of North Carolina at Chapel Hill, School of Medicine, Campus Box 7075, Chapel Hill, North Carolina 27599, USA

C. Wayne Smith
Speros P. Martel Section of Leukocyte Biology, Department of Pediatrics, Baylor College of Medicine, Texas Children's Clinical Care Ctr., Ste. 1130, 6621 Fannin, MC 3-2372, Houston, Texas 77030-2399, USA

Maurizio R. Soma
Institute of Pharmacological Sciences, University of Milan, Via Balzaretti 9, 20133 Milan, Italy

Bart Staels
Unité 325 INSERM, Département d'Athérosclérose, Institut Pasteur de Lille, 1 rue du Professeur Calmette, 59019 Lille, France

Daniel Steinberg
University of California, San Diego, Department of Medicine 0682, 9500 Gilman Drive, La Jolla, California 92093-0682, USA

George Steiner
Room NUW9-112, The Toronto Hospital (General Division), 200 Elizabeth Street, Toronto, Ontario M5G 2C4, Canada

Mark B. Taubman
Box 1269, Mount Sinai School of Medicine, One Gustave L. Levy Place, New York, NY 10029, USA

Gordon F. Tomaselli
Johns Hopkins School of Medicine, 720 North Rutland Ave., 844 Ross Building, Baltimore, Maryland 21205, USA

Diethelm Tschoepe
Diabetes Research Institute at the Heinrich Heine University Duesseldorf, Cellular Hemostasis and Clinical Angiology Group, Auf'm Hennekamp 65, 40225 Duesseldorf, Germany

Roger R. Williams
University of Utah, Cardiovascular Genetics Research Clinic, Cardiology Division, Department of Medicine, 410 Chipeta Way, Room 161, Salt Lake City, Utah 84108, USA

Peter W.F. Wilson
NHLBI, Framingham Heart Study, 5 Thurber Street, Framingham, Massachusetts 01701, USA

D.A. Wood
Imperial College School of Medicine at the National Heart and Lung Institute, Imperial College of Science, Technology and Medicine, University of London, Dovehouse Street, London SW3 6LY, United Kingdom

Kenneth Kun-yu Wu
Vascular Biology Research Center and Department of Medicine, University of Texas-Houston Medical School, 6431 Fannin St., MSB 5.016, Houston, Texas 77030, USA, and Vascular Biology and Atherothrombosis Program, Institute of Biomedical Sciences, Academia Sinica, Taipei, Taiwan

Lily Wu
University of Utah, Cardiovascular Genetics Research Clinic, Cardiology Division, Department of Medicine and, Department of Pathology, 410 Chipeta Way, Room 161, Salt Lake City, Utah 84108, USA

Jong K. Yun
Case Western Reserve University, School of Medicine, Molecular Cardiovascular Research Center, 10900 Euclid Ave., Cleveland, Ohio 44106, USA

Simona Zarini
Center for Cardiopulmonary Pharmacology, Institute of Pharmacological Sciences, School of Pharmacy, University of Milan, 20133 Milan, Italy

New Insights into the Role of HDL in the Development of Cardiovascular Disease

H. Bryan Brewer, Jr.

Introduction

Epidemiological studies have consistently demonstrated that plasma concentrations of high density lipoprotein (HDL) cholesterol are inversely correlated with the incidence of coronary heart disease (CHD) [1,2]. Although the mechanisms by which HDL protects against atherosclerosis remain to be definitively established, HDL has been postulated to facilitate the efflux of cholesterol from peripheral cells and transport the cholesterol back to the liver in a process termed reverse cholesterol transport [3]. The major apolipoprotein constituents of HDL are apoA-I and apoA-II. Plasma concentrations of apoA-I are inversely correlated with CHD, however the association of apoA-II levels with CHD has not been consistent [4,5]. A schematic overview of the proposed role of HDL in reverse cholesterol and lipoprotein metabolism is illustrated in Figure 1.

Routine screening of plasma HDL levels has been recommended by both the National Cholesterol Education Program [6] and the European Cholesterol Guidelines [7]. As HDL screening has become more extensive, asymptomatic individuals with abnormal plasma HDL levels have been identified with increasing frequency. This review will summarize recent studies on patients with hypoalphalipoproteinemias and hyperalphalipoproteinemias.

Hypoalphalipoproteinemia

Several epidemiological studies clearly established that low HDL is associated with an increased risk of CHD [1,2]. However, it is now known that not all individuals with low HDL cholesterol are at increased risk for premature CHD [8]. Several different genetic hypoalphalipoproteinemias do not have a marked increased risk of CHD including lecithin cholesterol acyltransferase (LCAT) deficiency [9], and selected kindreds with familial hypoalphalipoproteinemia [8]. Detailed metabolic studies in five kindreds with low HDL and no increased risk of CHD revealed that the low HDL levels were due to increased HDL catabolism with normal synthesis of both apoA-I and apoA-II [8].

Low HDL and increased triglycerides is a common lipoprotein phenotype in patients with established cardiovascular disease [10]. Aggressive treatment may reduce the risk of

1

A. M. Gotto, Jr. et al. (eds.), Multiple Risk Factors in Cardiovascular Disease, 1–7.
© 1998 *Kluwer Academic Publishers and Fondazione Giovanni Lorenzini. Printed in the Netherlands.*

coronary artery disease in these individuals. The identification of these individuals in the population represents a challenge for the physician since individuals with the genetic dyslipoproteinemia, familial hypertriglyceridemia, with low HDL and increased triglycerides have a similar lipoprotein phenotype but minimal increased risk of CHD [11]. A familial history of low HDL which cosegregates with CHD as well as the use of new noninvasive techniques including Ultrafast Computed Tomography [12] to detect coronary calcification maybe used to select those individuals with low HDL and hypertriglyceridemia which require treatment.

LIPOPROTEIN METABOLISM

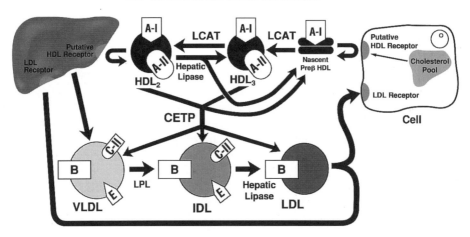

Figure 1. Overview of the metabolic pathways in lipoprotein metabolism. The major apoB containing lipoprotein particles include VLDL, IDL, and LDL. The hepatic apoB cascade involves the metabolic conversion of triglyceride rich VLDL secreted by the liver to LDL. VLDL triglycerides are hydrolyzed by lipoprotein lipase and remnants undergo stepwise delipidation with the formation of particles with a hydrated density of IDL and finally LDL. VLDL and IDL remnants are cleared from the plasma by interacting with the putative remnant and LDL receptors. Plasma LDL interacts with the LDL receptor on the liver and peripheral cells which initiates receptor mediated endocytosis and LDL degradation.

Disc-shaped nascent HDL are synthesized by both the liver and intestine. Nascent HDL removes excess cellular cholesterol and are converted to spherical lipoprotein particles with a hydrated density of HDL_3. Addition of cholesterol, phospholipids, and apolipoproteins from the metabolism of triglyceride rich lipoproteins and the uptake of cholesterol from peripheral tissues result in the conversion of lipoproteins in HDL_3 to particles with a hydrated density of HDL_2. Cholesterol in the lipoprotein particles is converted to cholesteryl esters by the enzyme lecithin cholesterol acyltransferase (LCAT). Cholesteryl esters are transferred to VLDL-IDL-LDL by the cholesterol ester transfer protein (CETP). Lipoproteins in HDL_2 are converted back to HDL_3 by the enzyme hepatic lipase.

Hyperalphalipoproteinemia

Several lines of evidence including epidemiological studies [1,2] have suggested that increased plasma HDL levels are associated with decreased CHD. In experimental animal studies, infusion of HDL+ very high density lipoprotein (VHDL) decreased atherosclerosis in cholesterol-fed rabbits [13]. Increased plasma HDL levels achieved by overexpressing human apoA-I in transgenic mice protect against the development of diet-induced atherosclerosis [14]. In addition, the atherosclerosis characteristic of apoE deficient mice was markedly decreased in the apoE deficient cross apoA-I transgenic mice overexpressing apoA-I [15]. In human studies, analysis of a kindred with markedly elevated HDL levels due to increased synthesis with normal catabolism of apoA-I is consistent with protection against CHD [16]. Based on these combined results it has been proposed that raising plasma HDL by dietary, pharmacologic, or genetic manipulation may be an effective strategy for the treatment of cardiovascular disease in man.

Recently, LCAT has been identified as a candidate gene for raising plasma HDL-cholesterol concentrations and decreasing atherosclerosis [17,18]. LCAT, a 63 kD plasma glycoprotein, is synthesized primarily in the liver [19], and is responsible for esterification of free cholesterol present in circulating plasma lipoproteins [3,20]. LCAT catalyzes the transfer of a fatty acid from the sn-2 position of phosphatidylcholine to the 3-hydroxyl group of cholesterol, yielding cholesteryl esters and lysolecithin [20]. In plasma, LCAT is found primarily associated with HDL [21] and to a lesser extent, it may also associate with apoB-containing non-HDL lipoproteins [22]. LCAT plays a central role in the maturation and metabolism of HDL as illustrated in Figure 1. LCAT mediates the esterification of free cholesterol which has been effluxed from peripheral cells and the cholesteryl esters are packaged into the core of the lipoprotein, converting discoidal particles into mature, spherical HDL [21,23]. HDL cholesteryl esters can then either be transported directly to the liver or transferred to apoB containing lipoproteins by the action of cholesteryl ester transfer protein (CETP) [24], for hepatic receptor mediated uptake and removal from the body [24-27]. LCAT in conjunction with CETP, hepatic lipase, and apoA-I play a central role in reverse cholesterol transport [3,20,28], a key process in the movement of cholesterol from peripheral cells to the liver.

To test the hypothesis that LCAT modulates plasma HDL concentrations as well as the development of atherosclerosis transgenic rabbits which overexpressed human LCAT were generated [17]. Rabbits expressing human LCAT demonstrated significant increases in plasma cholesterol, cholesteryl esters, phospholipids, and HDL-cholesterol . Of particular interest was the unexpected finding of a significant reduction in plasma non-HDL apoB containing lipoproteins [17]. To test the hypothesis that LCAT overexpression protected against atherosclerosis LCAT transgenic rabbits were placed for 16 weeks on a 0.3% cholesterol diet. When compared to controls, the plasma HDL-cholesterol and apoA-I concentrations were increased (p < 0.001) and the plasma non-HDL-lipoproteins decreased (p < 0.01) in LCAT transgenic rabbits after the high cholesterol diet. Thus, compared to controls, LCAT transgenic rabbits had increased HDL as well as decreased very low density lipoprotein (VLDL)/ intermediate density lipoprotein (IDL)/ low density lipoprotein (LDL).

Analysis of the aortas revealed that the LCAT transgenic rabbits had a 86% reduction in mean aortic lesion size when compared to control rabbits [18]. These results establish that LCAT overexpression in rabbits protects against the development of diet-induced atherosclerosis. LCAT represents an interesting candidate gene for gene therapy or drug development for atherosclerosis in man.

In the majority of cases elevated HDL appears to protect against premature CHD. However, several lines of evidence now indicate that elevated HDL may not always protect against CHD. LCAT transgenic mice like transgenic rabbits have increased plasma total cholesterol and HDL levels which correlated with plasma LCAT concentrations and activity [29]. High expressor transgenic mice had significant increases in plasma apoA-I, apoA-II, and apoE as well as the formation of two distinct HDL lipoproteins, apoE-rich HDL1 and apoA-I/apoA-II containing HDL [29]. These studies demonstrate that LCAT modulates mouse plasma HDL-cholesterol concentrations as well as HDL particle composition and heterogeneity *in vivo* resulting in hyperalphalipoproteinemia and a lipoprotein profile which would be anticipated to have a reduced risk of atherosclerosis.

To determine if LCAT overexpression protects against atherosclerosis in the LCAT transgenic mice, animals were placed on a high-fat high-cholesterol diet for 16 weeks [30]. When compared to control animals, LCAT transgenic mice had higher plasma HDL-cholesterol and apoA-I concentrations, but no significant differences in the plasma levels of the apoB containing lipoproteins [30]. In response to the atherogenic diet, mice overexpressing human LCAT had enhanced ($p < 0.002$) atherosclerosis when compared to controls [30]. Plasma LCAT concentrations were positively correlated with mean lesion size ($r=0.283$, $p < 0.02$), indicating that LCAT overexpression in mice resulted in enhanced, rather than reduced atherosclerosis as observed in the rabbit.

There are several differences in lipoprotein metabolism which may explain the results obtained on the protection against atherosclerosis in transgenic rabbits and mice. One important difference is the presence of CETP in the rabbit and its absence in the mouse. The exchange of cholesteryl ester from HDL to VLDL-IDL-LDL may represent a major pathway of reverse cholesterol transport in the rabbit and man which is missing in the mouse. In addition, the low plasma levels of the apoB containing lipoproteins in the LCAT transgenic rabbits which is not observed in LCAT transgenic mice may be of major importance in the protection against atherosclerosis in the LCAT transgenic rabbit.

In man, marked elevations of plasma HDL are observed in patients with CETP deficiency. To date the majority of patients with CETP deficiency have been reported from kindreds in Japan [31-33]. The marked increase in plasma HDL in patients with CETP deficiency has been shown by metabolic studies to be due to decreased catabolism of apoA-I and apoA-II [34]. Recently clinical studies in patients with CETP deficiency suggest an increased rather than a decreased risk of premature CHD [35,36].

Summary

Over the last decade a great of information has been acquired regarding the role of the plasma lipoproteins in the development of atherosclerosis. The importance of LDL in atherosclerosis has been clearly delineated and clinical studies as well as research has now turned to an analysis of the role of HDL and triglycerides in the development of CHD. There is growing evidence from animal and clinical studies that raising apoA-I and HDL may protect against atherosclerosis. Based on epidemiological and clinical studies elevated and decreased levels of plasma HDL are associated with decreased and increased risk of premature CHD respectively. However, not all patients with decreased plasma HDL or elevated levels of HDL are at risk or protected against atherosclerosis. New and improved methods of assessing atherosclerosis and risk will need to be developed in order to facilitate the physician in identifying those patients with abnormal HDL levels which require treatment.

References

1.   Miller GJ, Miller NE. Plasma high-density lipoprotein concentration and development of ischaemic heart-disease. Lancet 1975;1:16-19.

2.   Gordon DJ, Rifkind BM. High-density lipoprotein: The clinical implications of recent studies. N Engl J Med 1989;321:1311-16.

3.   Glomset JA, Janssen ET, Kennedy R, Dobbins J. Role of plasma lecithin:cholesterol acyltransferase in the metabolism of high density lipoproteins. J Lipid Res 1966;7:638-48.

4.   Miller NE. Associations of high-density lipoprotein subclasses and apolipoproteins with ischemic heart disease and coronary atherosclerosis. Am Heart J 1987;113:589-97.

5.   Rader DJ, Hoeg JM, Brewer HB, Jr. Quantitation of plasma apolipoproteins in the primary and secondary prevention of coronary artery disease. Ann Intern Med 1994;120:1012-25.

6.   Summary of the second report of the National Cholesterol Education Program (NCEP) Expert Panel on detection, evaluation, and treatment of high blood cholesterol in adults (Adult Treatment Panel II). JAMA 1993;269:3015-23.

7.   European Atherosclerosis Society. The recognition and management of hyperlipidemia in adults: A policy statement of the European Atherosclerosis Society. Eur Heart J 1988;9: 571-660.

8.   Rader DJ, Ikewaki K, Duverger N, et al. Very low high-density lipoproteins without coronary atherosclerosis. Lancet 1993;342:1455-58.

9.   Glomset JA, Assmann G, Gjone E, Norum KR. Lecithin:cholesterol acyltransferase deficiency and fish eye disease. In: Scriver CR, Beaudet AL, Sly WS, et al. The metabolic and molecular bases of inherited disease. 7th ed. New York: McGraw-Hill, Inc., 1995:1933-51.

10.   Schaefer EJ, Genest JJ, Jr., Ordovas JM, Salem DN, Wilson PWF. Familial lipoprotein disorders and premature coronary artery disease. Atherosclerosis 1994;108(Suppl.):S41-S54.

11.   Brunzell JD, Schrott HG, Motulsky AG, Bierman EL. Myocardial infarction in the familial forms of hypertriglyceridemia. Metabolism 1976;25:313-20.

12.   Hoeg JM, Feuerstein IM, Tucker EE. Detection and quantitation of calcific atherosclerosis by Ultrafast CT in children and young adults with homozygous familial hypercholesterolemia. Arterioscler Thromb 1994;14:1066-74.

13.   Badimon JJ, Badimon L, Fuster V. Regression of atherosclerotic lesions by high density lipoprotein plasma fraction in the cholesterol-fed rabbit. J Clin Invest 1990;85:1234-41.

14.   Rubin EM, Krauss RM, Spangler EA, Verstuyft JG, Clift SM. Inhibition of early atherogenesis in transgenic mice by human apolipoprotein AI. Nature 1991;353:265-67.

15.   Plump AS, Scott CJ, Breslow JL. Human apolipoprotein A-I gene expression increases high

density lipoprotein and suppresses atherosclerosis in the apolipoprotein E-deficient mouse. Proc Natl Acad Sci USA 1994;91:9607-11.

16.   Rader DJ, Schaefer JR, Lohse P, et al. Increased production of apolipoprotein A-I associated with elevated plasma levels of high-density lipoproteins, apolipoprotein A-I, and lipoprotein A-I in a patient with familial hyperalphalipoproteinemia. Metabolism 1993;42:1429-34.

17.   Hoeg JM, Vaisman BL, Demosky SJ, Jr., et al. Lecithin-cholesterol acyltransferase overexpression generates hyperalpha-lipoproteinemia and a nonatherogenic lipoprotein pattern in transgenic rabbits. J Biol Chem 1996;271:4396-4402.

18.   Hoeg JM, Santamarina-Fojo S, Berard AM, et al. Overexpression of lecithin:cholesterol acyltransferase in transgenic rabbits prevents diet-induced atherosclerosis. Proc Natl Acad Sci USA 1996;93:11448-53.

19.   McLean J, Wion K, Drayna D, Fielding C, Lawn R. Human lecithin-cholesterol acyltransferase gene: Complete gene sequence and sites of expression. Nucleic Acids Res 1986;14:9397-9406.

20.   Glomset JA. The plasma lecithin:cholesterol acyltransferase reaction. J Lipid Res 1968;9: 155-67.

21.   Francone OL, Gurakar A, Fielding C. Distribution and functions of lecithin:cholesterol acyltransferase and cholesteryl ester transfer protein in plasma lipoproteins. Evidence for a functional unit containing these activities together with apolipoproteins A-I and D that catalyzes the esterification and transfer of cell-derived cholesterol. J Biol Chem 1989;264: 7066-72.

22.   Chen CH, Albers JJ. Distribution of lecithin-cholesterol acyltransferase (LCAT) in human plasma lipoprotein fractions. Evidence for the association of active LCAT with low density lipoproteins. Biochem Biophys Res Commun 1982;107:1091-96.

23.   Castro GR, Fielding CJ. Early incorporation of cell-derived cholesterol into pre-beta-migrating high-density lipoprotein. Biochem 1988;27:25-29.

24.   Tall AR. Plasma cholesteryl ester transfer protein. J Lipid Res 1993;34:1255-1274.

25.   Goldstein JL, Brown MS, Anderson RG, Russell DW, Schneider WJ. Receptor-mediated endocytosis: Concepts emerging from the LDL receptor system. Annu Rev Cell Biol 1985;1: 1-39.

26.   Herz J, Hamann U, Rogne S, Myklebos O, Gausepohl H, Stanley KK. Surface location and high affinity for calcium of a 500 kDa liver membrane protein closely related to the LDL receptor suggest a physiological role as a lipoprotein receptor. EMBO J 1988;7:4119-27.

27.   Strickland DK, Ashcom JD, Williams S, Burgess WH, Migliorini M, Argraves WS. Sequence identity between alpha2-Macroglobulin receptor and low density lipoprotein receptor-related protein suggests that this molecule is a multifunctional receptor. J Biol Chem 1990;265: 17401-4.

28.   Miller NE, La Ville A, Crook D. Direct evidence that reverse cholesterol transport is mediated by high-density lipoprotein in rabbit. Nature 1985;314:109-11.

29.   Vaisman BL, Klein H-G, Rouis M, et al. Overexpression of human lecithin cholesterol acyltransferase leads to hyperalphalipoproteinemia in transgenic mice. J Biol Chem 1995;270: 12269-75.

30.   Berard AM, Remaley AT, Vaisman BL, et al. High plasma HDL concentrations associated with enhanced atherosclerosis in transgenic mice overexpressing lecithin cholesterol-acyltransferase. Nature Medicine 1997; in press

31.   Tall AR. Plasma cholesteryl ester transfer protein and high-density lipoproteins: new insights from molecular genetic studies. J Intern Med 1995;237:5-12.

32. Koizumi J, Mabuchi H, Yoshimura A, et al. Deficiency of serum cholesteryl-ester transfer activity in patients with familial hyperalphalipoproteinaemia. Atherosclerosis 1985;58: 175-86.
33. Kurasawa T, Yokoyama S, Miyake Y, Yamamura T, Yamamoto A. Rate of cholesteryl ester transfer between high and low density lipoproteins in human serum and a case with decreased transfer rate in association with hyperalphalipoproteinemia. J Biochem (Tokyo) 1985;98: 1499-1508.
34. Ikewaki K, Rader DJ, Sakamoto T, et al. Delayed catabolism of high-density lipoprotein apolipoproteins A-I and A-II in human cholesteryl ester transfer protein deficiency. J Clin Invest 1993;92:1650-58.
35. Hirano K-I, Yamashita S, Kuga Y, et al. Atherosclerotic disease in marked hyperalphalipoproteinemia: Combined reduction of cholesteryl ester transfer protein and hepatic triglyceride lipase. Arterioscler Thromb Vasc Biol 1995;15:1849-56.
36. Zhong S, Sharp DS, Grove JS, et al. Increased coronary heart disease in Japanese-American men with mutation in the cholesteryl ester transfer protein gene despite increased HDL levels. J Clin Invest 1996;97:2917-23.

MECHANISMS OF THE HYPOLIPIDEMIC ACTION OF FIBRATES

Johan Auwerx, Jean Dallongeville, Jean-Charles Fruchart, and Bart Staels

Pharmacological Action of Fibrates

Fibrates are generally effective in lowering elevated plasma triglycerides and cholesterol. The magnitude of lipid changes depends however upon the patients' pretreatment lipoprotein status [1], as well as upon the unique properties of each fibrate. The most pronounced effects of fibrates are a decrease in plasma triglyceride-rich lipoproteins and an increase in high density lipoprotein cholesterol (HDL-C) levels when baseline plasma concentrations are low [1]. The changes in the different lipoprotein fractions are reflected by changes in the concentrations of their major apolipoproteins. Fibrates efficiently reduce the apo C-III-containing particles of this lipoprotein class, which may be markers for increased risk for atherogenesis [2].

Evidence is available to implicate five major mechanisms underlying the above-mentioned modulation of lipoprotein phenotypes by fibrates:

(1) Induction of lipoprotein lipolysis (LPL). Part of the beneficial effects of fibrates on triglyceride-rich lipoprotein metabolism is likely due to an increased lipolysis. Increased triglyceride-rich lipoprotein lipolysis could be a reflection of changes in intrinsic LPL activity [3] or increased accessibility of triglyceride-rich lipoproteins for lipolysis by LPL [4]. Both increased plasma or tissue LPL activity [3] and reduced triglyceride-rich lipoprotein apo C-III content may significantly contribute to the hypolipidemic action of fibrates.

(2) Induction of hepatic fatty acid (FA) uptake and reduction of hepatic triglyceride production. In response to fibrates, there is an increase in FA uptake and conversion to acyl-CoA by the liver due to the induction of fatty acid transport protein (FATP) (Martin, Staels, and Auwerx, unpublished results) and acyl-CoA synthetase (ACS) [5] gene expression and activity. As a membrane transporter of long-chain fatty acids, FATP facilitates the passage of free fatty acids (FFA) across the plasma membrane. These FFA are subsequently esterified by the activity of ACS to acyl-CoA derivatives [5]. The induction of the β-oxidation pathway with a concomitant decrease in fatty acid synthesis by fibrates results in increased catabolism of these FAs resulting in a lower availability of fatty acids for triglyceride synthesis, a process which is also downregulated by fibrates [6].

(3) Increased removal of low density lipoprotein (LDL) particles. The interaction of the LDL particle with its receptor depends on the conformation of apo B-100 as well as on its structure. Small LDL possess a lower binding affinity for the LDL receptor than the

A. M. Gotto, Jr. et al. (eds.), Multiple Risk Factors in Cardiovascular Disease, 9–17.

intermediate or light forms. The above-mentioned modulation of the characteristics of plasma LDL after fibrates results in the formation of LDL with a higher affinity for the LDL receptor. Such particles are catabolized rapidly by the LDL receptor, leading to an average of 30% reduction in LDL-C levels in hypercholesterolemic patients.

(4) Reduction in neutral lipid (cholesteryl ester and triglyceride) exchange. This may result from decreased plasma levels of apo B-containing lipoprotein.

(5) Increase in HDL production and stimulation of reverse cholesterol transport. Fibrates increase the production of apo A-I and apo A-II in liver [7,8], which may contribute to the increase of plasma HDL concentrations and a more efficient reverse cholesterol transport.

Role of Transcription Factors in Mediating Fibrate Action

It has been known for several years that fibrates induce peroxisome proliferation in rodents. This process is linked to the induction of transcription of genes involved in peroxisomal β-oxidation, and is mediated by the activation of specific transcription factors, which have therefore been termed peroxisome proliferator activated receptors (PPARs).

THE PPAR FAMILY OF TRANSCRIPTION FACTORS

PPARs are members of the superfamily of nuclear hormone receptor proteins which are transcription factors transmitting the signal originating from lipid soluble factors, such as hormones, vitamins, and fatty acids, directly to the genome [9]. All nuclear receptors recognize and bind to derivatives of a specific DNA recognition sequence (PuGGTCA; Pu:any purine), termed response element. During evolution, mutation, duplication, and addition of flanking sequences have generated response elements distinctive for the various receptors. Once bound to its response element, the receptor complex can activate or repress the expression of a target gene. Transactivation or repression can occur through direct interaction with components of the transcription preinitiation complex or via specific proteins, adaptors, or coactivators, which bridge the receptor to the transcription machinery.

THE ROLE OF PPARS IN MEDIATING FIBRATE-ACTION ON LIPOPROTEIN METABOLISM IN MAN

In humans considerable progress has been made in elucidating the role of PPARs in mediating the regulation of genes involved in lipoprotein metabolism by fibrates.

Triglyceride-rich lipoprotein metabolism. The hypotriglyceridemic action of fibrates involves combined effects on LPL and apo C-III expression resulting in increased lipolysis. It is well established that fibrates increase post-heparin plasma LPL activity [3,10]. The induction of LPL expression occurs at the transcriptional level and is mediated by PPAR which binds to a PPRE which is present both in the human and the mouse LPL gene promoters. Interestingly, fibrate treatment increases LPL mRNA levels in liver a tissue which contains primarily PPARα, but not in adipose tissue, which contains primarily PPARγ [11]. In contrast, administration of thiazolidinediones, which are specific PPARγ ligands, results in increased LPL expression and activity only in adipose tissue, but not in liver or muscle [11]. These data indicate that the LPL PPRE can mediate the induction of LPL gene expression by both PPARα and γ.

In contrast to LPL, transcription of the apo C-III gene is inhibited by fibrates, resulting in a decreased production of apo C-III in the liver [12]. The repression of apo C-III gene expression by fibrates is mediated by a PPRE located in the apo C-III gene promoter [13] which has previously been shown to mediate transregulation by other members of the nuclear hormone receptor superfamily, such as the strong liver-specific transcription factor HNF-4. The repression of apo C-III gene expression by fibrates appears to be mediated via a dual mechanism acting through this site [13]. First, PPAR can compete for binding of HNF-4 to this site. Furthermore, fibrates decrease the expression levels of HNF-4. Both mechanisms would contribute to the lowered apo C-III gene transcription observed after fibrate treatment. Consistent with the repression of apo C-III expression, turn-over studies in humans indicate that fibrates reduce apo C-III synthesis. The fibrate induced reduction in apo C-III levels enhances the LPL-mediated effects on lipoprotein metabolism and results in both an increased catabolism of VLDL particles and an increased apo E-dependent clearance of VLDL remnants. Consequently, this dual action of fibrates on LPL and apo C-III gene expression may cause a reduction in plasma triglyceride concentrations and have thereby a beneficial effect on postprandial hypertriglyceridemia [14].

Recent animal studies suggest that fibrates exert their hypolipidemic action not only by enhancing the catabolism of triglyceride-rich lipoproteins but also by increasing the hepatic uptake of FFA [15]. The cellular uptake of long-chain fatty acids may be facilitated by fatty acid transporters, such as the fatty acid transporter protein (FATP) [16] and the fatty acid transporter (FAT) [17]. Preliminary studies indicate that the expression of these fatty acid transporters in rat liver is enhanced by fibrate treatment (Staels, Martin, Auwerx, unpublished results). While membrane transporters facilitate the passage of FFA across the plasma membrane, the acyl-CoA synthethase (ACS)-dependent esterification of these FFA to acyl-CoA derivatives prevents efflux from the cell [16]. This enzyme also activates the FFA for utilization in both catabolic (β-oxidation) and/or anabolic pathways (conversion into more complex cellular lipids). ACS gene expression and activity is induced by fibrates in a variety of tissues and cells via PPAR interacting with a PPRE located in the C-ACS promoter [5]. It is interesting to note that in rodents fibrate-induced ACS activity generates acyl-CoA esters which are predominantly used for β-oxidation [18]. Due to the increased activity of the peroxisomal β-oxidation pathway less acyl-CoA esters are available for triglyceride synthesis. A reduction in acetyl-CoA carboxylase [19] and FAS [20] activity inhibits de novo fatty acid synthesis thereby further diminishing the intracellular levels of FFA available for triglyceride synthesis. Moreover, fibrates have been reported not only to increase b-oxidation and decrease triglyceride synthesis [21], but also to decrease apo B and VLDL production [6,19]. As a consequence, a reduced secretion of VLDL particles together with the enhanced catabolism of triglyceride-rich particles most likely account for the hypolipidemic effect of fibrates. Further studies are required, however, to determine whether fibrates also regulate these genes in humans.

HDL metabolism. Studies in rodents have demonstrated that fibrates decrease HDL-C by lowering liver apo A-I and apo A-II gene expression [22,23]. In contrast, in man fibrates increase plasma levels of HDL and its major constituents apo A-I and apo A-II to a variable extent [24,25] and stimulate apo A-I production in human hepatocytes [8]. *In vitro* studies have demonstrated that the induction of human apo A-I gene expression after fibrates may be mediated by interaction of PPAR with a functional PPRE, localized in the A site of the apo A-I promoter. The lack of induction of apo A-I expression by fibrates in rodents is due to minor sequence differences between the human and rodent A-sites, which prevents the rodent A-site from binding to PPAR [8,26]. These *in vitro* observations have been confirmed by *in vivo* studies using transgenic mice overexpressing the human apo A-I gene under control of its homologous promoter containing the A-site [8]. In these mice, treatment with fibrates results in the transcriptional induction of human apo A-I gene expression, whereas the endogenous mouse apo A-I gene is repressed [8]. Furthermore, fibrate treatment increases plasma concentrations of HDL containing human apo A-I in these mice. Altogether these data indicate that fibrates have opposite effects on apo A-I gene expression in rodents and humans, due to differences in regulatory elements in their respective genes.

Human apo A-II plasma concentrations increase after fibrate treatment. This is a consequence of the induction of hepatic apo A-II synthesis by fibrates and is mediated through PPAR/RXR heterodimers which bind to an imperfect DR-1 in the apo A-II J site. Apo A-II production rate appears to be a determinant factor in the distribution of apo A-I among the LpA-I and Lp A-I:A-II particles [27], being inversely correlated with LpA-I levels. Therefore an increase in apo A-II production would result in a shift of apo A-I from Lp A-I to Lp A-I:A-II, resulting in lower Lp A-I and higher Lp A-I:A-II levels, which may be observed during fibrate treatment. The opposite effects of fibrates on apo A-I (increased [26]) and Lp A-I (decreased [28]) plasma levels are a reflection of the combined induction of apo A-I and apo A-II expression by fibrates.

Clinical Implications Use of Fibrates Treatment in Specific Lipoprotein Disorders

PRIMARY HYPERTRIGLYCERIDEMIA

Fibrates are first-line drugs for the treatment of primary hypertriglyceridemia. In these patients, fibrates most noticeably decrease plasma triglyceride-rich lipoproteins [29], but they also decrease, albeit to a lesser extent, total cholesterol, whereas HDL-C levels increase. The reduction in cholesterol and triglycerides is mainly due to the fall in VLDL, which is accompanied by changes in VLDL composition [30]. Fibrates predominantly reduce the concentrations of large VLDL subfractions [31], due to increased lipoprotein lipase activity [31]. The percent change in the concentration of large VLDL is inversely correlated with the changes in HDL and LDL [32].

Hypertriglyceridemic patients have low levels of dense LDL-C with an abnormal lipid composition [33], due to a decreased conversion of VLDL and a faster clearance of LDL. Treatment of hypertriglyceridemic subjects with fibrates normalizes the lipid composition of their LDL [29]. The cholesterol-ester content of LDL increases in all LDL subclasses resulting in large, less dense LDL particles [31,33]. These changes lead to a better interaction of LDL particles with the LDL receptor thereby improving LDL clearance.

HDL-C, which is low in patients with hypertriglyceridemia [34], increases after treatment with fibrates [29,30]. The lowering of the pool of triglyceride-rich lipoproteins upon treatment with fibrates decreases the availability of TG for CETP-mediated exchange with the cholesteryl ester (CE) of HDL. The resulting reduction in net CE transfer from HDL to triglyceride-rich lipoproteins [35], associated with unchanged lecithin:cholesterol acyl transferase (LCAT) activity will ultimately lead to an increase in cholesteryl ester and a decrease in triglyceride content of HDL. Although no direct correlation has been observed between the magnitude of changes in plasma triglycerides and HDL-C, the extent of HDL rise upon treatment with fibrates appears to depend on the distinct primary metabolic defects and on the levels of plasma triglyceride attained after treatment [36]. Improvement of LPL-mediated lipolysis of triglyceride-rich lipoproteins [31] and increased apo A-I and apo A-II synthesis may all contribute to the rise in HDL levels upon treatment with fibrates. Increased HDL levels after fibrate treatment are associated with increased LPL activity [31], although these observations are still somewhat controversial. In addition, fibrates attenuate the postprandial lipid response in hypertriglyceridemic subjects [37]. The improvement in postprandial lipemia, which is a cardiovascular risk factor [38], is attributed to the increase in LPL and hepatic lipase activity which favors clearance of triglyceride-rich lipoproteins of both endogenous and exogenous origin.

COMBINED HYPERLIPIDEMIA

It is estimated that fibrates reduce the ten-year probability for myocardial infarction in patients with primary combined hyperlipidemia [39]. Fibrates effectively lower plasma cholesterol, VLDL-C, and triglycerides and increase HDL-C in combined hypertriglyceridemia. The effect of fibrates on LDL-C are more evident than in patients with primary hypertriglyceridemia [40]. The reduction in total cholesterol is accounted for by the fall in both VLDL-C and LDL-C [41], whereas the reduction of triglyceride levels is associated with normalization of the typical atherogenic LDL subspecies profile in familial combined hyperlipidemia. Treatment with fibrates reduces the levels of dense LDL and LDL-triglyceride content [40]. Mean LDL peak particle size may increase to normal [40] or remain small [42]. The mean LDL flotation rate augments due to an increase in buoyant LDL [42].

PRIMARY HYPERCHOLESTEROLEMIA

Although fibrates are not considered to be first-line drugs in primary hypercholesterolemia [43,44], the new generation of fibrates efficiently reduce plasma cholesterol and LDL-C and increase HDL-C levels when used in monotherapy in patients with primary hypercholesterolemia [41,45]. The reduction in total cholesterol is accounted for by a fall in both VLDL-C and LDL-C [45]. Kinetic studies demonstrated that fibrates inhibit the formation of slowly metabolized LDL. Fibrates reduce the dense LDL but not the light LDL fraction and increase the mean cholesteryl ester content of LDL while the triglyceride content decreases [46], resulting in less dense and larger LDL subspecies [47], which are less susceptible to oxidation [33]. The affinity of LDL to cellular receptors was not affected by treatment. The increase in HDL-C is related to a lower CETP activity whereas LCAT activity is not affected. Also in patients with primary hypercholesterolemia, LPL activity increases upon treatment with fibrates resulting in a reduction of postprandial lipemia [48].

Conclusion

Fibrate is a lipid lowering agent with pleiotropic effects. As a consequence of its potent action on PPAR, LpL gene expression and activity increases in adipose tissue; apo C-III gene, in contrast, is inhibited. The combination of these effects result in activation of lipoprotein lipolysis. Finally, both apo A-I and apo A-II gene expression are stimulated.

Acknowledgements

Delphine Cayet, Eric Baugé and Odile Vidal are thanked for excellent technical help in research. Michael Briggs, Samir Deeb, Paul Grimaldi, Richard Heyman, Guy Mannaerts, Jim Paterniti, Senen Vilaro, and Walter Wahli are acknowledged for stimulating discussions, support, and suggestions. K. Schoonjans was supported by fellowships from ARC and IFN, J. Auwerx is a research director, and B. Staels is a research associate of the CNRS. This work was supported by INSERM U325, Institut Pasteur de Lille, Région Nord - Pas-de-Calais.

References

1.   Tikkanen MJ. Fibric acid derivatives. Curr Opin Lipidol 1992;3:29-33.
2.   Bard JM, Parra HJ, Camare R, et al. A multicenter comparison of the effects of simvastatin and fenofibrate therapy in severe primary hypercholesterolemia, with particular emphasis on lipoproteins defined by their apolipoprotein composition. Metabolism 1992;41:498-503.
3.   Heller F, Harvengt C. Effects of clofibrate, bezafibrate, fenofibrate, and probucol on plasma lipolytic enzymes in normolipidaemic subjects. Eur J Clin Pharmacol 1983;23:57-63.
4.   Goldberg AP, Applebaum-Bowden DM, Bierman EL, et al. Increase in lipoprotein lipase during clofibrate treatment of hypertriglyceridemia in patients on hemodialysis. N Engl J Med 1979;301:1073-76.
5.   Schoonjans K, Watanabe M, Suzuki H, et al. Induction of the acyl-coenzyme A synthetase gene by fibrates and fatty acids is mediated by a peroxisome proliferator response element in the C promoter. J Biol Chem 1995;270:19269-76.
6.   Lamb RG, Koch JC, Bush SR. An enzymatic explanation of the differential effects of oleate and gemfibrozil on cultured hepatocyte triacylglycerol and phosphatidylcholine biosynthesis and secretion. Biochim Biophys Acta 1993;1165:299-305.

7. Vu-Dac N, Schoonjans K, Kosykh V, et al. Fibrates increase human apolipoprotein A-II expression through activation of the peroxisome proliferator-activated receptor. J Clin Invest 1995;96:741-50.

8. Berthou L, Duverger N, Emmanuel F, et al. Opposite regulation of human versus mouse apolipoprotein A-I by fibrates in human apo A-I transgenic mice. J Clin Invest 1996;97:in press.

9. Evans RM. The steroid and thyroid hormone receptor superfamily. Science 1988;240:889-95.

10. Zimetbaum P, Frishman WH, Kahn S. Effects of gemfibrozil and other fibric acid derivatives on blood lipids and lipoproteins. J Clin Pharmacol 1991;31:25-37.

11. Schoonjans K, Staels B, Deeb S, Auwerx J. Fibrates and fatty acids induce lipoprotein lipase gene expression via the peroxisome proliferator activated receptor. Circulation 1995;92/8:I-495.

12. Staels B, Vu-Dac N, Kosykh V, et al. Fibrates down-regulate apolipoprotein C-III expression independent of induction of peroxisomal acyl co-enzyme A oxidase. J Clin Invest 1995;95:705-12.

13. Hertz R, Bishara-Shieban J, Bar-Tana J. Mode of action of peroxisome proliferators as hypolipidemic drugs, suppression of apolipoprotein C-III. J Biol Chem 1995;270:13470-75.

14. Auwerx J, Schoonjans K, Fruchart JC, Staels B. Transcriptional control of triglyceride metabolism; fibrates change the expression of the LPL and apo C-III genes by activating the nuclear receptor PPAR. Atherosclerosis 1995;in press.

15. Frenkel B, Mayorek N, Hertz R, Bar-Tana J. The hypochylomicronemic effect of beta, beta'-methyl-substituted hexadecanedioic acid (MEDICA 16) is mediated by a decrease in apolipoprotein C-III. J Biol Chem 1988;263:8491-97.

16. Schaffer JE, Lodish HF. Expression cloning and characterization of a novel long chain fatty acid transport protein. Cell 1994;79:427-36.

17. Abumrad NA, El-Maghrabi MR, Amri E-Z, Lopez E, Grimaldi PA. Cloning of a rat adipocyte membrane protein implicated in binding or transport of long-chain fatty acids that is induced during preadipocyte differentiation. J Biol Chem 1993;268:17665-68.

18. Aarsland A, Berge R. Peroxisome proliferating sulphur-and oxysubstituted fatty acid analogues are activated to acyl coenzyme A thioesters. Biochem Pharmacol 1990;41:53-61.

19. Asiedu DK, Al-Shurbaji A, Rustan AC, Björkhem I, Berge RK. Hepatic fatty acid metabolism as a determinant of plasma and liver triacylglycerol levels. Studies on tetradecylthioacetic and tetradecylthiopropionic acids. Eur J Biochem 1995;227:715-22.

20. Blake WL, Clarke SD. Suppression of rat hepatic fatty acid synthase and S14 transcription by dietary polyunsaturated fat. J Nutr 1990;120:1727-29.

21. Rustan AC, Christiansen EN, Drevor CA. Serum lipids, hepatic glycerolipid metabolism and peroxisomal fatty acid oxidation in rats fed omega-3 and omega-6 fatty acids. Biochem J 1992;283:333-39.

22. Staels B, Van Tol A, Andreu T, Auwerx J. Fibrates influence the expression of genes involved in lipoprotein metabolism in a tissue-selective manner in the rat. Arterioscl Thromb 1992;12:286-94.

23. Berthou L, Saladin R, Yaqoob P, et al. Regulation of rat liver apolipoprotein A-I, apolipoprotein A-II, and acyl-CoA oxidase gene expression by fibrates and dietary fatty acids. Eur J Biochem 1995;232:179-87.

24. Malmendier CL, Delcroix C. Effects of fenofibrate on high and low density lipoprotein metabolism in heterozygous familial hypercholesterolemia. Atherosclerosis 1985;55:161-69.

25. Mellies MJ, Stein EA, Khoury P, Lamkin G, Glueck CJ. Effects of fenofibrate on lipids,

lipoproteins and apolipoproteins in 33 subjects with primary hypercholesterolaemia. Atherosclerosis 1987;63:57-64.

26.   Vu-Dac N, Schoonjans K, Laine B, Fruchart JC, Auwerx J, Staels B. Negative regulation of the human apolipoprotein A-I promoter by fibrates can be attenuated by the interaction of the peroxisome proliferator-activated receptor with its response element. J Biol Chem 1994;269: 31012-18.

27.   Ikewaki K, Zech LA, Kindt M, Brewer HBJ, Rader DJ. Apolipoprotein A-II production rate is a major factor regulating the distribution of apolipoprotein A-I among HDL subclasses LpA-I and LpA-I:A-II in normolipidemic humans. Arter Thromb Vasc Biol 1995;15:306-12.

28.   Lussier-Cacan S, Bard J-M, Boulet L, et al. Lipoprotein composition changes induced by fenofibrate in dysbetalipoproteinemia type III. Atherosclerosis 1989;78:167-82.

29.   Sirtori C, Franceschini G, Gianfranceschini G, et al. Activity profile of gemfibrozil on the major plasma lipoprotein parameters. Eur J Epidemiol 1992;8:120-24.

30.   Bradford RH, Goldberg AC, Schonfeld G, Knopp RH. Double-blind comparison of bezafibrate versus placebo in male volunteers with hyperlipoproteinemia. Atherosclerosis 1992;92:31-40.

31.   Dachet C, Cavalerro E, Martin C, Girardot G , Jacotot B. Effect of gemfibrozil on the concentration and composition of very low density and low density lipoprotein subfractions in hypertriglyceridemic patients. Atherosclerosis 1995;113:1-9.

32.   Pauciullo P, Marotta G, Rubba P, et al. Serum lipoproteins, apolipoproteins and very low density lipoprotein subfractions during 6-month fibrate treatment in primary hypertriglyceridaemia. J Intern Med 1990;228:425-30.

33.   de Graaf J, Hendriks JC, Demacker PN, Stalenhoef AF. Identification of multiple dense LDL subfractions with enhanced susceptibility to in vitro oxidation among hypertriglyceridemic subjects. Normalization after clofibrate treatment. Arterioscl Thromb 1993;13:712-19.

34.   Avogaro P, Ghiselli G, Soldan S, Bittolo-Bon G. Relationship of triglycerides and HDL cholesterol in hypertriglyceridaemia. Atherosclerosis 1992;92:79-86.

35.   Mann CJ, Yen FT, Grant AM , Bihain BE. Mechanism of plasma cholesteryl ester transfer in hypertriglyceridemia. J Clin Invest 1991;88:2059-66.

36.   Weis S, Kudchodkar BJ, Clearfield MB, Lacko AG. The efficacy of gemfibrozil therapy for raising high density lipoprotein levels. Artery 1992;19:353-66.

37.   Ditschuneit HH, Fletchtner-Mors M, Hagel E, Ditschuneit H. Postprandial lipoprotein metabolism in obese patients with moderate hypertriglyceridaemia: Effect of gemfibrozil. J Intern Med Res 1992;20:197-210.

38.   Karpe F, Steiner G, Uffelman K, Olivecrona T, Hamsten A. Postprandial lipoproteins and progression of coronary atherosclerosis. Atherosclerosis 1994;106:83-97.

39.   Athyros VG, Papageorgiou AA, Avramidis MJ, Kontopoulos AG. Long-term effect of gemfibrozil on coronary heart disease risk profile of patients with primary combined hyperlipidaemia. Coron Artery Dis 1995;6:251-56.

40.   Bruckert E, Desager S, Chapman MJ. Ciprofibrate therapy normalises the atherogenic low-density lipoprotein subspecies profile in combined hyperlipidemia (published erratum appears in Atherosclerosis 1993;102(1):129). Atherosclerosis 1993;100:91-102.

41.   Cattin L, Da-Col PG, Feruglio FS, et al. Efficacy of ciprofibrate in primary type II and IV hyperlipidemia: The Italian multicenter study. Clin Ther 1990;12:482-88.

42.   Hokanson JE, Austin MA, Zambon A, Brunzell JD. Plasma triglyceride and LDL heterogenity in familial combined hyperlipidemia. Arterioscl Thromb 1993;13:427-34.

43.   Summary of the second report of the National Cholesterol Education Program (NCEP) expert

panel on detection, evaluation, and treatment of high blood cholesterol adults (adult treatment panel II). JAMA 1993;269:3015-23.

44.   Prevention of coronary heart disease: Scientific background and new clinical guidelines. Recommendations of the European Atherosclerosis Society prepared by international task force for preventions of coronary heart disease. Nut Metab Cardiovasc Dis 1992;2:113-56.

45.   Lupien PJ, Brun D, Gagne C, Moorjani S, Bielman P, Julien P. Gemfibrozil therapy in primary type II hyperlipoproteinemia: Effects on lipids, lipoproteins and apolipoproteins. Can J Cardiol 1991;7:27-33.

46.   Tilly-Kiesi M, Tikkanen MJ. Low density lipoprotein density and composition in hypercholesterolaemic men treated with HMG CoA reductase inhibitors and gemfibrozil. J Intern Med 1991;229:427-34.

47.   Tsai MY, Yuan J, Hunninghake DB. Effect of gemfibrozil on composition of lipoproteins and distribution of LDL subspecies. Atherosclerosis 1992;95:35-42.

48.   Simpson HS, Williamson CM, Olivecrona T, et al. Postprandial lipemia, fenofibrate and coronary artery disease. Atherosclerosis 1990;85:193-202.

LIPID LOWERING DRUGS AND THE ARTERIAL WALL

R. Paoletti, F. Bernini, A. Corsini, and M. Soma

Introduction

In the last decade a new class of agents which specifically inhibit 3-hydroxy-3-methylglutaryl coenzyme A (HMG-CoA) reductase, the rate limiting enzyme in cholesterol biosynthesis, was developed [1]. A number of clinical studies have demonstrated that HMG-CoA reductase inhibitors (vastatins) can induce regression of vascular atherosclerosis [2-4], decrease the incidence of coronary heart disease (CHD) [2,3], and improve survival in CHD patients [5].

In patients with atherosclerosis it is presumed that any beneficial effects of vastatins would be linked to their hypolipidemic properties, thus suggesting that the hypolipidemic effect is the main mechanism for preventing the development of atherosclerosis [6,7]. However, since mevalonic acid (MVA), the product of the enzyme reaction, is the precursor of numerous metabolites, inhibition of HMG-CoA reductase has the potential to result in pleiotropic effects [8-11]. Indeed, MVA is not only the precursor of cholesterol, but also of a number of nonsteroidal isoprenoid compounds essential for normal cellular activity such as dolichol, heme A, ubiquinone, and isopentenyladenosine [8,9]. MVA is also the source of the covalently modifying prenyl group(s) (farnesol and geranylgeraniol) of a limited set of isoprenylated proteins involved in signal transduction and in the control of cell proliferation [9,12,13]. Other mechanisms, therefore, potentially contribute to the beneficial antiatherosclerotic effect of HMG-CoA reductase inhibitors [14,15]. This possibility is supported by experimental evidence indicating that some vastatins can interfere with major events involved in the formation of atherosclerotic lesions independently of their hypocholesterolemic properties [16-19].

In the present article we summarize our experience in investigating the direct antiatherosclerotic properties of vastatins.

Effect of Vastatins on Cholesterol Metabolism in Macrophages

Modified LDL, like acetylated LDL (AcLDL), deliver to macrophages, after lysosomal degradation, large amounts of unesterified cholesterol which stimulate the activity of the microsomal enzyme acyl-CoA:cholesterol acyltransferase (ACAT) with consequent intracellular accumulation of esterified cholesterol [20]. This process may induce lipid accumulation in the arterial wall, a major event of atherogenesis [21].

A. M. Gotto, Jr. et al. (eds.), Multiple Risk Factors in Cardiovascular Disease, 19–24.

Several compounds have been reported to reduce cholesterol esterification in cells. Some act directly by inhibiting ACAT activity [22], others indirectly by reducing lipoprotein degradation and their cholesteryl ester hydrolysis in the lysosomes [23,24], by slowing down intracellular cholesterol movement [25,26] or inhibiting scavenger receptor expression and cellular influx of modified lipoproteins [27,28]. Depending on the mechanism involved each agent may have different effects on cellular cholesterol content, localization, and on esterified to free form ratio. ACAT inhibitors may increase free cholesterol content of the plasma membrane, with minor effect on total cellular cholesterol [29]. Free cholesterol accumulation in lysosomes is observed with compounds active on intracellular cholesterol movement [25,26]. Accumulation of cholesteryl esters in these organelles is achieved with agents inhibiting the activity of lysosomal enzymes [23,24]. Finally, a decrease of total cellular cholesterol is observed with compounds inhibiting the expression of scavenger receptors [28]. Recently it was reported that vastatins are able to inhibit cholesterol esterification and deposition induced by AcLDL in human macrophages [30] and mouse peritoneal macrophages (MPM) [31,32]. Since this inhibition did not occur neither in cell-free homogenates nor in cholesterol preloaded cells, but was observed only when vastatins were simultaneously incubated with AcLDL, it was concluded that these drugs are not direct inhibitors of ACAT. Results obtained in our laboratory showed that inhibition of cholesterol esterification in MPM by vastatins could be fully reversed by exogenous mevalonate or by geranylgeraniol (a mevalonate metabolite), and took place in the presence of an excess of exogenous cholesterol [31]. These results provided the first evidence that mevalonate pathway plays an essential role in the process of esterification of excess cholesterol delivered to macrophages by modified LDL.

In our laboratory we also showed that HMG-CoA reductase inhibitors reduce *in vitro* cholesterol accumulation elicited by AcLDL in mouse peritoneal macrophages by inhibiting the endocytosis of these lipoproteins by cells [22]. Inhibition ^{125}I AcLDL degradation and fluorescent DI-acLDL internalization offered direct evidence for this conclusion.

The mechanism involved in fluvastatin action on AcLDL endocytosis needs clarification. The effect is not related to a decreased expression of the scavenger receptors since no decrease of cellular binding at 4°C could be detected. Although we cannot exclude an inhibitory effect of vastatins on the endocytosis of other ligands, the effect on AcLDL seems not due to a nonspecific depression of cellular endocytotic functions since in the condition in which AcLDL degradation was reduced, a slight but significant increase of native LDL degradation was. Our results show that the inhibition by fluvastatin of AcLDL catabolism is reversed by mevalonate and its isoprenoid derivative geranylgeraniol. This result suggests the involvement of nonsterol products of the mevalonate pathway in AcLDL endocytosis. Interestingly, data from our laboratory indicate that the effects of fluvastatin are more pronounced in cholesterol loaded cells. This result may be explained by the lower HMG-CoA reductase activity in cholesterol-rich cells as compared to unloaded cells [9]. This observation suggests the possibility that the mevalonate pathway in the arterial lesions may represent a selective target for pharmacological intervention.

Effect of Vastatin on Myocyte Migration and Proliferation

Two additional key events in the atherogenic cascade are the migration and proliferation of arterial myocytes, [21,33-35]. MVA and other intermediates (isoprenoids) of cholesterol biosynthesis are essential for these processes [9,11,36], hence it is conceivable that vastatins can affect directly migration and proliferation of arterial myocytes

Our results show that treatment of cultured arterial myocyte smooth muscle cells (SMC) with vastatins inhibits their proliferation. This effect was overcome by simultaneous exposure of SMC to exogenous MVA. One critical end product of MVA is cholesterol that, in proliferating cells, is required for cell membrane formation [9,37]. It is unlikely, however, that inhibition of cholesterol synthesis explains the actions of fluvastatin and simvastatin on SMC proliferation. In fact, cells were stimulated to growth by exposure to a medium containing 10% fetal calf serum which provides an exogenous source of cholesterol. Thus, inhibition of cell proliferation by vastatins likely resulted from inhibition of production of one or more isoprenoids intermediates of MVA metabolism. Recently, several proteins that are involved in growth factor signal transduction have been shown to be lipid-modified by the covalent attachment of MVA-derived isoprenoid group (prenylation) such as geranylgeraniol or farnesol [9,12,13,38,39]. Function and localization of these proteins are dependent on their covalent modification by these specific lipids [12,13,38].

Vastatins inhibit the biosynthesis of these two isoprenoids and one possible mechanism by which fluvastatin and simvastatin inhibit cell growth may be the interference with signaling pathways that require prenylated proteins. The fact that geranylgeraniol can, under these experimental conditions, partially prevent vastatins-induced inhibition of cell growth in the absence of other prenyl intermediates suggests that proteins modified by this isoprene, rather than, or in addition to, those that have been farnesylated, are responsible for inducing cell proliferation. The characterization of some of these proteins (such as nuclear lamin B [40], ras protein [41], and heterotrimeric and low molecular weight guanine nucleotide-binding proteins [42]) provides new insights into the link between the MVA pathway, signal transduction, and cell cycle progression.

According to these findings, in our experiments squalene failed to overcome the inhibitory effect of simvastatin and therefore it is unlikely that the putative regulator(s) of cell proliferation is squalene or any distal sterol intermediate in the cholesterol synthetic pathway [11]. We also observed that fibrinogen-induced SMC migration suggest a direct relationship between the MVA synthetic pathway and this cellular process.

Our *in vivo* data, according to *in vitro* observations, show that vastatins, albeit with different potencies, decreased neointimal proliferation in normocholesterolemic rabbits without affecting plasma cholesterol levels. Similarly, Gellman et al. [18] have shown that the action of lovastatin in reducing intimal hyperplasia after balloon angioplasty of the femoral artery in hypercholesterolemic rabbits appears to be unrelated to cholesterol lowering. Zhu et al. [17] also have shown that lovastatin can halt the progression of the aortic plaque, independently of cholesterol levels in experimentally induced atherosclerosis in rabbits. Recently, Bocan et al. [19] did not find any correlation between the lipid lowering effects of various HMG-CoA reductase inhibitors and their beneficial effect on atherosclerotic lesion formation in cholesterol-fed rabbits. All together, these studies suggest that vastatins can directly affect atheroma formation irrespective of plasma lipid changes probably through local inhibition of HMG-CoA reductase activity within cells of the vascular wall. Indeed, our *in vivo* data demonstrate that the mechanism underlying the antiproliferative effect of vastatins is really related to the local inhibition of MVA synthesis in SMC, since local delivery of MVA fully prevented the inhibitory effect of fluvastatin [36].

Conclusion

In conclusion, HMG-CoA reductase inhibitors may exert a direct antiatherosclerotic effect on the arterial wall independently of their lipid lowering properties. This activity, which affects major processes involved in the formation of atherosclerotic lesions, is linked to the local modulation of the MVA pathway and could translate into a more significant prevention of cardiovascular disease.

References

1.   Endo A. The discovery and development of HMG-CoA reductase inhibitors. J Lipid Res 1992;33:1569-82.
2.   Brown BG, Zhao X-Q, Sacco DE, Albers JJ. Lipid lowering and plaque regression. New insights into prevention of plaque disruption and clinical events in coronary disease. Circulation 1993;87:1781-91.
3.   Jukema JW, Bruschke AVG, van Boven AJ, et al. Effects of lipid lowering by pravastatin on progression and regression of coronary artery disease in symptomatic men with normal to moderately elevated serum cholesterol levels. The Regression Growth Evaluation Statin Study (REGRESS). Circulation 1995;91:2528-40.
4.   MAAS Investigators. Effect of simvastatin on coronary atheroma: The Multicentre Anti-Atheroma Study (MAAS). Lancet 1994;344:633-38.
5.   Scandinavian Simvastatin Survival Study Group. Randomised trial of cholesterol lowering in 4444 patients with coronary heart disease: The Scandinavian Simvastatin Survival Study (4S). Lancet 1994;344:1383-89.
6.   Hunninghake DB. HMG-CoA reductase inhibitors. Curr Opin Lipidol 1992;3:22-28.
7.   Feussner G. HMG-CoA reductase inhibitors. Curr Opin Lipidol 1994;5:59-68
8.   Grunler J, Ericsson J, Dallner G. Branch-point reactions in the biosynthesis of cholesterol, dolichol, ubiquinone and prenylated proteins. Biochim Biophys Acta 1994;1212:259-77.
9.   Goldstein JL, Brown MS. Regulation of the mevalonate pathway. Nature 1990;343:425-30.
10.   Bernini F, Didoni G, Bonfadini G, Bellosta S, Fumagalli R. Requirement for mevalonate in acetylated LDL induction of cholesterol esterification in macrophages. Atherosclerosis 1993; 104:19-26.
11.   Corsini A, Mazzotti M, Raiteri M, et al. Relationship between mevalonate pathway and arterial myocyte proliferation: In vitro studies with inhibitors of HMG-CoA reductase. Atherosclerosis 1993;101:117-25.
12.   Maltese WA. Posttranslational modification of proteins by isoprenoids in mammalian cells. FASEB J 1990;4:3319-28.
13.   Casey PJ. Biochemistry of protein prenylation. J Lipid Res 1992;33:1731-40.

14.   Corsini A, Raiteri M, Soma MR, Bernini F, Fumagalli R, Paoletti R. Pathogenesis of atherosclerosis and the role of drug intervention: Focus on HMG-CoA reductase inhibitors. Am J Cardiol 1995; in press.

15.   Corsini A, Maggi FM, Catapano AL. Pharmacology of competitive inhibitors of HMG-CoA reductase. Pharm Res 1995;31:9-27.

16.   Soma MR, Donetti E, Parolini C, et al. HMG-CoA reductase inhibitors: In vivo effects on carotid intimal thickening in normocholesterolemic rabbits. Arterioscl Thromb 1993;13:571-78.

17.   Zhu BQ, Sievers RE, Sun YP, Isenberg WM, Parmley WW. Effect of lovastatin on suppression and regression of atherosclerosis in lipid-fed rabbits. J Cardiovasc Pharmacol 1992;19:246-55.

18.   Gellman J, Ezekowitz MD, Sarembock IJ, et al. Effect of lovastatin on intimal hyperplasia after balloon angioplasty. A study in an atherosclerotic hypercholesterolemic rabbit. J Am Coll Cardiol 1991;17:251-59.

19.   Bocan TMA, Mazur MJ, Mueller SB, et al. Antiatherosclerotic activity of inhibitors of 3-hydroxy-3-methylglutaryl coenzyme A reductase in cholesterol-fed rabbits: a biochemical and morphological evaluation. Atherosclerosis 1994;111:127-42.

20.   Brown MS, Goldstein JL, Krieger M, Ho YK, Anderson RGW. Reversible accumulation of cholesteryl esters in macrophages incubated with acetylated lipoproteins. J Cell Biol 1979;82:597-613.

21.   Ross R. The pathogenesis of atherosclerosis: A perspective for the 1990s. Nature 1993;362:801-9.

22.   Sliskovic DR, White AD. Therapeutic potential of ACAT inhibitors as lipid lowering and anti-atherosclerotic agents. Trends Pharmacol Sci 1991;12:194-99.

23.   Goldstein JL, Brown MS, Ho YK, Innerarity TL, Mahley RW. Cholesteryl ester accumulation in macrophages resulting from receptor-mediated uptake and degradation of hypercholesterolemic canine b-very low density lipoproteins. J Biol Chem 1980;255:1839-48.

24.   Bernini F, Catapano AL, Corsini A, Fumagalli R, Paoletti R. Effects of calcium antagonists on lipids and atherosclerosis. Am J Cardiol 1989;64:129I-134I.

25.   Liscum L, Faust JR. The intracellular transport of low density lipoprotein-derived cholesterol is inhibited in Chinese hamster ovary cells cultured with 3-b-[2-(diethylamino)ethoxy]androst-5-en-17-one. J Biol Chem 1989;264:11796-806.

26.   Butler JD, Blanchette-Mackie J, Goldin E, et al. Progesterone blocks cholesterol translocation from lysosomes. J Biol Chem 1992;267:23797-805.

27.   Bottalico LA, Wager RE, Agellon LB, Assoian RK, Tabas I. Transforming growth factor-β1 inhibits scavenger receptor activity in THP-1 human macrophages. J Biol Chem 1991;266:22866-71.

28.   Geng Y-J, Hansson GJ. Interferon-τ inhibts scavenger receptor expression and foam cell formation in human monocyte-derived macrophages. J Clin Invest 1992;89:1322-30.

29.   Xu X-X, Tabas I. Lipoprotein activate acyl-coenzyme A: cholesterol acyltransferase in macrophages only after cellular cholesterol pools are expanded to a critical threshold level. J Biol Chem 1991;266:17040-48.

30.   Kempen HJM, Vermeer M, de Wit E, Havekes LM. Vastatins inhibit cholesterol ester accumulation in human monocyte-derived macrophages. Arterioscl Thromb 1991;11:146-53.

31.   Bernini F, Didoni G, Bonfadini G, Bellosta S, Fumagalli R. Requirement for mevalonate in acetylated LDL induction of cholesterol esterification in macrophages. Atherosclerosis 1993;104:19-26.

32.   Bernini F, Scurati N, Bonfadini G, Fumagalli R. HMG-CoA reductase inhibitors reduce acetyl LDL endocytosis in mouse peritoneal macrophages. Arterioscl Thromb Vasc Biol 1995;15: 1352-58.

33.   Wissler RW. Update on the pathogenesis of atherosclerosis. Am J Med 1991;91(Suppl.1B): 1B-3S-1B-9S

34.   Schwartz CJ, Valente AJ, Sprague EA. A modern view of atherogenesis. Am J Cardiol 1993; 71:9B-14B.

35.   Ip JH, Fuster V, Badimon L, Badimon J, Chesebro JH. Syndromes of accelerated atherosclerosis: Role of vascular injury and smooth muscle cell proliferation. J Am Coll Cardiol 1990;15:1667-87.

36.   Soma MR, Parolini C, Donetti E, Fumagalli R, Paoletti R. Inhibition of isoprenoid biosynthesis and arterial smooth muscle cell proliferation. J Cardiovasc Pharmacol 1995; 25(Suppl.4):S20-S24.

37.   Chen HW. Role of cholesterol metabolism in cell growth. Fed Proc 1984;43:126-30.

38.   Casey PJ, Moomaw JF, Zhang FL, Higgins JB, Thissen JA. Prenylation and G protein signaling. In: Bardin CW (editor). Recent Progress in Hormone Research. Vol. 49 San Diego: Academic Press Inc., 1994:215-33.

39.   Farnsworth CC, Gelb MH, Glomset JA. Identification of geranylgeranyl-modified proteins in HeLa cells. Science 1990;247:320-22.

40.   Farnsworth CC, Wolda SL, Gelb MH, Glomset JA. Human lamin B contains a farnesylated cysteine residue. J Biol Chem 1989;264:20422-29.

41.   Casey PJ, Solsky PA, Der CJ, Buss JE. p21ras is modified by a farnesyl isoprenoid. Proc Natl Acad Sci USA 1989;86:8323-27.

42.   Glomset JA, Farnsworth CC. Role of protein modification reactions in programming interactions between ras-related GTPases and cell membranes. Ann Rev Cell Biol 1994;10: 181-205.

Antonio M. Gotto, Jr.

Introduction

The last half of the 20th century has seen remarkable progress in understanding the relation between dyslipidemia and coronary heart disease (CHD) and in initiating both public health and specific therapeutic strategies to take advantage of this knowledge. One of the earliest achievements in lipidology was the introduction of classification schemes based on knowledge concerning the physiology and pathophysiology of the plasma lipoproteins [1-6]. As the human and animal evidence linking lipids to atherosclerosis risk grew, the "lipid hypothesis" emerged, postulating that lowering serum cholesterol would decrease the incidence of CHD events.

Large diet trials investigated the efficacy of modifying fat and cholesterol intake in reducing heart disease risk. In the Wadsworth–Veterans Administration (VA) study, 846 male patients of a veterans' hospital in Los Angeles, 55 years of age or older, were randomized either to a diet in which polyunsaturated fat was substituted for saturated fat or to the usual hospital diet [7]. Some of these patients had evidence of CHD; follow-up lasted for up to 8 years. Although there was no significant difference between the two diet groups in the primary endpoint of sudden CHD death or definite myocardial infarction (MI), total events, defined as sudden CHD death, definite MI, definite cerebral infarction, ruptured aneurysm, and amputations, were fewer in the experimental group than in the control (48/424 versus 70/422, $p < 0.05$). Critics continue to debate whether the results of the Wadsworth–VA study also suggested an increase of cancer in the treatment group.

Early drug interventions were evaluated in patients with established coronary disease in the Coronary Drug Project (CDP) [8]. In this study, 8,341 men, 30-64 years of age, were randomized to either placebo or one of five treatment arms: conjugated estrogens 2.5 mg/day, conjugated estrogens 5.0 mg/day, clofibrate 1.8 g/day, dextrothyroxine sodium 6.0 mg/day, or niacin 3.0 g/day. Patients were followed up for 5 years (total 5-8.5 years). Three of the interventions, namely, dextrothyroxine and both dosages of high-dose estrogen, had to be terminated because of an increase of adverse effects in the group receiving the drug or hormone. Niacin treatment was associated with a significant reduction in definite, nonfatal MI (5-year rates were 8.9% versus 12.2%), although there were side effects associated with niacin treatment. At the end of the 5-year follow-up, clofibrate failed to produce significant clinical benefit in patients on this treatment. There was also evidence that

25

A. M. Gotto, Jr. et al. (eds.), Multiple Risk Factors in Cardiovascular Disease, 25–33.
© 1998 Kluwer Academic Publishers and Fondazione Giovanni Lorenzini. Printed in the Netherlands.

clofibrate treatment was associated with increased incidence of nonfatal cardiovascular events.

The Lipid Research Clinics Coronary Primary Prevention Trial (LRC-CPPT) tested the lipid hypothesis in 3,806 asymptomatic men with primary hypercholesterolemia, who were randomized to receive 24 g/day of cholestyramine or placebo; the mean follow-up was 7.4 years [9]. Cholestyramine treatment was associated with a 19% reduction in CHD events, defined as a combination of nonfatal MI and/or CHD death ($p < 0.05$).

In the 1980s, the results of several trials of various lipid-lowering interventions were used in a national cholesterol consensus statement by the NIH [10]. This statement recommended desirable and undesirable levels of blood cholesterol and specific therapeutic regimens for various levels of risk, and was the basis for establishing a public health campaign as well as for widespread screening to detect hypercholesterolemia in the general population. The guidelines of the first Adult Treatment Panel of the National Cholesterol Education Program (NCEP) were released in October 1987 [11]. Approximately 1 month after the release of these guidelines, the positive results of the Helsinki Heart Study with gemfibrozil were reported [12]. In this 5-year, primary-prevention trial, 4,081 asymptomatic men with non-high density lipoprotein (HDL) cholesterol of 200 mg/dL or higher were randomized to receive either 600 mg gemfibrozil twice daily or placebo. There was a 34% reduction in definite MI, sudden cardiac death, or unwitnessed deaths from CHD ($p < 0.02$). In a refined analysis of these results, primary-prevention patients with the combination of elevated cholesterol, elevated triglyceride, and relatively low levels of HDL cholesterol derived the most benefit with gemfibrozil therapy (71% risk reduction) [13,14].

An issue of great controversy has been whether lipid-regulating interventions might increase deaths from noncardiovascular causes. In the LRC-CPPT, there was only a nonsignificant 7% decrease in all-cause mortality in the cholestyramine group, reflecting an increased number of noncardiovascular deaths in that group [9]. Analysis of long-term follow-up of the subjects in the CDP who received nicotinic acid showed an 11% decrease in overall mortality rate compared with the placebo group (p=0.0004) after 15 years, nearly 9 of which were after the discontinuation of the study drug [15]. The smaller Stockholm Ischaemic Heart Disease Secondary-Prevention Study [16] reported a decrease in all-cause mortality in post-MI patients treated with a combination of nicotinic acid and clofibrate (82 deaths/276 in control versus 61/279 in intervention group, $p < 0.05$). However, benefit seemed to be limited to patients with triglyceride levels greater than 133 mg/dL, and was most pronounced in patients whose triglyceride fell by 30% or more.

Evidence of Clinical Benefit from the Statin Trials

Two large-scale clinical studies in the 1990s have provided compelling evidence for the safety of lipid regulation. The Scandinavian Simvastatin Survival Study (4S), a randomized trial in which the only primary endpoint was total mortality rate, showed that lipid lowering was associated with a significant reduction in this endpoint [17]. Over a median 5.4-year follow-up, 4,444 men and women, aged 35-69, with a history of MI or angina pectoris and total cholesterol of 212-310 mg/dL were treated with either 20 mg/day of the HMG-CoA reductase inhibitor simvastatin or placebo. Simvastatin dosage was titrated over the course of the study to reduce total cholesterol to between 116 and 201 mg/dL; thus, 37% of patients in the simvastatin group received 40 mg/day and 2 patients received only 10 mg/day. A 25% reduction in total cholesterol and a 35% reduction in low density lipoprotein (LDL) cholesterol in the simvastatin group coincided with a 30% reduction in risk for dying of any cause (p=0.0003). Subanalysis of the causes of death showed that simvastatin treatment was not associated with increased deaths from non-CHD causes (67/2223 in the placebo versus 71/2221 in the simvastatin group), thus establishing that the primary effect of simvastatin therapy on mortality was in reducing CHD deaths (189 coronary deaths in the placebo versus 111 in the simvastatin group, a 42% risk reduction). Simvastatin therapy was also associated with a 34% reduction in the risk for having one or more major coronary events (p < 0.00001) and a 37% reduction in the risk for undergoing revascularization procedures. CHD benefit was found across all quartiles of baseline total, LDL, and HDL cholesterol, with similar benefit in each quartile [18].

The results of the West of Scotland Coronary Prevention Study (WOSCOPS) extend a similar benefit to an asymptomatic population [19]. In this trial, 6,595 men, 45-64 years old, with no history of MI were randomized to receive 40 mg/day of pravastatin or placebo. Five percent had evidence of angina pectoris. Pravastatin therapy led to a 20% reduction in total plasma cholesterol and a 26% reduction in LDL cholesterol. This study also reported significant reductions in clinical events. There was a 31% reduction in the risk for nonfatal MI or CHD death (p < 0.001) and a 33% reduction in definite plus suspected deaths from MI (p=0.033). The all-cause mortality rate was reduced by 22% (p=0.051). Together with the results of 4S, the WOSCOPS results should alleviate many concerns about the safety of lipid lowering as an appropriate strategy for managing CHD risk whether in primary or secondary prevention.

Extending the Benefit to Patients with "Average" Cholesterol Concentrations

In trials such as 4S or WOSCOPS, patients were at relatively high risk for CHD due either to pre-existing symptomatic disease or to severe elevations in total and LDL cholesterol. Less clearly established was whether benefit could be obtained in CHD patients with mild to moderate elevations in total and LDL cholesterol, who represent the majority of the population with CHD. The Cholesterol and Recurrent Events (CARE) trial provides compelling evidence that such benefit may be substantial [20]. In CARE, 4,159 men and women, post-MI, were treated either with pravastatin, 40 mg/d, or with placebo. The mean LDL cholesterol concentration in CARE was 139 mg/dL; pravastatin treatment reduced LDL cholesterol by 32%. After a mean follow-up of 5 years, pravastatin-treated patients were at a 24% lower risk for having a recurrent event (defined as either nonfatal MI or CHD death, P=0.003). Also, the benefit was greater among women than men in CARE (46% risk reduction versus 20% risk reduction, P=0.05 for interaction). This finding reinforces the importance of lipid-lowering therapy in secondary prevention.

Only two trials have examined the effect of cholesterol lowering on vascular disease progression in patients without severe elevations in LDL cholesterol. The first, the Harvard

Atherosclerosis Reversibility Project (HARP), reported no angiographic benefit of treatment with pravastatin in this population [21]. However, in the Lipoprotein and Coronary Atherosclerosis Study (LCAS), disease progression was slowed in patients without severely elevated LDL cholesterol and with angiographic evidence of CHD. In LCAS, 429 men and women were randomized to treatment either with fluvastatin, 20 mg/bid, or with placebo; the trial length was approximately 2.5 years. The primary endpoint was the change in minimum lumen diameter (ΔMLD). At the end of follow-up, ΔMLD was –0.028 mm in fluvastatin-treated patients versus –0.100 mm in the control group (P < 0.01) [22].

Regression Trials: Vascular Benefit of Lipid Lowering

A large number of trials with vascular endpoints have reported the benefit of cholesterol lowering on altering the course of disease. A number of important findings have come to light as a result of these "regression" studies. One important observation is that atherosclerotic disease continues to progress if left untreated. As was demonstrated in LCAS and other studies, treatment of patients with evidence of CHD usually does not lead to substantial reductions in coronary stenosis, but, in general, decreases the rate of progression. Although the changes in coronary blockage caused by lipid-regulating therapy are relatively small, they may be associated with unexpectedly large reductions in CHD events [23]. Indeed, evidence from some of these studies showed that progression of CHD blockage carries with it a markedly increased risk for experiencing a CHD event. The results of the Program on the Surgical Control of the Hyperlipidemias (POSCH), in which the lipid-regulating intervention was partial ileal bypass surgery, demonstrate this point. In POSCH, 838 men and women, 30-64 years of age, with prior MI and hypercholesterolemia, were randomized either to surgical intervention or to the control. Mean follow-up was 9.7 years. The results of POSCH confirmed that aggressive lipid management could inhibit the progression of atherosclerotic disease, but failed to show a statistically significant difference in all-cause mortality, which was its primary endpoint. However, the lengthy follow-up period allowed the investigators to demonstrate that angiographic changes were predictive of future events [24].

The Culprit Lesion and Lesion Stabilization

Another important observation that came from the angiographic studies is that the most dangerous atherosclerotic lesion is typically not one causing 80-90% obstruction but a less severe lesion that causes an obstruction of 70% or less and has a lipid-rich core and a weakened fibrous cap [23]. The concept of the "culprit lesion" suggested that the manipulation of lesion composition rather than lesion stenosis may be a mediating factor in the sizable clinical benefits seen in the regression trials.

At least four hypotheses have been proposed to describe the unexpectedly high reduction in CHD events observed as a result of aggressive lipid reduction in the regression trials. The proposed mechanisms of benefit of lipid lowering include a reduction of an inflammatory response associated with atherosclerosis, the protective antioxidant effects of lipid lowering, restoration of endothelial function, and the improvement of myocardial ischemia.

Plaque stabilization is centered on the concept that ischemic events may be prevented by altering the lipid-filled lesion in which the connective tissue is degraded, perhaps by the production of metalloproteinases. In such lesions, smooth muscle cells are rare, and inflammatory cells, in particular activated macrophages and T cells, are common [25]. Of particular interest is the preventive and therapeutic value of inhibiting smooth muscle cell proliferation, which has been implicated in the 30-40% increased risk for restenosis post-angioplasty and in the production of degradative metalloproteinases under cytokine stimulation. However, smooth muscle cells may also be essential in maintaining the structural integrity of atherosclerotic lesions through their production of extracellular matrix proteins and collagen, suggesting that inhibition of such proliferation may be detrimental at certain stages of plaque development [26].

Although *in vitro* studies of oxidized lipoproteins have implicated them as mediating injury to the vascular wall, their role in atherogenesis *in vivo* is less clear. Oxidized lipoproteins may play a role in the inflammatory reaction associated with plaque formation, involving increased leukocyte chemotaxis and facilitation of foam cell formation [27]. This immunologic reaction may be decreased by aggressive cholesterol lowering. In the KAPS study, pravastatin therapy was associated with increased lipoprotein resistance to oxidation [28].

The presence of atherosclerotic disease is associated with a paradoxical vasoconstricting response to vasodilators such as endothelium-derived relaxing factor (EDRF) or acetylcholine. A study by Anderson et al. showed that lovastatin, in conjunction with probucol, a cholesterol-lowering agent with putative antioxidant effects, could improve endothelial function, as measured by vessel response to acetylcholine [29]. Egashira et al. similarly demonstrated that pravastatin therapy was associated with improved acetylcholine-induced vasodilatation [30].

As a complement to restoring endothelial function, the benefits of managing myocardial ischemia and improving response of the stenotic vessel to increased myocardial demand are also under investigation [31]. Rapid improvement in myocardial perfusion, as detected by positron-emission tomography (PET) scanning, has also been reported, and the studies of Gould et al. showed the potential benefit of a very aggressive program of lifestyle modification [32].

Refining Treatment Guidelines

As the end of the century approaches, several avenues in atherosclerosis research have begun to be explored. One such avenue is the refinement of existing treatment guidelines. Based on the results of the regression trials and secondary-prevention trials such as 4S and CARE, various groups have indicated the need for more aggressive implementation of lipid-lowering therapy and risk factor modification in all eligible patients [33]. However, according to the U.S. National Heart, Lung, and Blood Institute (NHLBI) 1995 Cholesterol Awareness Surveys, only 29% of the patients with established CHD are currently undergoing pharmacologic treatment for hypercholesterolemia, in spite of the very slight evidence of any harm and the great deal of evidence of benefit in such patients [34].

The current guidelines of the U.S. National Cholesterol Education Program (NCEP) recommend a target LDL cholesterol value of 100 mg/dL or less in patients with established CHD [35]. The target goal in primary prevention depends on the overall risk status of the patient. The use of a target goal has been questioned by Thompson et al. [36] on the basis of a combined analysis of the results of 11 angiographic trials, which concluded that changes in percent diameter stenosis were correlated with percent reductions in LDL cholesterol ($r=0.74$, $p < 0.0005$) but not with LDL cholesterol concentrations during these trials. However, in the Post-CABG trial, aggressive therapy to an LDL cholesterol target below 100 mg/dL with lovastatin yielded greater angiographic benefit than a more moderate strategy [37]. The controversy about whether one should aim for a given percent reduction in LDL cholesterol or for a target value is still widely debated and may not be resolved even with more refined analyses of the major statin trials.

Furthermore, risk assessment may be refined by identifying other markers for CHD risk, such as paraoxonase [38]. Trials will also be needed to test whether raising HDL cholesterol [39] and/or lowering triglyceride concentrations will independently decrease CHD risk. Postprandial lipemia and insulin resistance as risk factors or markers for CHD risk may also gain increasing importance [40,41]. The increased CHD risk conferred by elevated lipoprotein[a] (Lp[a]) levels also warrants closer investigation [42]. There is also renewed interest in the roles of triglyceride and low HDL cholesterol as CHD risk factors [43]. These emerging factors, taken together with others such as obesity, smoking, and diabetes, have given rise to the concept of global risk, in which the synergistic interaction of multiple risk factors is considered in making treatment decisions.

Refining treatment guidelines will likely be one of the most important challenges facing atherosclerosis researchers in the new century. The priority centers on identifying the goals of therapy: should LDL cholesterol reduction continue to be the primary target for all patients, and, in patients with relatively low levels of LDL cholesterol but who also have low levels of HDL cholesterol and/or elevated triglyceride, should the treatment target these two other lipid risk factors? At present the majority of data support reducing LDL cholesterol as the primary goal of therapy; however, the effects of modifying these other lipid fractions may be determined by future research.

Conclusion

The intimate relation between lipid disorders and CHD risk is supported by so much evidence as to be virtually incontrovertible. The challenge remains to uncover the mechanisms that mediate that relation. The preponderance of evidence supports the current strategy of aggressive management of hypercholesterolemia to reduce CHD morbidity and mortality. As the mechanisms underlying the pathology of this disease become better understood, new treatment strategies and refinements of existing therapies and management protocols may present themselves. Investigating these new directions is crucial if we are to continue to reverse the worldwide toll of CHD morbidity and mortality.

References

1. Fredrickson DS, Levy RI, Lees RS. Fat transport in lipoproteins—an integrated approach to mechanisms and disorders. N Engl J Med 1967;276:34-44.
2. Fredrickson DS, Levy RI, Lees RS. Fat transport in lipoproteins—an integrated approach to mechanisms and disorders (continued). N Engl J Med 1967;276:94-103.
3. Fredrickson DS, Levy RI, Lees RS. Fat transport in lipoproteins—an integrated approach to mechanisms and disorders (continued). N Engl J Med 1967;276:148-56.
4. Fredrickson DS, Levy RI, Lees RS. Fat transport in lipoproteins—an integrated approach to mechanisms and disorders (continued). N Engl J Med 1967;276:215-25.
5. Fredrickson DS, Levy RI, Lees RS. Fat transport in lipoproteins—an integrated approach to mechanisms and disorders (continued). N Engl J Med 1967;276:273-81.
6. Fredrickson DS, Lees RS. System for phenotyping hyperlipidemia. Circulation 1965;31:321-27.
7. Dayton S, Pearce ML, Hashimoto S, Dixon WJ, Tomiyasu U. A controlled clinical trial of a diet high in unsaturated fat in preventing complications of atherosclerosis. Circulation 1969; 40(Suppl.2):II-1-II-63.
8. Coronary Drug Project Research Group. Clofibrate and niacin in coronary heart disease. JAMA 1975;231(4):360-81.
9. Lipid Research Clinics Program: The Lipid Research Clinics Coronary Primary Prevention Trial results. I. Reduction in incidence of coronary heart disease. JAMA 1984;251:351-64.
    Lipid Research Clinics Program: The Lipid Research Clinics Coronary Primary Prevention Trial results. II. The relationship of reduction in incidence of coronary heart disease to cholesterol lowering. JAMA 1984;251:365-74.
10. NIH Consensus Development Conference on Lowering Blood Cholesterol to Prevent Heart Disease. Lowering blood cholesterol to prevent heart disease: NIH consensus development conference statement. Arteriosclerosis 1985;5:404-12.
11. Expert Panel. Report of the National Cholesterol Education Program Expert Panel on detection, evaluation, and treatment of high blood cholesterol in adults. Arch Intern Med 1988; 148:36-69.
12. Frick MH, Elo O, Haapa K, et al. Helsinki Heart Study: primary-prevention trial with gemfibrozil in middle-aged men with dyslipidemia. Safety of treatment, changes in risk factors, and incidence of coronary heart disease. N Engl J Med 1987;317(20):1237-45.
13. Huttunen JK, Manninen V, Mänttäri M, et al. The Helsinki Heart Study: central findings and clinical implications. Ann Med 1991;23:155-59.
14. Manninen V, Tenkanen L, Koskinen P, et al. Joint effects of serum triglyceride and LDL cholesterol and HDL cholesterol concentrations on coronary heart disease risk in the Helsinki Heart Study: Implications for treatment. Circulation 1992;85(1):37-45.
15. Canner PL, Berge KG, Wenger NK, et al., for the Coronary Drug Project Research Group. Fifteen year mortality in Coronary Drug Project patients: Long-term benefit with niacin. J Am Coll Cardiol 1986;8(6):1245-55.
16. Carlson LA, Rosenhamer G. Reduction of mortality in the Stockholm Ischaemic Heart Disease Secondary Prevention Study by combined treatment with clofibrate and nicotinic acid. Acta Med Scand 1988;223:405-18.
17. Scandinavian Simvastatin Survival Study Group. Randomised trial of cholesterol lowering in 4444 patients with coronary heart disease: The Scandinavian Simvastatin Survival Study (4S). Lancet 1994;344:1383-89.

18.   Scandinavian Simvastatin Survival Study Group. Baseline serum cholesterol and treatment effect in the Scandinavian Simvastatin Survival Study (4S). Lancet 1995;345:1274-75.

19.   Shepherd J, Cobbe SM, Ford I, et al., for the West of Scotland Coronary Prevention Study Group. Prevention of coronary heart disease with pravastatin in men with hypercholesterolemia. N Engl J Med 1995;333(20):1301-7.

20.   Sacks FM, Pfeffer MA, Moye LA, et al., for the Cholesterol and Recurrent Events Trial Investigators. The effect of pravastatin on coronary events after myocardial infarction in patients with average cholesterol levels. N Engl J Med 1996;335:1001-9.

21.   Sacks FM, Pasternak RC, Gibson CM, Rosner B, Stone PH, for the Harvard Atherosclerosis Reversibility Project (HARP). Effect on coronary atherosclerosis of decrease in plasma cholesterol concentrations in normocholesterolaemic patients. Lancet 1997;344:1182-86.

22.   Herd JA, Ballantyne CM, Farmer JA, et al., for the LCAS investigators. Effects of fluvastatin on coronary atherosclerosis in patients with mild to moderate cholesterol elevations (Lipoprotein and Coronary Atherosclerosis Study [LCAS]). Am J Cardiol 1997;80:278-86.

23.   Brown BG, Zhao X-Q, Sacco DE, Albers JJ. Lipid lowering and plaque regression: new insights into prevention of plaque disruption and clinical events in coronary disease. Circulation 1993;87(6):1781-91.

24.   Buchwald H, Matts JP, Fitch LL, et al., for the Program on the Surgical Control of the Hyperlipidemias (POSCH) Group. Changes in sequential coronary arteriograms and subsequent coronary events. JAMA 1992;268(11):1429-33.

25.   Libby P. Molecular bases of the acute coronary syndromes. Circulation 1995;91(11):2844-50.

26.   Weissberg PL, Clesham GJ, Bennett MR. Is vascular smooth muscle cell proliferation beneficial? Lancet 1996;347:305-7

27.   Steinberg D, Witztum JL. Lipoproteins and atherogenesis: Current concepts. JAMA 1990;264 (23):3047-51.

28.   Salonen R, Nyssonen K, Porkkala-Sarataho E, Salonen JT. The Kuopio Atherosclerosis Prevention Study (KAPS): Effect of pravastatin treatment on lipids, oxidation resistance of lipoproteins, and atherosclerotic progression. Am J Cardiol 1995;76:34C-39C.

29.   Anderson TJ, Meredith IT, Yeung AC, Frei B, Selwyn AP, Ganz P. The effect of cholesterol-lowering and antioxidant therapy on endothelium-dependent coronary vasomotion. N Engl J Med 1995;332(8):488-93.

30.   Egashira K, Hirooka Y, Kai H, et al. Reduction in serum cholesterol with pravastatin improves endothelium-dependent coronary vasomotion in patients with hypercholesterolemia. Circulation 1994;89(6):2519-24.

31.   Yeung AC, Raby KE, Ganz P, Selwyn AP. New insights into the management of myocardial ischemia. Am J Cardiol 1992;70:8G-13G.

32.   Gould KL, Ornish D, Scherwitz L, et al. Changes in myocardial perfusion abnormalities by positron emission tomography after long-term, intense risk factor modification. JAMA 1995; 274(11):894-901.

33.   Smith SC Jr, Blair SN, Criqui MH, et al., the Secondary Prevention Panel. Preventing heart attack and death in patients with coronary disease. Circulation 1995;92(1):2-4.

34.   LaRosa JC. Cholesterol Agonistics. Ann Intern Med 1996;124:505-8.

35.   National Cholesterol Education Program: Second report of the Expert Panel on Detection, Evaluation, and Treatment of High Blood Cholesterol in Adults (Adult Treatment Panel II). Circulation 1994;89:1329-445.

36.   Thompson GR, Hollyer J, Waters DD. Percentage change rather than plasma level of LDL-cholesterol determines therapeutic response in coronary heart disease. Curr Opin Lipidol

1995;6(6):386-88.

37. The Post Coronary Artery Bypass Graft Trial Investigators. The effect of aggressive lowering of low-density lipoprotein cholesterol levels and low-dose anticoagulation on obstructive changes in saphenous-vein coronary-artery bypass grafts. N Engl J Med 1997;336:153-62.

38. Hegele RA, Brunt H, Connelly PW. A polymorphism of the paraoxonase gene associated with variation in plasma lipoproteins in a genetic isolate. Arterioscler Thromb Vasc Biol 1995;15: 89-95.

39. Barter PJ, Rye K-A. High density lipoproteins and coronary heart disease. Atherosclerosis 1996;121:1-12.

40. Ebenbichler, CF, Kirchmair R, Egger C, Patsch JR. Postprandial state and atherosclerosis. Curr Opin Lipidol 1995;6:286-90.

41. Reaven GM. Role of insulin resistance in human disease (Syndrome X): An expanded definition. Annu Rev Med 1993;44:121-31.

42. Loscalzo J. Lipoprotein(a). A unique risk factor for atherothrombotic disease. Arteriosclerosis 1990;10:672-79.

43. Assman G, Schulte H. Relation of high-density lipoprotein cholesterol and triglycerides to incidence of atherosclerotic coronary artery disease (the PROCAM experience). Am J Cardiol 1992;70:733-37.

ROLE OF THE FIBRINOLYTIC AND THE COAGULATION SYSTEM IN THE FORMATION AND DISORDERS OF BLOOD VESSELS

Peter Carmeliet and Désiré Collen

Introduction

The blood coagulation, the fibrinolytic (or plasminogen/plasmin), and matrix metallo-proteinase systems constitute families of proteinases that have been extensively characterized at the structural level. Previous biochemical, genetic, and epidemiologic studies suggested that they determine the balance between the formation and dissolution of blood clots and contribute to the pathogenesis of various cardiovascular disorders such as thrombosis, atherosclerosis, and restenosis. Two recently developed technologies, gene targeting and gene transfer, that allow manipulation of the genetic balance of these proteinase systems in a controllable manner *in vivo* have allowed more definitive elucidation of the biological role of these systems. This review summarizes the insights that have been obtained from the gene targeting studies and discusses the use of adenovirus-mediated transfer of fibrinolytic genes to study and possibly to develop novel strategies for the treatment of restenosis and thrombosis.

The Coagulation System

Tissue factor (TF) initiates the coagulation cascade by functioning as a cellular receptor and cofactor for activation of factor VII to factor VIIa [1]. This complex activates factor X directly or indirectly via activation of factor IX, resulting in the generation of thrombin-mediated conversion of fibrinogen to fibrin [2]. Anticoagulation is mediated by thrombin, which, when bound to its cellular receptor thrombomodulin, functions by activating protein C. Anticoagulation is further provided by tissue factor pathway inhibitor, which controls the activity of the tissue factor/factor VIIa complex and factor Xa, and by antithrombin III, which interacts with thrombin, factor Xa, and factor IXa in a heparin-dependent manner [2].

The Plasminogen System

The plasminogen system is composed of an inactive proenzyme plasminogen (Plg) that can be converted to plasmin by either of two plasminogen activators (PA), tissue-type PA (t-PA) or urokinase-type PA (u-PA) [3]. This system is controlled at the level of plasminogen

A. M. Gotto, Jr. et al. (eds.), Multiple Risk Factors in Cardiovascular Disease, 35–44.

activators by plasminogen activator inhibitors (PAIs), of which PAI-1 is believed to be physiologically the most important [4], and at the level of plasmin by alpha$_2$-antiplasmin [3]. Due to its fibrin-specificity, t-PA is primarily involved in clot dissolution, whereas u-PA binds a cellular receptor, the urokinase receptor (u-PAR), and has been implicated in pericellular proteolysis during cell migration and tissue remodeling [5]. Plasmin degrades fibrin and other extracellular matrix proteins, directly or indirectly via activation of matrix-degrading proteinases.

The Matrix Metalloproteinase System

Matrix metalloproteinases (MMPs) have been subdivided in categories based on their sequence homology and substrate specificity: the collagenases-1 to -3 (MMP-1, MMP-8, MMP-13) which cleave the native helix of fibrillar collagens type I, II, and III; the gelatinases-A and -B (MMP-2 and MMP-9) which degrade collagen type IV, V, VII, and X, and elastin, and which may act synergistically with collagenases by degrading denatured collagens (gelatins); the stromelysins-1 and -2 (MMP-3 and MMP-10) and matrilysin (MMP-7) which break down the proteoglycan core proteins, laminin, fibronectin, elastin, gelatin, and nonhelical regions of collagen type II, IV, V, IX, and X, and which may superactivate MMP-1 and MMP-9; the macrophage metalloelastase (MMP-12) which primarily degrades insoluble elastin in addition to type IV collagen, fibronectin, laminin, entactin, and proteoglycans; and the membrane-type metalloproteinases (MT1-MMP and MT2-MMP) which activate gelatinase-A [6]. Their action is inhibited by tissue-inhibitors of MMPs (TIMPs). Most MMPs are secreted as zymogens, requiring extracellular activation. *In vitro*, organomercurial compounds, proteinases (including plasmin, trypsin, kallikrein, cathepsin G, or neutrophil elastase), oxygen radicals, or association with the cell surface can activate pro-MMPs, but it is not known whether any of these mechanisms are operational *in vivo* [7].

Formation of Blood Vessels

Blood vessels initially develop as endothelial lined channels primarily through processes called vasculogenesis (*in situ* differentiation of hemangioblasts to endothelial cells that become aligned in a primitive vascular plexus) and angiogenesis (sprouting of preexisting vessels) [8]. These fragile primitive blood vessels require structural support to accommodate the increased blood pressure during further embryogenesis, which is provided by the accumulation and differentiation of early smooth muscle cells around the endothelial cells. Whereas recent targeting studies of, amongst others, the vascular endothelial growth factor [9], have revealed a central role in the development of these endothelial lined channels, the molecular mechanisms involved in the development of the smooth muscle wall remained largely elusive. Recently, novel insights were derived from the targeted inactivation of the tissue factor gene [10]. Indeed, tissue factor deficiency resulted in impaired development of the primitive smooth muscle cell layer around the fragile endothelial lined channels in the yolk sac, which play an essential role in transferring the maternally derived nutrients from the yolk sac to the rapidly growing embryo. At a time when the blood pressure increased during embryogenesis (day 9 of gestation), the immature tissue factor-deficient blood vessels ruptured, formed micro-aneurysms and "blood lakes" and failed to sustain proper circulation between the yolk sac and embryo. Secondarily, the embryo became wasted and died due to generalized necrosis. Only in advanced stages of deterioration did the immature blood vessels become leaky, resulting in bleeding into the intracoelomic cavity. Embryonic lethality due to abnormal vessel fragility was also observed by two other studies [11,12]. An unresolved question is how tissue factor exerts this morphogenic action, i.e. via intracellular signaling as suggested previously [11], via adhesion, and/or via fibrin formation. Indeed, factor VII-deficient mice develop normally till birth and die early postnatally due to massive hemorrhaging [13]. Since transfer of maternal factor VII to the embryo appears to be infinitesimally small, and since intraembryonic injection of thrombin failed to induce fibrin thrombi, and the factor VIIa inhibitor rNAPc2 failed to induce the typical tissue factor deficient-like vascular fragility, the role of tissue factor in early embryonic development may depend less on fibrin formation than previously anticipated [13].

Other coagulation factors appear also to be involved in morphogenetic processes during early embryogenesis, possibly in vascular development. Indeed, deficiency of factor V [14] and the thrombin receptor [15] both resulted in approximately 50% of the homozygous deficient embryos in abnormal yolk sac vasculature around a similar developmental stage as tissue factor-deficient embryos. The leakage of blood from the defective blood vessels in tissue factor-deficient embryos ("vascular" bleeding) contrasts with the postnatal bleeding in mice deficient of factor VII [13], factor VIII [16], fibrinogen [17] and in the surviving fraction of factor V-deficient mice [14], which occurs due to defective clot formation following trauma of normally developed blood vessels ("hemostatic" bleeding). Thus, it appears from these targeting studies that several coagulation factors (tissue factor, factor V, thrombin receptor) participate in morphogenic processes in addition to hemostasis, whereas other coagulation factors (factor VIII, fibrinogen) play a predominant or essential role in hemostasis via clot formation. This raises an interesting question whether tissue factor and the thrombin receptor, which are expressed during restenosis and atherosclerosis, also play a similar (nonhemostatic) role in these processes.

Thrombosis and Thrombolysis

FIBRIN DEPOSITS AND PULMONARY PLASMA CLOT LYSIS IN TRANSGENIC MICE

Deficient fibrinolytic activity, e.g. resulting from increased plasma PAI-1 levels or reduced plasma t-PA or plasminogen levels, might participate in the development of thrombotic events [18]. Fibrin surveillance in the different knock out mice was analyzed in quiescent conditions and after challenge. In unstressed conditions, u-PA-deficient mice developed occasional minor fibrin deposits in liver and intestines and excessive fibrin deposition in chronic non healing skin ulcerations, whereas in t-PA-deficient mice, no spontaneous fibrin deposits were observed [19]. Mice with a single deficiency of plasminogen (Plg) or a combined deficiency of t-PA and u-PA, however, revealed extensive intra- and extra-vascular fibrin deposits in several organs ([19-21]; P. Carmeliet et al., unpublished observations). Interestingly, mice with a combined deficiency of t-PA and u-PAR did not display such excessive fibrin deposits, suggesting that sufficient plasmin proteolysis can occur in the absence of u-PA binding to u-PAR [22].

After traumatic or inflammatory challenge, mice with a single deficiency of t-PA or u-PA were significantly more susceptible to venous thrombosis, e.g. following local injection of proinflammatory endotoxin in the footpad [19] or after hypoxia in the pulmonary vasculature (Pinsky et al., personal communication). Significant fibrin and matrix deposition was present in Plg-deficient mice following skin wounds [23] or during experimental glomerulonephritis [24]. Similar to Plg-deficient patients, Plg-deficient mice also suffered increased and prolonged arterial thrombosis, but only after injury [25]. The requirement of injury for arterial thrombosis in Plg-deficient mice may be related to the fact that mice, in contrast to men, do not normally develop vasculopathies such as atherosclerosis, which can provide highly thrombogenic surfaces via plaque rupture.

The increased thrombotic susceptibility of t-PA-deficient and of combined t-PA:u-PA- or Plg-deficient mice can be explained by their significantly reduced rate of spontaneous lysis of ^{125}I-fibrin labeled pulmonary plasma clots [19,20]. On the contrary, PAI-1-deficient mice were virtually protected against development of venous thrombosis following injection of endotoxin, consistent with their ability to lyse these plasma clots at a significantly higher rate than wild type mice [26,27]. The increased susceptibility of u-PA-deficient mice to thrombosis associated with inflammation or injury, might be due to their impaired macrophage function. Indeed, thioglycollate-stimulated macrophages (which are known to express cell-associated u-PA) isolated from u-PA-deficient mice, lacked plasminogen-dependent breakdown of ^{125}I-labeled fibrin (fibrinolysis) or of ^{3}H-labelled subendothelial matrix (mostly collagenolysis), whereas macrophages from t-PA-deficient or PAI-1-deficient mice did not [19,28].

ADENOVIRUS-MEDIATED TRANSFER OF T-PA OR PAI-1

More recently, we have used adenoviral-mediated transfer of fibrinolytic system components in these "knock-out" mice in an attempt to revert their phenotypes. Intravenous injection of adenoviruses, expressing a recombinant PAI-1-resistant human t-PA (rt-PA) gene, in t-PA-deficient mice increased plasma rt-PA levels 100 to 1000-fold above normal and restored their impaired thrombolytic potential in a dose-related way [29]. Conversely, adenovirus-mediated transfer of recombinant human PAI-1 in PAI-1-deficient mice resulted in 100- to 1000-fold increased plasma PAI-1 levels above normal and efficiently reduced the increased thrombolytic potential of PAI-1-deficient mice (Carmeliet et al., unpublished observations).

Neointima Formation

Vascular interventions for the treatment of atherothrombosis induce "restenosis" of the vessel within three to six months in 30 to 50 % of treated patients. This may result from remodeling of the vessel wall (such as occurs predominantly after balloon angioplasty) and/or accumulation of cells and extracellular matrix in the intimal layer (such as occurs predominantly after intraluminal stent application). Proteinases may participate in proliferation and migration of smooth muscle and/or endothelial cells, and in extensive matrix remodeling during this wound healing response. Two proteinase systems have been implicated, the plasminogen (or fibrinolytic) system and the metalloproteinase system, which in concert can degrade most extracellular matrix proteins. In contrast to the constitutive expression of t-PA by quiescent endothelial cells [3] and of PAI-1 by uninjured vascular smooth muscle cells [30], u-PA and t-PA activity in the vessel wall are significantly increased after injury, coincident with the time of smooth muscle cell proliferation and migration [31]. This increase in plasmin proteolysis is counterbalanced by increased expression of PAI-1 in injured smooth muscle and endothelial cells and by its release from accumulating platelets.

U-PA-MEDIATED PLASMIN PROTEOLYSIS PROMOTES NEOINTIMA FORMATION

We have used two experimental models of arterial injury, one based on the use of an electric current and the other on the use of an intraluminal guidewire to examine the molecular mechanisms of neointima formation in mice deficient in fibrinolytic system components [32]. The electric current injury model differs from mechanical injury models in that it induces a more severe injury across the vessel wall resulting in necrosis of all smooth muscle cells. This necessitates wound healing to initiate from the adjacent uninjured borders and to progress into the central necrotic region. Microscopic and morphometric analysis revealed that the rate and degree of neointima formation and the neointimal cell accumulation after injury was similar in wild type, t-PA-deficient and u-PAR-deficient arteries [33,34]. However, neointima formation in PAI-1-deficient arteries occurred at earlier times post-injury [35]. In contrast, both the degree and the rate of arterial neointima formation in u-PA-deficient, Plg-deficient, and combined t-PA:u-PA-deficient arteries was significantly reduced until 6 weeks after injury [25]. Similar genotypic differences were obtained after mechanical injury, which more closely mimics the injury in patients. Evaluation of the mechanisms responsible for these genotype-specific differences in neointima formation revealed that proliferation of medial and neointimal smooth muscle cells was only marginally different between the genotypes. Impaired migration of smooth muscle cells could be a significant cause of reduced neointima formation in mice lacking u-PA-mediated plasmin proteolysis since smooth muscle cells migrated over a shorter distance from the uninjured border into the central injured region in Plg-deficient than in wild type arteries [25,33]. Although our results demonstrate that migration of smooth muscle cells requires plasmin proteolysis, it is possible that PAI-1 may also influence cellular migration by a novel mechanism in cell adhesion through interaction with the $\alpha_v\beta_3$-integrin receptor [36]. That u-PAR-deficient arteries developed a similar degree of neointima suggests that sufficient pericellular plasmin proteolysis can still occur in the absence of binding of u-PA to its cellular receptor. Somewhat surprisingly, no genotypic differences were obtained in reendothelialization, suggesting a cell-type specific requirement of plasmin proteolysis for cellular migration [25].

INHIBITION OF NEOINTIMA FORMATION BY ADENOVIRUS-MEDIATED PAI-1 GENE TRANSFER

The involvement of plasmin proteolysis in neointima formation was supported by intravenous injection in PAI-1-deficient mice of a replication-defective adenovirus that expresses human PAI-1, which resulted in more than 100- to 1000-fold increased plasma PAI-1 levels and in a similar degree of inhibition of neointima formation as observed in u-PA-deficient mice [35]. Proteinase-inhibitors have been suggested as anti-restenosis drugs. Our studies suggest that strategies aimed at reducing u-PA-mediated plasmin proteolysis may reduce intimal thickening. However, antifibrinolytic strategies should be targeted at inhibiting plasmin proteolysis and not at preventing the interaction of u-PA with its receptor.

TRANSPLANT ATHEROSCLEROSIS IN PLASMINOGEN-DEFICIENT MICE

More recently, (in a collaboration with V. Shi and E. Haber), we analyzed the role of the plasminogen system in a mouse model of transplant arteriosclerosis that mimics in many ways the accelerated arteriosclerosis in coronary arteries of transplanted cardiac allografts in men [37]. In this model, host-derived leukocytes infiltrate beneath the endothelium and form a predominantly leukocyte-rich neointima by 15 days after transplantation, whereas, at later times, smooth muscle cells, derived from the donor graft, accumulate in the neointima. Since previous targeting studies have shown that migration of leukocytes and smooth muscle cells is dependent on plasmin proteolysis, carotid arteries from B.10A(2R) wild type mice were transplanted in C57Bl6:129 Plg-deficient mice. Initial analysis suggests that neointima formation within 45 days after transplantation is reduced in these mice, suggesting a significant role for plasmin proteolysis in this process. Whether cellular migration, proliferation or matrix remodeling are affected, remains to be determined.

Atherosclerosis

Epidemiologic, genetic, and molecular evidence suggests that impaired fibrinolysis resulting from increased PAI-1 or reduced t-PA expression or from inhibition of plasminogen activation, may contribute to the development and/or progression of atherosclerosis [38-40], presumably by promoting thrombosis or matrix deposition. Indeed, PAI-1 plasma levels are elevated in patients with ischemic heart disease, angina pectoris, and recurrent myocardial infarction [40]. Recent genetic analyses revealed a link between polymorphisms in the PAI-1 promoter and the susceptibility of atherothrombosis. A possible role for increased plasmin proteolysis in atherosclerosis is, however, suggested by the enhanced expression of t-PA and u-PA in plaques [41,42]. Plasmin proteolysis might indeed participate in plaque neovascularization, induction of plaque rupture or in ulceration and formation of aneurysms. A causative role of the plasminogen system in these processes has, however, not been conclusively demonstrated.

Atherosclerosis was studied in mice deficient in apolipoprotein E (apoE) and in t-PA, u-PA, or PAI-1, and fed a cholesterol-rich diet for 5 to 25 weeks [43]. No differences in the size or predilection site of plaques were observed between mice with a single deficiency of apoE or with a combined deficiency of apoE and t-PA or of apoE and u-PA. However, significant genotypic differences were observed in the destruction of the media with resultant erosion, transmedial ulceration, medial smooth muscle cell loss, dilatation of the vessel wall, and aneurysm formation. At the ultrastructural level, macrophages appeared to degrade the elastin fibers which were eroded, fragmented, and subsequently completely degraded. Only after macrophages crossed the internal elastic lamina, they left behind a trail of disorganized collagen bundles and glycoprotein-rich matrix which appeared totally degraded and scattered. Thus, macrophage-mediated elastolysis (which dilates but does not rupture the vessel wall) appeared to precede subsequent collagenolysis (which ruptures the vessel wall). Whereas both apoE-deficient and apoE:t-PA-deficient mice developed severe media destruction, apoE:u-PA-deficient mice were virtually completely protected. Plaque macrophages expressed abundant amounts of u-PA mRNA, antigen and activity at the base of the plaque and in the media, similar as in the atherosclerotic, aneurysmatic arteries in patients. Consistent with the notion that plasmin is unable to degrade elastin and collagen by itself, plasmin promoted degradation of elastin and collagen via activation of matrix metalloproteinases (MMPs) such as stromelysin-1 (MMP-3), gelatinase-B (MMP-9), the macrophage metalloelastase (MMP-12), and the mouse interstitial collagenase (MMP-13). The expression of these metalloproteinases was induced *in situ* in advanced atherosclerotic plaques by macrophages which also expressed increased amounts of u-PA. Taken together, these results implicate an important role of u-PA in maintenance of the structural integrity of the atherosclerotic vessel wall. Its importance in amplifying degradation of all matrix components in the vessel wall likely relates to its ability to trigger activation of several matrix metalloproteinases. These studies also provide the first *in vivo* evidence for a role of plasmin in activation of proMMPs in pathophysiological conditions.

In contrast, mice with a combined deficiency of apoE and PAI-1 developed normal fatty streak lesions but, subsequently, revealed a transient delayed progression to fibroproliferative plaques. Whether the increased plasmin proteolytic balance in these mice might prevent matrix accumulation and, consequently, delay plaque progression, or whether more abundant plasmin increased activation of latent TGF-β with its pleiotropic role on smooth muscle cell function and matrix accumulation, remains to be determined. Taken together, these targeting studies identify a specific role for u-PA in the destruction of the media that may precede aneurysm formation, and for PAI-1 in plaque progression, possibly by promoting matrix deposition.

Myocardial Infarction

Although t-PA has been widely used as a therapeutic thrombolytic agent, the involvement of the plasminogen system in healing of the ischemic myocardium has not been explored. Initial studies (in collaboration with M. Daemen and J. Smeets, Maastricht, the Netherlands) suggest, however, that the plasminogen system is importantly involved in this process. Indeed, following ligation of the left anterior descending coronary artery, wild type or t-PA-deficient mice heal their ischemic myocardium within two weeks via scar formation, i.e. the ischemic myocardium becomes infiltrated by leukocytes, endothelial cells, and fibroblasts with resultant deposition of collagen. In a fraction of these mice, rupture of the ischemic myocardium occurs shortly after infarction, possibly related to excessive plasmin proteolysis by infiltrating wound cells. In sharp contrast, mice lacking u-PA or Plg fail to heal the ischemic myocardium which remains largely devoid of infiltrating leukocytes, endothelial cells, and fibroblasts and collagen deposition and myocardial wall rupture do not appear to occur. Mural thrombosis in the ventricular cavity occurred, however, regularly in Plg-deficient but not in wild type mice. How these morphologic observations correlate with expression of fibrinolytic or matrix metalloproteinase enzymes and whether cardiac function is affected differently in the various genotypes remains to be determined.

References

1. Edgington TS, Mackman N, Brand K, Ruf W. The structural biology of expression and function of tissue factor. Thromb Haemost 1991;66(1):67-79.
2. Furie B, Furie BC. The molecular basis of blood coagulation. Cell 1988;53(4):505-18.
3. Collen D, Lijnen HR. Basic and clinical aspects of fibrinolysis and thrombolysis. Blood 1991; 78(12):3114-24.
4. Schneiderman J, Loskutoff DJ. Plasminogen activator inhibitors. Trends Cardiovasc Med 1991;1:99-102.
5. Vassalli JD. The urokinase receptor. Fibrinolysis 1994;8(Suppl.1):172-81.
6. Murphy G. Matrix metalloproteinases and their inhibitors. Acta Orthop Scand (Suppl 256) 1995;66:55-60.
7. Murphy G, Atkinson S, Ward R, Gavrilovic J, Reynolds JJ. The role of plasminogen activators in the regulation of connective tissue metalloproteinases. Ann N Y Acad Sci 1992; 667:1-12.
8. Risau W. Differentiation of endothelium. FASEB J 1995;9(10):926-33.
9. Carmeliet P, Ferreira V, Breier G, et al. Abnormal blood vessel development and lethality in embryos lacking a single vascular endothelial growth factor allele. Nature 1996;380:435-39.
10. Carmeliet P, Mackman N, Moons L, et al. Role of tissue factor in embryonic blood vessel development. Nature 1996;383:73-75.
11. Bugge TH, Xiao Q, Kombrinck KW, et al. Fatal embryonic bleeding events in mice lacking tissue factor, the cell-associated initiator of blood coagulation. Proc Natl Acad Sci USA 1996; 93(13):6258-63.
12. Toomey JR, Kratzer KE, Lasky NM, Stanton JJ, Broze GJ, Jr. Targeted disruption of the murine tissue factor gene results in embryonic lethality. Blood 1996;88(5):1583-87.
13. Rosen E, Chan JY, Esohe I, et al. Factor VII deficient mice develop normally but suffer fatal perinatal bleeding. Nature 1997; in press.
14. Cui J, O'Shea KS, Purkayastha A, Saunders TL, Ginsburg D. Fatal haemorrhage and incomplete block to embryogenesis in mice lacking coagulation factor V. Nature 1996;384 (6604):66-68.
15. Connolly AJ, Ishihara H, Kahn ML, Farese RV, Jr., Coughlin SR. Role of the thrombin receptor in development and evidence for a second receptor. Nature 1996;381(6582):516-19.
16. Bi L, Lawler AM, Antonarakis SE, High KA, Gearhart JD, Kazazian HH, Jr. Targeted disruption of the mouse factor VIII gene produces a model of haemophilia A. Nat Genet 1995; 10(1):119-21.
17. Suh TT, Holmback K, Jensen NJ, et al. Resolution of spontaneous bleeding events but failure

of pregnancy in fibrinogen-deficient mice. Genes Dev 1995;9(16):2020-33.

18. Aoki N. Hemostasis associated with abnormalities of fibrinolysis. Blood Rev 1989;3(1):11-17.

19. Carmeliet P, Schoonjans L, Kieckens L, et al. Physiological consequences of loss of plasminogen activator gene function in mice. Nature 1994;368(6470):419-24.

20. Ploplis VA, Carmeliet P, Vazirzadeh S, et al. Effects of disruption of the plasminogen gene on thrombosis, growth, and health in mice. Circulation 1995;92(9):2585-93.

21. Bugge TH, Flick MJ, Daugherty CC, Degen JL. Plasminogen deficiency causes severe thrombosis but is compatible with development and reproduction. Genes Dev 1995;9(7):794-807.

22. Bugge TH, Flick MJ, Danton MJ, et al. Urokinase-type plasminogen activator is effective in fibrin clearance in the absence of its receptor or tissue-type plasminogen activator. Proc Natl Acad Sci USA 1996;93(12):5899-904.

23. Romer J, Bugge TH, Pyke C, et al. Impaired wound healing in mice with a disrupted plasminogen gene. Nat Med 1996;2(3):287-92.

24. Kitching AR, Holdsworth SR, Ploplis V, et al. Plasminogen and plasminogen activators protect against renal injury in crescentic glomerulonephritis. J Exp Med 1997;5:963-68.

25. Carmeliet P, Moons L, Ploplis V, Plow EF, Collen D. Impaired arterial neointima formation in mice with disruption of the plasminogen gene. J Clin Invest 1997;99:200-208.

26. Carmeliet P, Kieckens L, Schoonjans L, et al. Plasminogen activator inhibitor-1 gene-deficient mice. I. Generation by homologous recombination and characterization. J Clin Invest 1993;92:2746-55.

27. Carmeliet P, Stassen JM, Schoonjans L, et al. Plasminogen activator inhibitor-1 gene-deficient mice. II. Effects on hemostasis, thrombosis and thrombolysis. J Clin Invest 1993;92:2756-60.

28. Carmeliet P, Bouche A, De Clercq C, et al. Biological effects of disruption of the tissue-type plasminogen activator, urokinase-type plasminogen activator, and plasminogen activator inhibitor-1 genes in mice. Ann N Y Acad Sci 1995;748:367-81.

29. Carmeliet P, Stassen JM, Meidell R, Collen D, Gerard R. Adenovirus-mediated gene transfer of rt-PA restores thrombolysis in t-PA deficient mice. Blood 1997;90(4):1527-34.

30. Simpson AJ, Booth NA, Moore NR, Bennett B. Distribution of plasminogen activator inhibitor (PAI-1) in tissues. J Clin Pathol 1991;44(2):139-43.

31. Clowes AW, Clowes MM, Au YP, Reidy MA, Belin D. Smooth muscle cells express urokinase during mitogenesis and tissue-type plasminogen activator during migration in injured rat carotid artery. Circ Res 1990;67(1):61-67.

32. Carmeliet P, Moons L, Stassen JM, et al. A model for arterial neointima formation using perivascular electric injury in mice. Am J Pathol 1997;150:761-77.

33. Carmeliet P, Moons L, Herbert J-M, et al. Urokinase-type but not tissue-type plasminogen activator mediates arterial neointima formation in mice. Circ Res 1997; in press.

34. Carmeliet P, Moons L, Dewerchin M, et al. Urokinase receptor independent role of the urokinase-type plasminogen activator during vascular wound healing. J Cell Biol (under revision).

35. Carmeliet P, Moons L, Lijnen R, et al. Inhibitory role of plasminogen activator inhibitor-1 in arterial wound healing and neointima formation. A gene targeting and gene transfer study in mice. Circulation 1997; in press.

36. Stefansson S, Lawrence DA. The serpin PAI-1 inhibits cell migration by blocking integrin alpha V beta3 binding to vitronectin. Nature 1996;383(6599):441-43.

37. Shi C, Russell ME, Bianchi C, Newell JB, Haber E. Murine model of accelerated transplant

arteriosclerosis. Circ Res 1994;75(2):199-207.

38. Schneiderman J, Sawdey MS, Keeton MR, et al. Increased type 1 plasminogen activator inhibitor gene expression in atherosclerotic human arteries. Proc Natl Acad Sci USA 1992;89 (15):6998-7002.

39. Wiman B. Plasminogen activator inhibitor 1 (PAI-1) in plasma: Its role in thrombotic disease. Thromb Haemost 1995;74(1):71-76.

40. Hamsten A, Eriksson P. Fibrinolysis and atherosclerosis: An update. Fibrinolysis 1994;8 (Suppl.1):253-62.

41. Lupu F, Heim DA, Bachmann F, Hurni M, Kakkar VV, Kruithof EK. Plasminogen activator expression in human atherosclerotic lesions. Arterioscler Thromb Vasc Biol 1995;15(9):1444-55.

42. Schneiderman J, Bordin GM, Engelberg I, et al. Expression of fibrinolytic genes in atherosclerotic abdominal aortic aneurysm wall. A possible mechanism for aneurysm expansion. J Clin Invest 1995;96(1):639-45.

43. Carmeliet P, Moons L, Lijnen R, et al. Urokinase-generated plasmin induces atherosclerotic aneurysm formation via activation of matrix malloproteinases. Nature Genetics 1997; under revision.

Evolving Understanding of Coronary Thrombosis and New Insights into Therapeutic Strategies[1]

Valentin Fuster

I was asked to describe the processes leading to coronary thrombosis and myocardial infarction (MI) based on the most recent studies of vascular biology and to outline evolving strategies for prevention. A major challenge for the 1990s is to better understand such processes to prevent "heart attacks," the term for the combined disorders of MI and sudden related death. It is estimated that more than 1.5 million MI occur annually in the United States, and at least 500,000 infarctions result in death, usually suddenly [1]; accordingly, MI is the most frequent cause of mortality in the United States, as well as in most Western countries [2,3]. However, even the optimal use of thrombolytic therapy for MI — the advance on which the greatest attention has been focused — could prevent only 25,000 deaths acutely, or 5% of the total, because most deaths occur suddenly before any type of treatment can be initiated [4].

The Lesions of Atherosclerosis-Thrombosis

According to the criteria set for the by the American Heart Association Committee on Vascular Lesions, plaque progression can be subdivided into the five phases shown in Figure 1 [5,6].

Phase 1 consists of a small lesion of the kind commonly present in people under the age of 30. Such lesions may progress over a period of years and are categorized as three types. Type I lesions consist of macrophage-derived foam cells that contain lipid droplets. Type II lesions consist of both macrophages and smooth muscle cells with extracellular lipid deposits, and type III lesions consist of smooth muscle cells surrounded by extracellular connective tissue, fibrils, and lipid deposits.

Phase 2 consists of a plaque that, although not necessarily stenotic may be prone to disruption because of its high lipid content. The lesion is categorized morphologically as one of two variants. Type IV plaques consists of confluent cellular lesions with a great deal of extracellular lipid, intermixed with fibrous tissue, whereas type Va possess an extracellular lipid core covered by a thin fibrous cap. Phase 2 can evolve into acute phase 3 and 4, and

[1]Parts of this manuscript are a modification of two recent publications by V. Fuster et al. Lancet 1996;348(Suppl.):s7-s10 and Thrombosis and Haemostasis 1997;78(1):247-255.

A. M. Gotto, Jr. et al. (eds.), Multiple Risk Factors in Cardiovascular Disease, 45–59.

either of these can evolve into fibrotic phase 5.

Phase 3 consists of the acute "complicated" type VI lesions; disruption of a type IV or Va lesion leads to the formation of a mural thrombus which may or may not completely occlude the artery. Changes in geometry of the disrupted plaque, and organization of the mural thrombus by connective tissue, can lead to the more occlusive and fibrotic type Vb or Vc lesions of phase 5. Such type Vb or Vc lesions may cause angina. However, because the preceding stenosis and ischemia can give rise to a protective collateral circulation, a final occlusion may be silent or clinically inapparent.

The acute "complicated" type VI lesion of phase 4, rather than being characterized by a small mural thrombus (as in phase 3), consists of an occlusive thrombus and results in an acute coronary syndrome.

Both phase 3 and phase 4 can develop into the occlusive and fibrotic type Vb or Vc lesions of phase 5.

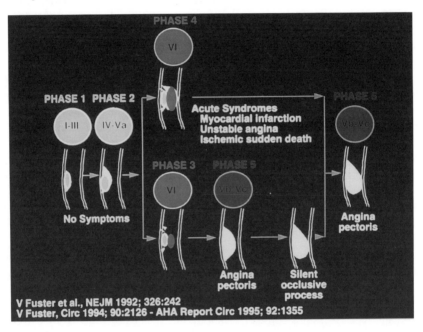

Figure 1. Phases and lesion morphology of the progression of coronary atherosclerosis according to gross pathological and clinical findings. Modified with permission from V. Fuster et al. [5].

Disruption of the Vulnerable Plaque [7]

Over the last few years, pathologic studies have revealed that such type IV and Va lesions are commonly composed of an abundant crescentic mass of lipids, intermixed or separated from the vessel lumen by a discrete component of extracellular matrix (Figures 2 and 3)

[5,8,9]. Interestingly, it has become apparent that arteriographically mild coronary lesions may be associated with significant progression to severe stenosis or total occlusion [9-11]. These lesions may account for as many as two-thirds of the patients in whom unstable angina or other acute coronary syndromes develop (Figure 4) [8,9]. This unpredictable and episodic progression is most likely caused by disruption of type IV and V lesions with subsequent thrombus formation, which changes the plaque geometry and leads to intermittent plaque growth and acute occlusive coronary syndromes [9,12].

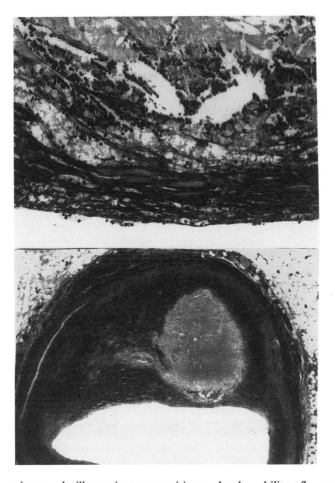

Figure 2. Photomicrographs illustrating composition and vulnerability of coronary plaques. A vulnerable plaque, containing a core of soft atheromatous gruel that is separated from the vascular lumen by a thin cap of fibrous tissue. The fibrous cap is infiltrated by foam cells that can be clearly seen at high magnification, indicating ongoing disease activity. Such a thin and macrophage-infiltrated cap is probably weak and vulnerable, and it was indeed disrupted nearby. With permission from E. Falk et al. [9].

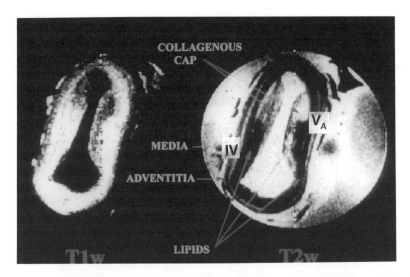

Figure 3. Nuclear magnetic resonance images of vulnerable or unstable lesions. T2w image identifies a collagenous cap on both plaques. In the type V lesions (right), the cap completely covers the lipid core. In the type IV lesions (left), the plaque is only partially covered, and infiltration of fat is more diffuse. Modified with permission from V. Fuster et al. [5].

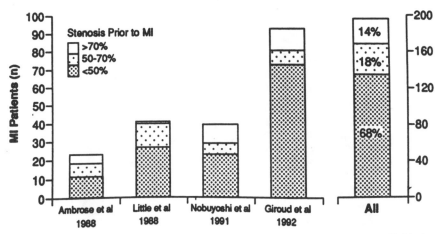

Figure 4. Bar graph showing stenosis severity and associated risk of myocardial infarction (MI). MI evolves most frequently from plaques that are only mildly to moderately obstructive months to years before infarction. The bar graph is constructed from data published by J. Ambrose et al. (J Am Coll Cardiol 1988;12:56-62), W.C. Little et al., (Circulation 1988;78(5 Pt.1):1157-1166), M. Nobuyoshi et al. (J Am Coll Cardiol 1991;18:904-910), and D. Giroud et al. (Am J Cardiol 1988;12:56-62). Modified with permission from E. Falk et al. [9].

Plaques that undergo disruption tend to be relatively soft and have a high concentration of cholesteryl esters, rather than of free cholesterol monohydrate crystals. In addition to this rather "passive" phenomenon of plaque disruption, a better understanding of an "active" phenomenon related to macrophage activity is evolving.

"Passive" plaque disruption related to physical forces occurs most frequently where the fibrous cap is thinnest, most heavily infiltrated by foam cells and, therefore, weakest. For eccentric plaques, this is often the shoulder or between the plaque and the adjacent vessel wall [8]. Pathoanatomic examination of intact and disrupted plaques and *in vitro* mechanical testing of isolated fibrous caps from aorta, indicate that vulnerability to rupture depends on three factors (Figure 5) [5,9]: 1) circumferential wall stress or cap "fatigue," which in part relates to a combination of the thickness and collagen content of the fibrous cap covering the core, blood pressure and the radius of the lumen [13]; thus, long-term repetitive cyclic stresses may weaken a material and increase its vulnerability to fracture, ultimately leading to sudden and unprovoked (i.e. untriggered) mechanical failure; 2) location, size and consistency of the atheromatous core; and 3) blood flow characteristics, particularly impact of flow on the proximal aspect of the plaque (i.e. configuration and angulation of the plaque, etc).

- Mild to Medium Size - Not Severely Stenotic
- Significant Lipid Core and Fibrous Cap
- Inflamation (Macrophages)
- Wall Stress:

1. Circumferential Wall Stress (σ) = $\dfrac{\text{Pressure (P) x Radium (r)}}{\text{Cap Thickness (h)}}$

2. Localized Wall Stress - Structural Configuration
3. Blood Flow Rheology - External Configuration
   Degree of Stenosis (Shear Stress)
   Angulation (Flow Separation or Oscillatory Flow)
4. Lipid Density (Crystals) - Regression

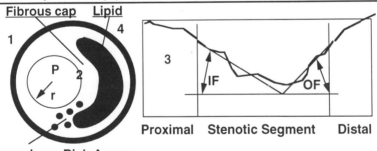

Fibrous cap   Lipid

Macrophage-Rich Areas

Proximal   Stenotic Segment   Distal

Figure 5. Pathogenesis of vulnerable or unstable lipid-rich lesion types IV and Va. Composite modified from Richardson et al. [8], Loree et al. (Circ Res 1992;71:850), MacIssac et al. [13], and Taeymans et al. (Circulation 1992;85:78). IF = inflow angle; OF = outflow angle.

As mentioned, an "active" phenomenon of plaque disruption is probably important. Thus, atherectomy specimens from patients with acute coronary syndromes revealed macrophage-rich areas [14]. Macrophages can degrade extracellular matrix by phagocytosis or by secreting proteolytic enzymes such as plasminogen activators and a family of matrix metalloproteinases (MMPs: collagenases, gelatinases, and stromelysins) that may weaken the fibrous cap, predisposing it to rupture. Indeed, the MMPs and their cosecreted tissue inhibitors of metalloproteinases (TIMP-1 and TIMP-2) are critical for vascular remodeling. Moreover, we have observed that human monocyte-derived macrophages grown in culture are capable of degrading cap collagen, while expressing MMP-1 (interstitial collagenase) and inducing MMP-2 (gelatinolytic) activity in the culture medium that can be prevented by MMP inhibitors (Figure 6) [9,15]. Several studies have now identified MMPs in human coronary plaques and lipid-filled macrophages (foam cells) that may be particularly active in destabilizing plaques, thus predisposing them to rupture [16,17].

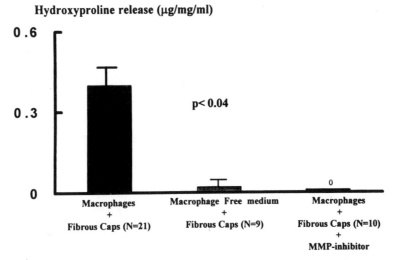

Figure 6. Data supporting the role of monocyte-derived macrophages and matrix-degrading metalloproteinases (MMPs) in inducing collagen breakdown in fibrous caps of human atherosclerotic plaques. Bar graph showing that incubation of fibrous caps with macrophages results in hydroxyproline release into the supernatant (indicative of collagen breakdown), a process inhibited by an MMP inhibitor. With permission from E. Falk et al. [15].

Acute Thrombosis

As recently reviewed [18], disruption of a vulnerable or unstable plaque with a subsequent change in plaque geometry and thrombosis results in a type VI or complicated lesion (Figure 1). Such a rapid change in atherosclerotic plaque may result in acute occlusion or subocclusion with clinical manifestations of unstable angina or other acute coronary syndromes [5,6]. More frequently, however, such rapid changes appear to result in mural thrombus without evident clinical symptoms which, by self-organization, may be a main contributor to the progression of atherosclerosis [5,6]. More specifically, at the time of coronary plaque disruption, a number of local and thrombogenic factors may influence the degree and the duration of thrombus deposition (Table 1) [5,19,20]; such a thrombus may then be either partially lysed or become replaced in the process of organization by the vascular repair response [6,21].

Table 1. Thrombotic Complications of Plaque Disruption: Local and Systemic Thrombogenic Risk Factors

---

Local Factors

- Degree of plaque disruption (i.e. fissure, ulcer)

- Degree of stenosis (i.e. change in geometry)

- Tissue substrate (i.e. lipid-rich plaque)

- Surface of residual thrombus (i.e. recurrence)

- Vasoconstriction (i.e. platelets, thrombin)

Systemic Factors

- Catecholamines (i.e. smoking, stress, cocaine)

- Renin-angiotensin (i.e. DD genotype)

- Cholesterol, lipoprotein(a) and other metabolic states (i.e. homocystinemia, diabetes)

- Fibrinogen, impaired fibrinolysis (i.e. plasminogen activator inhibitor-1), activated platelets and clotting (i.e. Factor VII, thrombin generation [fragment 1+2] or activity [fibrinopeptide A])

High risk: presumably by the presence of several local or systemic thrombogenic risk factors at the time of plaque disruption, indicates acute occlusive labile thrombus versus fixed mural thrombus (unstable angina and non-Q wave and Q wave myocardial infarction).
Low risk: presumably by the paucity of thrombogenic risk factors at the time of plaque disruption, indicates only mural thrombus (progressive atherogenesis). With permission from V. Fuster [3].

SUBSTRATE DEPENDENT THROMBOSIS [18]

In regard to the composition of human atherosclerotic plaques, there is a significant heterogeneity, even in the same individual, and plaque disruption exposes various vessel wall components to blood. Data on the thrombogenicity of disrupted atherosclerotic lesions are limited. The thrombogenicity of human atherosclerotic plaques was evaluated by exposure to flowing blood at high shear rate. The evaluated aortic plaques included normal intima (disease-free), fatty streaks, sclerotic plaques, fibrolipid plaques, and atheromatous lipid rich core. The lipid core abundant in cholesterol ester, displayed the highest thrombogenicity (Figure 7) [22].

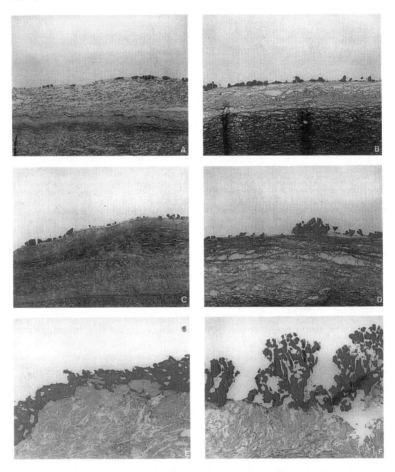

Figure 7. Representative photomicrographs from the different types of substrates exposed to flowing blood. Longitudinal section of an intimal segment of human atherosclerotic plaque showing: (A) rich cellular layer without lipid infiltration; (B) foam cell-rich matrix; (C) collagen-rich matrix; (D) collagen-poor matrix without cholesterol crystals; (E) and (F) acellular collagen-poor soft core with abundant cholesterol crystals. Note the formation of larger thrombi on atheromatous core (E and F). Trichrome x 100. With permission from A. Fernandez-Ortiz et al. [22].

TISSUE FACTOR DEPENDENT THROMBOSIS [18]

A small-molecular-weight glycoprotein--tissue factor (TF)-- initiates the extrinsic clotting cascade and is considered a major regulator of coagulation, hemostasis, and thrombosis. TF forms a high-affinity complex with coagulation factors VII/VIIa; TF-VIIa complex activates factors IX and X thereby leading to thrombin generation [23]. TF antigen is normally present only in the arterial adventitia. However, each of the major cell types in plaques (smooth muscle cells, macrophages, and endothelial cells) are capable of TF expression. TF antigen is found in the cells of atherosclerotic plaques and extracellularly in the lipid rich core and fibrous matrix as well [24]. We examined the role of TF in the thrombogenicity of various types of atherosclerotic plaques and their components. As in previous studies [22], *in vitro* examination revealed that platelet deposition was significantly greater on lipid-rich atheromatous core than on all other substrates (Figure 8) [25]. The lipid-rich core also exhibits the most intense TF staining when compared to other arterial components. This observation suggests that TF is an important determinant of the thrombogenicity of human atherosclerotic lesions after spontaneous or mechanical plaque disruption. Colocalization of directional coronary atherectomy specimens from patients with unstable angina demonstrated a strong relationship between TF and macrophages (Figures 9,10) [26]. Finally, a positive relationship was also observed between TF antigen content and activity in human coronary artery plaque tissue [27]. As a result of these recent observations, it appears that TF content and activity in the atheromatous gruel is mediated by macrophages, thus, suggesting a cell-mediated thrombogenicity in patients with acute coronary syndromes following plaque disruption.

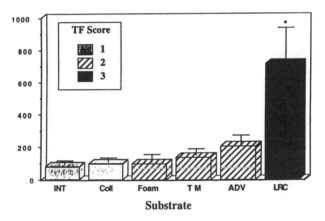

Figure 8. Platelet deposition and tissue factor activity. Platelet deposition data are expressed as Mean ± SEM; TF staining intensity is expressed as the average of the independent observers. Note the positive correlation between platelet-thrombus formation and TF score on the exposed human substrates (p < 0.01). INT = normal intima, COLL = collagen-rich matrix, FOAM = foam cell-rich matrix, TM = normal tunica media, ADV = adventitia, and LRC = lipid-rich core (*p=0.0002), ANOVA). With permission from V. Toschi et al. [25].

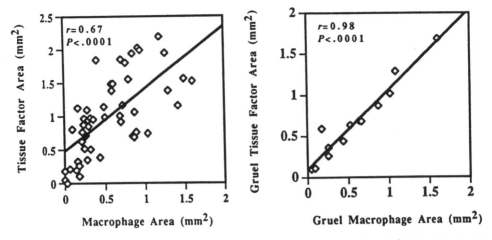

Figure 9. Left: scatterplot showing association of macrophage area (mm²) identified with KP1 immunostaining and tissue factor area (mm²) identified with a polyclonal antibody in coronary atherectomy specimens from 50 patients with acute coronary syndromes. Right: scatterplot showing association of lipid-rich macrophage area (mm²) identified with trichrome staining and lipid-rich tissue factor area (mm²) identified with a polyclonal antibody in coronary atherectomy specimens from 50 patients with acute coronary syndromes. With permission from P.R. Moreno et al. [26].

Antithrombotic Approaches to Prevention

Approaches toward retardation or even reversal of atherosclerotic lesions in humans for prevention of plaque disruption and acute coronary events include the better control of risk factors, such as reducing plasma cholesterol levels. Nevertheless, if atherosclerotic plaque disruption cannot be prevented, a beneficial effect of antiplatelet and anticoagulant agents has been observed in the prevention of acute coronary events.

The best-suited, least toxic, and most widely used antithrombotic agent in acute and chronic coronary artery disease is aspirin. It has been shown to be effective in unstable angina and acute myocardial infarction during and after coronary revascularization, in the secondary prevention of chronic coronary and cerebrovascular disease, and in primary prevention, particularly in high-risk groups [5,18,19]. Aspirin interferes with only one of the three pathways of platelet activation, the one dependent of thromboxane A_2. The other two pathways, one dependent on ADP and collagen and the other on thrombin, remain unaffected, as does the coagulation system. On the other hand, current anticoagulant agents interfere only partially with the coagulation system and do not affect platelet activation. It is not surprising, therefore, that aspirin, or anticoagulants cannot completely prevent coronary thrombotic events, although the relative antithrombotic effectiveness of both types of antithrombotic agents is clinically similar.

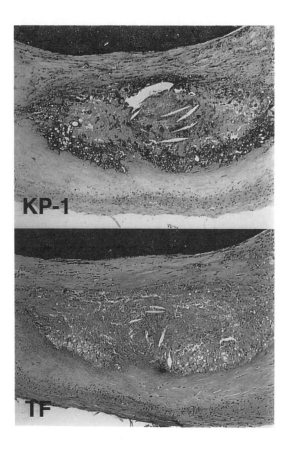

Figure 10. Photomicrographs of immunohistochemically stained adjacent tissue sections of human coronary artery showing: (top) a "vulnerable" macrophage-rich (KP-1+) atherosclerotic plaque and (bottom) staining for TF antigen which is observed mainly in the necrotic, lipid-rich core of the plaque. PAP method; original magnification x 40.

Combination therapy with a platelet inhibitor (aspirin or ticlopidine) and an anticoagulant agent (intravenous heparin, subcutaneous low-molecular-weight heparin or oral warfarin) may have an additive effect. Thus far, such therapy (aspirin and heparin/warfarin) is being considered only for the short term (< 1 week to 3 months) in patients at high-risk for thrombotic events, such as those with acute myocardial infarction or unstable angina. The long-term (3 years) postmyocardial study CHAMP is randomizing patients to receive either 160 mg/day of aspirin or 80 mg of aspirin plus coumadin to achieve an INR of 1.5-2.5. Results of this study may settle some of the unanswered questions regarding the use of anticoagulants and antiplatelet agents for long-term secondary prevention of acute myocardial infarction. As we reported, the combination of fixed very low-dose anticoagulants and antiplatelet agents in the long-term secondary prevention of acute myocardial infarction has been discouraging in the CARS study involving 9,000 patients [28]. Similar discouraging results with very low-dose anticoagulants have been reported by the SPAF III investigators on atrial fibrillation [29] and by the study group on coronary artery bypass grafts for the prevention of graft disease and occlusion [30].

Table 2 outlines some of the newer antithrombotic approaches being investigated for the treatment of acute coronary syndromes or at the time of PTCA [18]. These antithrombotics are used intravenously and act by either blocking the early stage of thrombin-related platelet activation, such as the specific antithrombins hirudin and hirulog, or by blocking the late stage of receptor glycoprotein IIb/IIIa-related platelet activation. Other intravenous agents such as TF inhibitors [31], as well as subcutaneous and oral antithrombins and receptor glycoproteins IIb/IIIa blockers, are new exploratory antithrombotic strategies for the prevention of coronary thrombosis.

Table 2. New Antithrombotics, ACS, Clinical Trials, 1997

Agents	Unstable Angina	MI	PCTA-Occlusion
Hirudin	GUSTO-IIA [32][1]	GUSTO-IIA [32][1]	HELVETICA[1]
	GUSTO-IIB [33][1]	TIMI-9A [34][1]	
	OASIS[2]	HIT III [35][1]	
	(6 Mo:ASA+A/C)	GUSTO-IIB [33][1]	
		TIMI 9B [36][1]	
		OASIS (non ST↑)[2]	
Hirulog	TIMI-8[1]	HERO (SK)[3]	PTCA[1]
IIb/IIIa	CANADIAN (Pilot) [37][3]	PARADIGM II[2]	IMPACT-II PTCA[38][1]
Block.	PRISM [39][3]		RESTORE [40][1]
	PRISM PLUS [39][3]		CAPTURE [38][1]
	PARAGON[2]		EPIC (& Resten) [41][3]
	PURSUIT[2]		EPILOG (Resten) [42][3]
			ERASER (Stent)[2]

[1] Questionable; [2] Ongoing; [3] Definitive-Benefit.

References

1.   American Heart Association. Heart and Stroke Facts: 1996 Statistical Supplement. Dallas, Texas: American Heart Association National Center, 1996.
2.   Cooper ES. Prevention: The key to progress. AHA Medical/Scientific Statement. Circulation 1993;24:629-32.
3.   WHO-MONICA Project. Myocardial infarction and coronary deaths in the World Health Organization Monica Project: Registration procedures, event rates, and care-facility rates in 38 populations from 21 countries in four continents. Circulation 1994;90:583-612.
4.   Muller JE, Abela GS, Nesto RW, Tofler GH. Triggers, acute risk factors and vulnerable plaques: The lexicon of a new frontier. J Am Coll Cardiol 1994;23:809-13.
5.   Fuster V. Mechanisms leading to myocardial infarction: Insights from studies of vascular biology. Lewis A. Conner Memorial Lecture. Circulation 1994;90:2126-46.
6.   Stary HC, Chandler AB, Dinsmore RE, et al. A definition of advanced types of atherosclerotic lesions and a histological classification of atherosclerosis: A report from the Committee on Vascular Lesions of the Council on Arteriosclerosis, American Heart Association. Circulation 1995;92:1355-74.
7.   Fuster V. Human Lesion Studies. Ann NY Acad Science 1997;811:207-25.
8.   Richardson PD, Davies MJ, Born GV. Influence of plaque configuration and stress distribution on fissuring of coronary atherosclerotic plaques. Lancet 1989;2(8669):1462-63.
9   Falk E, Shah PK, Fuster V. Coronary plaque disruption. Circulation 1995;92:657-71.
10.   Ambrose JA, Tannenbaum M, Alexpoulos D, et al. Angiographic progression of coronary artery disease and the development of myocardial infarction. J Am Coll Cardiol 1988;12:56-62.
11.   Little WC, Constantinescu M, Applegate RJ, et al. Can coronary angiography predict the site of a subsequent myocardial infarction in patients with mild-to-moderate coronary artery disease. Circulation 188;78(5 Pt.1):1157-66.
12.   Davies MJ. Stability and instability: Two faces of coronary atherosclerosis. Circulation 1994; 2013-19.
13.   MacIssac AL, Thomas JD, Topol EJ. Toward the quiescent coronary plaque. J Am Coll Cardiol 1993;22:1228-41.
14.   Moreno PR, Falk E, Palacios IF, Newell JB, Fuster V, Fallon JT. Macrophage infiltration in acute coronary syndromes. Implications for plaque rupture. Circulation 1994;90(2):775-78.
15.   Shah PK, Falk E, Badimon JJ, et al. Human monocyte-derived macrophages induce collagen breakdown in fibrous caps of atherosclerotic plaques. Potential role of matrix-degrading metalloproteinases and implications for plaque rupture. Circulation 1995;92:1565-69.
16.   Galis ZS, Sukhova GK, Lark MW, Libby P. Increased expression of matrix metalloproteinase and matrix degrading activity in vulnerable regions of human atherosclerotic plaques. J Clin Invest 1994;94(6):2493-503.
17.   Galis ZS, Sukhova GK, Kranzhofer R, Clark S, Libby P. Macrophage foam cells from experimental atheroma constitutively produce matrix-degrading proteinases. Proc Natl Acad Sci USA 1995;92(2):402-6.
18.   Fuster V, Fallon JT, Nemerson Y. Coronary thrombosis. The Lancet 1996;348(Suppl.):s7-s10.
19.   Fuster V, Badimon L, Badimon JJ, Chesebro JH. The pathogenesis of coronary artery disease and the acute coronary syndromes. N Engl J Med 1992;326:310-18.
20.   Burke AP, Farb A, Malcolm GT, Liang YH, Smialek J, Virmani R. Coronary risk factors and

plaque morphology in men with coronary disease who died suddenly. N Engl J Med 1997: 336(18):1276-81.

21. Ross R. The pathogenesis of atherosclerosis: A perspective for the 1990s. Nature 1993;362: 801-9.

22. Fernandez-Ortiz A, Badimon JJ, Falk E, et al. Characterization of the relative thrombogenicity of atherosclerotic plaque components: Implications for consequences of plaque rupture. J Am Coll Cardiol 1994;23:1562-69.

23. Banner DW, D'Arcy A, Chene C, et al. The crystal structure of the complex of blood coagulation factor VIIa with soluble tissue factor. Nature 1996;380(6569):41-46.

24. Thiruvikraman SV, Guha A, Roboz J, Taubman MB, Nemerson Y, Fallon JT. In situ localization of tissue factor in human atherosclerotic plaques by binding of digoxigenin labeled factors VIIa and X. Lab Inv 1996;75:451-61.

25. Toschi V, Gallo R, Lettino M, et al. Tissue factor predicts the thrombogenicity of human atherosclerotic plaque components. Circulation 1997;95:594-99.

26. Moreno PR, Bernardi VH, Lopez-Cuellar J, et al. Macrophages, smooth muscle cells and tissue factor in unstable angina: Implications for cell mediated thrombogenicity in acute coronary syndromes. Circulation 1996;94:3090-97.

27. Marmur JDE, Thiruvikraman SV, Fyfe BS, et al. The identification of active tissue factor in human coronary atheroma. Circulation 1996;94:1226-32.

28. Coumadin Aspirin Reinfarction Study (CARS) Investigators. A randomized, double-blind study of fixed low-dose warfarin plus aspirin in post-myocardial infarction patients. The Lancet 1997;in press.

29. Stroke Prevention in Atrial Fibrillation Investigators. Adjusted-dose warfarin versus low-intensity, fixed-dose warfarin plus aspirin for high-risk patients with atrial fibrillation: Stroke Prevention in Atrial Fibrillation III randomised clinical trial. Lancet 1996;348:633-38.

30. The Post Coronary Artery Bypass Graft Trial Investigators. The effect of aggressive lowering of low-density lipoprotein cholesterol levels and low-dose anticoagulation on obstructive changes in saphenous-vein coronary artery bypass grafts. N Engl J Med 1997;336:152-62.

31. Badimon JJ, Lettino M, Toschi V, et al. Inhibitory effects of TFPA on thrombus formation triggered by lipid-rich human atherosclerotic plaques. Circulation 1995;92(Suppl.I):I-693.

32. The Global Use of Strategies in Open Occluded Coronary Arteries (GUSTO) IIa Investigators. Randomized trials of intravenous heparin versus recombinant hirudin for acute coronary syndromes. Circulation 1994;90:1631-37.

33. The Global Use of Strategies to Open Occluded Coronary Arteries (GUSTO) IIb Investigators. A comparison of recombinant hirudin with heparin for the treatment of acute coronary syndromes. N Engl J Med 1996;35:775-82.

34. Antmann EM for the TIMI 9A Investigators. Hirudin in acute myocardial infarction. Safety report from the thrombolysis and thrombin inhibition in myocardial infarction (TIMI) 9A trial. Circulation 1994;90:1624-30.

35. Neuhaus K-L, v. Essen R, Tebbe U, et al. Safety Observations from the pilot phase of the randomized r-hirudin for improvement of thrombolysis (HIT-III) study. Circulation 1994;90:1638-42.

36. Antmann EM for the TIMI 9B Investigators. Hirudin in acute myocardial infarction. Thrombolysis and thrombin inhibition in myocardial infarction (TIMI) 9B trial. Circulation 1996;349:911-21.

37. Theroux P, Kouz S, Roy L, et al. for the investigators. Platelet membrane receptor glycoprotein IIb/IIIa antagonism in unstable angina. The Canadian Lamifiban Study.

Circulation 1996;94:899-905.

38.   The IMPACT-II Investigators. Randomised placebo-controlled trial of effect of eptifibatide on complications of percutaneous coronary intervention: IMPACT-II. Lancet 1997;349:1422-28.

The CAPTURE Investigators. Randomised placebo-controlled trial of abciximab before and after during coronary intervention in refractory unstable angina: The CAPTURE study. Lancet 1997;347:1429-35.

39.   The PRISM and PRISM PLUS Studies. Presented at the American College of Cardiology Scientific Sessions. 1997.

40.   The HERO Study. Presented at the American College of Cardiology and European Society of Cardiology Scientific Sessions. 1996.

41.   Tolop EJ, Califf RM, Weisman HF, et al. on behalf of the EPIC Investigators. Randomised trial of coronary intervention with antibody against platelet IIb/IIIa integrin for reduction of clinical restenosis: Results at six months. Lancet 1994;343:881-86.

The EPIC Investigators. Use of a monclonal antibody directed against the platelet glycoprotein IIb/IIIa receptor in high risk coronary angioplasty. N Eng J Med 1994;330:956-61.

42.   The EPILOG Investigators. Platelet glycoprotein IIb/IIIa receptor blockade and low-dose heparin during percutaneous coronary revascularization. N Eng J. Med 1997;336:1689-96.

PLATELET ACTIVATION AND CAROTID ARTERIAL ATHEROTHROMBOSIS

Kenneth Kun-yu Wu

Introduction

Blood platelets play a major role in atherosclerosis and thrombosis [1]. They are critical for the pathogenesis of human carotid atherosclerosis, thromboembolism, and thrombotic stroke. A key event in all these processes is platelet activation by matrix proteins notably collagen and by inducers at the arterial damage site. Platelet activation results in drastic changes which include the following key events: 1) membrane phospholipid changes facilitating coagulation reaction and thrombin generation; 2) conformation changes in glycoprotein II_b-III_a rendering it functionally active for fibrinogen binding and platelet aggregation; 3) activation of arachidonic acid metabolism with the synthesis and release of thromboxane A_2 (TXA_2); and 4) intracellular changes leading to release of biologically active compounds from dense-granule (ADP, serotonin) and alpha-granules. Alpha-granular products comprise growth factors, coagulation factors, β-thromboglobulin (β-TG), platelet factor 4 (PF-4), and P-selectin.

ADP, thrombin, and TXA_2 recruit new platelets and amplify platelet activation and aggregation. TXA_2 and serotonin are vasoconstrictive agents and are important in ischemia. P-selectin is secreted on to the platelet membrane and maybe involved in platelet-neutrophil interaction. Growth factors such as platelet-derived growth factors play a key part in smooth muscle cell migration and proliferation. Hence, platelet activation leads to platelet aggregation and causes or contributes to vasoconstriction, internal hyperplasia, atherosclerosis, and thrombosis.

Platelet activation generally occurs on and at the vicinity of damaged arterial wall. However, clinical studies provide evidence to indicate that platelet aggregates and activated platelets are detectable in circulating blood of patients with various arterial atherothrombotic disorders [1,2]. Methods used to determine platelet activation in patients evolve from platelet aggregation and platelet aggregate ratios developed in the 1970s to βTG, PF-4, and TXB_2 (urinary 2,3-dinor-TXb$_2$) in the 1980s and platelet surface markers by flow cytometry in the 1990s (Table 1). Despite the use of diverse techniques over a more than 20-year span, the results are consistent and certain conclusions may be reached: 1) patients with myocardial infraction (MI) or thrombotic stroke are more prone to have platelet aggregates and activated platelets in circulating blood than healthy subjects and 2) platelet preparations obtained from patients with MI or stroke are more reactive *in vitro* in response to

A. M. Gotto, Jr. et al. (eds.), Multiple Risk Factors in Cardiovascular Disease, 61–65.
© 1998 Kluwer Academic Publishers and Fondazione Giovanni Lorenzini. Printed in the Netherlands.

mechanical stirring ("spontaneous" platelet aggregation), chemical stimulation, or shear stress.

Table 1. Laboratory Assays for Platelet Activation and Aggregation

1970s	• Platelet aggregation
	Spontaneous aggregation
	Induced aggregation
	• "Circulating" platelet aggregates
	• Platelet α-granule releasates
	β-thromboglobulin
	Platelet factor 4
1980s	• Thromboxane B_2 and metabolites
	Serum TXB_2
	Urine 2,3-dinor-TXB_2
	Plasma or urine 11-dehydro-TXB_2
1980s-90s	• Activated platelet membrane markers by flow cytometry
	Conformational active glycoprotein II_b-III_a
	P-selectin (GMP-140, or PADGM)
	• Platelet aggregates by flow cytometry
	Sizing of platelet aggregates by flow cytometry using GPIb MoAb
	• Platelet-neutrophil aggregates
	Dual label with P-selectin and GPIb Ab's

We previously reported spontaneous platelet aggregation in patients with stroke and demonstrated by a formalin fixation method a corresponding increase of circulating platelet aggregates in these patients [3-5]. It has recently been shown in a prospective study that post-MI patients who exhibited persistent positive spontaneous platelet aggregation increased risk for recurrent MI and MI-related mortality by several fold [6].

We have recently shown by flow cytometry the persistent presence of activated platelets and platelet-neutrophil aggregates in patients with atherothrombotic stroke but not in patients with lacunar stroke [7]. Furthermore, our results indicate that the atherothrombotic stroke patients' platelets are more prone to developing large platelet aggregates when subjected to a pathological level of shear stress (140 dynes/cm^2) [7]. These results suggest that platelets from certain subjects are more prone to be activated, and the tendency of platelet hyperreactivity increases the risk of stroke or MI.

Platelet Activation and Carotid Arterial Wall Thickness

There is less information regarding platelet activation in subclinical human atherosclerosis. Correlation of plasma level of βTG and PF4 with carotid arterial wall thickness was investigated in cross-sectional cases and controls in Atherosclerosis Risk in Communities (ARIC) study. Fifteen thousand eight hundred subjects, aged 45-64 at the time of entry, were recruited by probability sampling from four U.S. communities [8]. Carotid arterial wall thickness was determined in each subject by high-resolution B-mode ultrasonography according to a standardized procedure and the results were interpreted blindly by experienced readers. The procedure had a high degree of reproducibility [9]. Blood samples for βTG and PF4 measurements were prepared in a special antiplatelet and anticoagulant cocktail according to standardized procedures [10,11]. The repeatability of βTG was acceptable whereas that of PF4 was low [12]. Four hundred fifty-nine subjects were identified as cases with increased carotid arterial wall thickness. The thickness is at > 90th percentile of all participants. Four hundred fifty-nine subjects whose carotid arterial wall thickness was < 70th percentile of the participant population and who are age-, sex-, and race-matched with cases were included as controls. The mean values of βTG and PF4 were significantly higher in cases than in controls [13]. However, when analyzed by quartiles using conditional logistic regression, only βTG values exhibited a statistically significant association with arterial wall thickness. The quartile determination revealed a potential threshold effect. The odds ratio (OR) determined by multivariate logistic regression analysis was significantly higher for the upper most quartiles of βTG (> 27 mg/ml) compared to the lower three quartiles. The OR was 1.7 (95% confidential interval 1.1-2.5) in men and women, 2.3 in white men (95% CI 1.2-4.2), 1.4 in white women (95% CI 0. 6-3.0), and 1.0 in blacks (95% CI 0.4-2.5). This study indicates that plasma βTG levels are independently associated with early atherosclerosis in middle-aged adults, especially white men and may be useful as a marker for early atherosclerosis. In this study, plasma fibrinogen levels were also independently associated with carotid arterial wall thickness.

A Finnish population-based study also revealed an independent association of fibrinogen with carotid arterial wall thickness in middle-aged subjects [14]. Interestingly, this study showed an association of platelet hyperaggregability with progression of arterial wall thickness during a two-year follow-up [15].

Factors Contributing to Platelet Activation in Arterial Atherothrombotic Disorders

The mechanism for increased platelet aggregability and for increased circulating activated platelets in patients with atherosclerosis and its sequel has not been elucidated.

It may be speculated that three factors may contribute to increased platelet activation: 1) arterial wall injury, 2) circulating inducers of platelet activation, and 3) genetic predisposition. Arterial wall injury is accompanied by the availability of ADP, thrombin, and TXA_2 which may induce circulating platelet activation. This possibility seems low especially in early atherosclerosis. A number of risk factors for cardiovascular diseases are associated with increased platelet activation. Diabetes mellitus, cigarette smoking, and hypercholesterolemia are among better investigated examples. These risk factors plus other less well-defined platelet activating agents may contribute to platelet activation which in turn may contribute to arterial atherothrombosis.

Although the concept that platelet gene polymorphism may contribute to platelet reactivity is emerging, evidence to support this is limited. A number of polymorphism sites have been shown in platelet glycoprotein II_b-III_a, glycoprotein I_b, and glycoprotein I_aII_a genes. A recent report has shown that a glycoprotein III_a polymorphism may be associated with coronary heart disease [16]. This is an interesting report. However, this area requires further investigations to confirm that gene polymorphisms at $GPIII_a$ as well as other sites are independently associated with atherothrombotic disorders and are independent risk factors for these disorders. In addition, platelet functional correlation with gene polymorphism must be established.

Prospectives

Clinical trials with aspirin and ticlopidine have unequivocally established the importance of platelet function in human arterial atherothrombotic disorders. Response to antiplatelet agents appears heterogenous. There have not been established markers to serve as a guide for therapeutic efficacy. Population-based epidemiological studies and clinical trials will provide valuable information regarding the usefulness of certain platelet activation markers for identifying high risk patients and monitoring therapeutic efficacy.

Elucidation of genetic and environmental factors that contribute to platelet activation is essential for further understanding of population heterogeneity of platelet activation potentials and for the understanding the structure-function relationship of certain functional important platelet gene polymorphism. Several population-based studies have begun to evaluate the association of platelet gene polymorphism with MI or stroke. The results should shed light on the mechanism by which platelet activation occurs in patients with arterial atherothrombotic disorders.

Acknowledgments

The author wishes to thank Angela Wang for secretarial assistance. The work is supported in part by a program project grant from Institute of Neurological Diseases and Stroke (NS-23327) and a research contract from National Heart Lung and Blood Institute (HC-55022) of National Institutes of Health, U.S.A.

References

1. Wu KK. Platelet activation mechanisms and markers in arterial thrombosis. J Intern Med 1996;239:17-34.
2. Grand Round. Platelet activation and arterial thrombosis. Lancet 1994;344:991-95.
3. Wu KK, Hoak JC. A new method for the quantitative detection of platelet aggregates in patients with arterial insufficiency. Lancet 1974;II:924-26.
4. Wu KK, Hoak JC. Spontaneous platelet aggregation in arterial insufficiency mechanisms and implication. Thromb Haemost 1976;35:702-11.
5. Wu KK, Hoak JC. Increased platelet aggregates in patients with transient ischemic attacks. Stroke 1975;6:521-24.
6. Trip MD, Cats VM, vanCapelle FJL, Vreeken J. Platelet hyperactivity and prognosis in survivors of myocardial infraction. New Eng J Med 1990;323:1549-54.
7. Konstantopoulos K, Grotta JC, Sills C, Wu KK, Hellums JD. Shear-induced platelet aggregation in normal subjects and stroke patients. Thromb Haemost 1995;74:1329-34.
8. The ARIC Investigators. The Atherosclerosis Risk in Communities (ARIC) Study: Design and objectives. Am J Epidemiol 1989;129:687-702.
9. Heiss G, Sharrett AR, Branes R, Chambless LE, Szklo M, Alzola C, and the ARIC Investigators. Carotid atherosclerosis measured by B-mode ultrasound in populations: Associations with cardiovascular risk factors in the ARIC study. Am J Epidemiol 1991;134:250-56.
10. Papp AC, Hatzakis H, Bracey A, Wu KK. ARIC Hemostasis Study-I. Development of blood collection and processing system suitable for multicenter hemostatic studies. Thromb Haemost 1989;61:15-19.
11. Wu KK, Papp AC, Patsch W, Rock R, Eckfeldt J, Sharrett AR. ARIC Hemostasis Study-II. Organizational plan and feasibility study. Thromb Haemost 1990;64:521-25.
12. Nguyen ND, Ghaddar HM, Stinson V, Chambless LE, Wu KK. ARIC Hemostasis Study-IV. Intra-individual variability and reliability coefficient of hemostatic factors. Thromb Haemost 1995;73:256-60.
13. Ghaddar HM, Certes J, Salomaa V, et al. Correlation of specific platelet activation markers with carotid arterial wall thickness. Thromb Haemost 1995;74:943-48.
14. Salonen R, Seppanen K, Rauramaa R, Salonen JT. Prevalence of carotid atherosclerosis and serum cholesterol levels in Eastern Finland. Arteriosclerosis 1988;8:788-92.
15. Salonen R, Salonen J. Progression of carotid atherosclerosis and its determinants: A population-based ultrasonography study. Atherosclerosis 1990;81:33-40.
16. Weiss EJ, Bray PF, Tayback M, et al. A polymorphism of a platelet glycoprotein receptor as an inherited risk factor for coronary thrombosis. New Eng J Med 1996;334:1090-94.

TISSUE FACTOR AND THE REGULATION OF ARTERIAL THROMBOSIS

Mark B. Taubman

Introduction

Thrombosis is integral to the development and progression of atherosclerosis, leading to arterial occlusion and resulting in myocardial infarction, unstable angina, and sudden death [1,2]. Plaque rupture, occurring at fissures in "unstable" lipid-rich lesions, is thought to be a major precipitant of acute arterial thrombosis [1-4], exposing circulating blood to thrombogenic plaque proteins. Thrombosis may also occur on the luminal surface of severely stenotic vessels possessing heavily calcified, "stable" plaques, in some cases as a complication of arterial bypass surgery, balloon angioplasty, atherectomy, or coronary artery stenting [5-7]. Thrombus is comprised chiefly of platelets and fibrin. This discussion will focus predominantly on the role of tissue factor in mediating fibrin deposition in atherosclerosis.

Discussion

Tissue factor (TF) is a transmembrane glycoprotein that initiates coagulation [8-11]. TF binds to factor VII/VIIa, and the resulting complex acts as a catalyst for the conversion of factors IX and X to IXa and Xa respectively, triggering the clotting cascade. This ultimately leads to the generation of thrombin, which in turn cleaves fibrinogen to fibrin. Cross-linked fibrin is one of two major ingredients of the thrombus, the other being platelets. Circulating platelets adhere to the surface of injured vessels as well as directly to the fibrin clot.

There is increasing evidence that TF is a major component of the atherosclerotic plaque and its exposure during plaque rupture is likely responsible for many acute thrombotic coronary events. In normal human coronary and internal mammary arteries and aortas, TF mRNA and antigen are found in abundance only in the adventitia [12,13]. TF mRNA and antigen are undetectable in normal arterial endothelium and either undetectable or present at low levels in the media. In carotid endarterectomies [13], TF mRNA and protein were absent from the plaque endothelium, but were present in mesenchymal-like intimal cells (presumably smooth muscle cells [SMC]), in foam cells, and monocytes adjacent to cholesterol clefts, and in the extracellular matrix. In human coronary atherectomy specimens [14], TF antigen was present in 33% of de novo lesions (n=43) and in 6% of restenotic lesions (n=18). Moreno and colleagues [15] detected TF antigen in

A. M. Gotto, Jr. et al. (eds.), Multiple Risk Factors in Cardiovascular Disease, 67–74.

virtually all samples from 50 coronary atherectomies. Using a semiquantitative analysis, TF content (expressed as percentage of sample containing TF) was found to be larger in samples from patients with unstable angina ($42 \pm 3\%$) than stable angina ($18 \pm 4\%$). TF predominated in cellular areas containing macrophages and SMC in patients with unstable angina, whereas TF was found mostly in acellular areas in patients with stable angina.

We recently examined TF activity (Xa generation) in homogenized specimens from human coronary atherectomies [16]. Significant TF activity was detected in 84%. TF antigen was detected immunohistochemically in cellular and acellular areas in 86%. Thrombus was present in 19/43 lesions with detectable TF antigen, in contrast to 0/7 lesions without detectable TF antigen. One problem with examining coronary atherectomy specimens is that only small fragments are available for examination. To get a better perspective on the distribution of TF in plaques, we examined atherosclerotic human coronary and carotid arteries. In addition to staining with antibodies to TF, we also employed a highly sensitive binding assay using digoxigenin-labeled Factors VIIa (DigVIIa) and X (DigX) [17]. After reacting with tissue sections, digoxigenin-labeled factors were then identified with antibody to digoxigenin. The binding of digoxigenin-labeled factors was specific, in that binding of DigVIIa was Ca^{2+}-dependent and blocked by an excess of Factor VIIa or by preincubation with antibody to TF, and binding of DigX did not occur in the absence of Factor VIIa. TF was detected in all atherosclerotic plaques using either antibody to TF or digoxigenin-labeled factors. Of particular note was the intense staining of the lipid-rich core. TF staining and DigVIIa binding were also noted in macrophages surrounding the core and in plaque SMC, as well as in relatively acellular, fibrotic regions of advanced plaques. The arterial media showed minimal staining. The endothelium overlying the plaque also stained for TF. The finding of abundant TF in the lipid-rich core is consistent with studies in which thrombus formation and platelet deposition were examined on plaque components exposed to circulating blood in a perfusion chamber [18]. The lipid-rich core was found to be most thrombogenic [19-21].

The most likely source of TF in the lipid-rich core and in the extracellular matrix of acellular, fibrotic regions of atherosclerotic plaques are macrophages recruited to the developing plaque. It remains to be determined whether the bulk of this extracellular TF derives from cell debris or is actively extruded from the cell surface. Intimal SMC provide a second, and probably lesser, source of TF in the chronic atherosclerotic plaque. However, studies in animal models suggest that the SMC may be the predominant source of TF in acute arterial injury.

In normal rabbit and rat aorta, endothelial denudation with a balloon catheter results in the rapid deposition of a monolayer of platelets with no associated fibrin formation, even when medial smooth muscle injury is present [22]. In contrast, fibrin deposition occurs rapidly when previously injured rabbit arteries, possessing a neointima, are subjected to a second injury ("double injury") [23]. Induction of TF in arterial SMC has been reported in rabbit [24,25] and porcine [26] models of arterial injury. We have examined TF expression and fibrin deposition in rat aortic and carotid arteries using single and double injury. Fibrinogen was seen on the luminal surface after the first and second injury. Fibrin deposition and microthrombi were not seen at any time after single injury, but were present on the luminal surface following the second injury. In uninjured rat aortic media, TF mRNA was undetectable by blot or *in situ* hybridization. Two hours after balloon injury, medial TF mRNA levels increased markedly, returning to baseline after 24 hours [27]. TF antigen was not detectable in the endothelium or media of normal vessels or during the first 4 hours after injury. In contrast, medial TF was abundant at 24 hours and then slowly diminished. Subsequently, TF antigen accumulated in the developing intimal plaque, with high levels detectable 2 weeks after single injury [17]. Staining of whole mount preparations showed minimal TF antigen on the surface of uninjured or singly-injured vessels. In contrast, the second injury was associated with rapid and marked exposure (within 5 minutes) of TF antigen overlying the intimal SMC.

These studies allow one to hypothesize that TF induced in the medial SMC of normal arteries, and subsequently in the SMC of the developing neointima, is protected from the circulation by the presence of an intact internal elastic lamina, the rapid deposition of a platelet monolayer, and ultimately by re-endothelialization and the secretion of extracellular matrix. The second injury denudes the endothelium and subendothelial matrix and exposes active intimal TF to circulating blood, leading to activation of coagulation and fibrin deposition.

The significance of TF induction in acute injury remains to be determined. In rabbits subjected to arterial injury and mechanical stenosis, antibodies to TF inhibited the variations in cyclical flow [24], thought to result in part from thrombus formation and dislodgement. TF antibody also inhibited thrombus formation in a rabbit femoral artery eversion graft preparation in 4/5 animals [28]. An active-site inactivated factor VIIa (DEGR-VIIa) or tissue factor pathway inhibitor (TFPI) inhibited angiographic restenosis and intimal hyperplasia in an atherosclerotic rabbit balloon injury model [29]. Exogenously administered TFPI has been shown to inhibit venous thrombosis in rabbits [30] and to attenuate stenosis in balloon-injured hyperlipidemic pigs [31]. These studies have provided evidence that the induction of TF in arterial SMC is not only critical for thrombosis but may play a role in mediating the extent of intimal hyperplasia and stenosis.

The above studies suggest that TF may be an important target for regulating arterial thrombosis and the progression of atherosclerosis. As such, it is critical to understand how TF synthesis is regulated in vascular cells. Considerable information has been obtained concerning the regulation of TF in cell culture (reviewed in [8]). These studies have provided many insights into the agents potentially responsible for TF induction *in vivo*. In endothelial and monocyte cultures, TF mRNA or procoagulant activity is induced by tumor necrosis factor [32-34], bacterial endotoxin [35,36], interleukin 1 [37], a-thrombin [38], oxidized-LDL [39,40], allogeneic lymphocytes [41], complement components [42], and immune complexes [43]. TF expression in endothelial cells is also regulated by shear stress [44]. The regulation of TF gene expression in endothelial cells and monocytes has been extensively studied and shown to involve cooperative activation of several elements on the human TF promoter, and in particular the NFkB binding site (reviewed in [45]).

We have focused on the regulation of TF in vascular SMC. TF mRNA is rapidly induced in cultured rat aortic SMC by serum, PDGF, epidermal growth factor, angiotensin II, and a-thrombin, with levels peaking within 60-90 minutes and returning to baseline within

4 hours [46]. Serum, PDGF, and a-thrombin also induces TF mRNA and protein in human aortic and coronary artery SMC, although peak levels occur 2-4 hours after treatment [47]. The induction of TF in SMC and endothelial cells by thrombin suggests a positive feedback whereby thrombin, generated as a consequence of TF activation, can perpetuate a procoagulant state. The induction of TF in rat and human SMC appears to be due largely to increases in transcription [48]. In human SMC, PDGF-induced TF transcription peaks at 30 minutes, as determined by nuclear run-off analysis. In contrast, TF mRNA half-life, as determined from decay curves generated in the presence of actinomycin D, is not substantially altered by PDGF treatment, suggesting that changes in mRNA stability do not play an important role in regulating TF mRNA accumulation in SMC.

We have examined the cellular distribution of TF antigen in human SMC, using both anti-TF antibodies and digoxigenin-labeled clotting factors. Both techniques suggest that TF antigen predominates in the perinuclear cytoplasm 2-6 hours after agonist treatment. At later time points, TF antigen appears most abundant in patches at the cell surface. Measurements of TF activity suggest a different distribution from that detected immunohistochemically. When human SMC monolayers are assayed for surface activity (Xa generation) in a parallel plate flow chamber, similar to that used for endothelial cells [44], TF activity peaks at 4-6 hours and returns to baseline within 16 hours [47]. Peak levels of surface TF activity represent less than 20% of the activity measured in cell lysates. The remainder of the TF may exist in an intracellular pool, as predicted by immunostaining, or be "encrypted" on the cell surface [49-55]. The appearance of discrete patches of TF antigen seen at the cell surface does not correlate with the presence of surface TF activity, as measured in the flow chamber. These patches may represent coalescence of surface TF, localized in caveolae, into structures earmarked for internalization and degradation, as suggested by Mulder and colleagues [54]. Alternatively, they may represent TF-containing vesicles capable of budding from the cell surface into the extracellular space [49,56]. This latter possibility is particularly intriguing as a source of the extracellular TF found in atherosclerotic plaques. The studies in cell culture suggest that the induction of TF mRNA and protein and the presence of active TF on the surface of arterial SMC in response to growth agonists is transient. This may be an important adaptive mechanism for limiting the procoagulant potential of SMC in the arterial wall.

In summary, TF antigen and activity are found in abundance in advanced human atherosclerotic plaques. In chronic atherosclerosis, the macrophage is likely to be the major source of TF within the plaque. TF is also induced in medial SMC in response to balloon injury and subsequently accumulates in the developing neointima. The exposure of TF to circulating blood may be responsible for the thrombotic complications associated with plaque rupture and acute arterial injury. In addition, the expression of TF and the resulting activation of the coagulation cascade may indirectly play a role in intimal hyperplasia and plaque progression. TF must therefore be viewed as a potential target for inhibiting the thrombotic complications of atherosclerosis. Among the agents currently being examined for their effects on thrombus formation and intimal hyperplasia are TFPI (reviewed in [57]) and direct factor Xa inhibitors, such as tick anticoagulant peptide (TAP) and leech anticoagulant peptide (ATS) [58,59]. Continued analysis of TF gene regulation may also lead to molecular approaches for inhibiting TF production by vascular cells.

Acknowledgements

The author would like to thank Alison D Schecter, Peter L.A. Giesen, John T Fallon, and Yale Nemerson for their contribution to research described in this manuscript. This research was supported in part by National Institutes of Health Grants HL43302 and HL29019.

References

1. Fuster V, Badimon L, Badimon JJ, Chesebro JH. The pathogenesis of coronary artery disease and the acute coronary syndromes (2). N Engl J Med 1992;326(5):310-18.
2. Fuster V, Badimon L, Badimon JJ, Chesebro JH. The pathogenesis of coronary artery disease and the acute coronary syndromes (1). N Engl J Med 1992;326(4):242-50.
3. Gersh BJ, Chesebro JH, Braunwald E, et al. Coronary artery bypass graft surgery after thrombolytic therapy in the Thrombolysis in Myocardial Infarction Trial, Phase II (TIMI II). J Am Coll Cardiol 1995;25(2):395-402.
4. Davies MJ, Thomas AC. Plaque fissuring--the cause of acute myocardial infarction, sudden ischaemic death, and crescendo angina. Br Heart J 1985;53(4):363-73.
5. Nath FC, Muller DW, Ellis SG, et al. Thrombosis of a flexible coil coronary stent: Frequency, predictors and clinical outcome. J Am Coll Cardiol 1993;21(3):622-27.
6. Losordo DW, Rosenfield K, Pieczek A, Baker K, Harding M, Isner JM. How does angioplasty work? Serial analysis of human iliac arteries using intravascular ultrasound. Circulation 1992;86(6):1845-58.
7. Carrozza JP, Jr., Baim DS. Complications of directional coronary atherectomy: Incidence, causes, and management. Am J Cardiol 1993;72(13):47E-54E.
8. Edgington TS, Mackman N, Brand K, Ruf W. The structural biology of expression and function of tissue factor. Thromb Haemost 1991;66(1):67-79.
9. Nemerson Y. Tissue factor and hemostasis. Blood 1988;71(1):1-8.
10. Rapaport SI, Rao LV. The tissue factor pathway: How it has become a "prima ballerina." Thromb Haemost 1995;74(1):7-17.
11. Nemerson Y. Tissue factor: Then and now. Thromb Haemost 1995;74(1):180-84.
12. Drake AT, Morrissey HJ, Edgington ST. Selective cellular expression of tissue factor in human tissues. Am J Pathol 1989;134(5):1087-97.
13. Wilcox JN, Smith KM, Schwartz SM, Gordon D. Localization of tissue factor in the normal vessel wall and in the atherosclerotic plaque. Proc Natl Acad Sci USA 1989;86(8):2839-43.
14. Annex BH, Denning SM, Channon KM, et al. Differential expression of tissue factor protein in directional atherectomy specimens from patients with stable and unstable coronary syndromes. Circulation 1995;91(3):619-22.
15. Moreno PR, Bernardi VH, Lopez-Cuellar J, et al. Macrophages, smooth muscle cells, and tissue factor in unstable angina. Implications for cell-mediated thrombogenicity in acute coronary syndromes. Circulation 1996;94(12):3090-97.
16. Marmur JD, Thiruvikraman SV, Fyfe BS, et al. Identification of active tissue factor in human coronary atheroma. Circulation 1996;94(6):1226-32.
17. Thiruvikraman SV, Guha A, Roboz J, Taubman MB, Nemerson Y, Fallon JT. In situ localization of tissue factor in human atherosclerotic plaques by binding of digoxigenin-

labeled factors VIIa and X. Lab Invest 1996;75(4):451-61.

18.   Badimon L, Badimon JJ, Galvez A, Chesebro JH, Fuster V. Influence of arterial damage and wall shear rate on platelet deposition. Ex vivo study in a swine model. Arteriosclerosis 1986;6(3):312-20.

19.   Fernandez-Ortiz A, Badimon JJ, Falk E, et al. Characterization of the relative thrombogenicity of atherosclerotic plaque components: Implications for consequences of plaque rupture. J Am Coll Cardiol 1994;23(7):1562-69.

20.   Mailhac A, Badimon JJ, Fallon JT, et al. Effect of an eccentric severe stenosis on fibrin(ogen) deposition on severely damaged vessel wall in arterial thrombosis. Relative contribution of fibrin(ogen) and platelets. Circulation 1994;90(2):988-96.

21.   Badimon JJ, Weng D, Chesebro JH, Fuster V, Badimon L. Platelet deposition induced by severely damaged vessel wall is inhibited by a boroarginine synthetic peptide with antithrombin activity. Thromb Haemost 1994;71(4):511-16.

22.   Clowes AW, Clowes MM, Gown AM, Wight TN. Localization of proteoheparan sulfate in rat aorta. Histochemistry 1984;80(4):379-84.

23.   Groves MH, Rathbone-Kinlough LR, Richardson M, Jorgensen L, Moore S, Mustard FJ. Thrombin generation and fibrin formation following injury to rabbit neointima. Lab Invest 1982;46(6):605-12.

24.   Pawashe AB, Golino P, Ambrosio G, et al. A monoclonal antibody against rabbit tissue factor inhibits thrombus formation in stenotic injured rabbit carotid arteries. Circulation Res 1994;74(1):56-63.

25.   Speidel CM, Eisenberg PR, Ruf W, Edgington TS, Abendschein DR. Tissue factor mediates prolonged procoagulant activity on the luminal surface of balloon-injured aortas in rabbits. Circulation 1995;92(11):3323-30.

26.   Gallo R, Fallon JT, Toschi V, et al. Bi-phasic increase of tissue factor activity after angioplasty in porcine coronary arteries. Circulation 1995;92:I-354 (Abstract).

27.   Marmur JD, Rossikhina M, Guha A, et al. Tissue factor is rapidly induced in arterial smooth muscle after balloon injury. J Clin Invest 1993;91(5):2253-59.

28.   Jang IK, Gold HK, Leinbach RC, Fallon JT, Collen D, Wilcox JN. Antithrombotic effect of a monoclonal antibody against tissue factor in a rabbit model of platelet-mediated arterial thrombosis. Arterioscler Thromb 1992;12(8):948-54.

29.   Jang Y, Guzman LA, Lincoff AM, et al. Influence of blockade at specific levels of the coagulation cascade on restenosis in a rabbit atherosclerotic femoral artery injury model. Circulation 1995;92(10):3041-50.

30.   Holst J, Lindblad B, Bergqvist D, et al. Antithrombotic effect of recombinant truncated tissue factor pathway inhibitor (TFPI1-161) in experimental venous thrombosis--a comparison with low molecular weight heparin. Thromb Haemost 1994;71(2):214-19.

31.   Oltrana L, Speidel CM, Recchia D, Abendschein DR. Inhibition of tissue factor-mediated thrombosis markedly attenuates stenosis after balloon-induced arterial injury in hyperlipidemic minipigs. Circulation 1994;90:I-344.

32.   Conway EM, Bach R, Rosenberg RD, Konigsberg WH. Tumor necrosis factor enhances expression of tissue factor mRNA in endothelial cells. Thromb Res 1989;53(3):231-41.

33.   Nawroth PP, Stern DM. Modulation of endothelial cell hemostatic properties by tumor necrosis factor. J Exp Med 1986;163(3):740-45.

34.   Scarpati EM, Sadler JE. Regulation of endothelial cell coagulant properties. Modulation of tissue factor, plasminogen activator inhibitors, and thrombomodulin by phorbol 12-myristate 13-acetate and tumor necrosis factor. J Biol Chem 1989;264(34):20705-13.

35.   Crossman DC, Carr DP, Tuddenham EG, Pearson JD, McVey JH. The regulation of tissue factor mRNA in human endothelial cells in response to endotoxin or phorbol ester. J Biol Chem 1990;265(17):9782-87.

36.   Moore KL, Andreoli SP, Esmon NL, Esmon CT, Bang NU. Endotoxin enhances tissue factor and suppresses thrombomodulin expression of human vascular endothelium in vitro. J Clin Invest 1987;79(1):124-30.

37.   Bevilacqua MP, Pober JS, Majeau GR, Cotran RS, Gimbrone MA, Jr. Interleukin 1 (IL-1) induces biosynthesis and cell surface expression of procoagulant activity in human vascular endothelial cells. J Exp Med 1984;160(2):618-23.

38.   Brox JH, Osterud B, Bjorklid E, Fenton JWd. Production and availability of thromboplastin in endothelial cells: The effects of thrombin, endotoxin and platelets. Br J Haematol 1984;57(2):239-46.

39.   Drake TA, Hannani K, Fei HH, Lavi S, Berliner JA. Minimally oxidized low-density lipoprotein induces tissue factor expression in cultured human endothelial cells. Am J Pathol 1991;138(3):601-7.

40.   Brand K, Banka CL, Mackman N, Terkeltaub RA, Fan ST, Curtiss LK. Oxidized LDL enhances lipopolysaccharide-induced tissue factor expression in human adherent monocytes. Arterioscl Thromb 1994;14(5):790-97.

41.   Carlsen E, Gaudernack G, Filion-Myklebust C, Pettersen KS, Prydz H. Allogenic induction of thromboplastin synthesis in monocytes and endothelial cells. Biphasic effect of cyclosporin A. Clin Exp Immunol 1989;76(3):428-33.

42.   Muhlfelder TW, Niemetz J, Kreutzer D, Beebe D, Ward PA, Rosenfeld SI. C5 chemotactic fragment induces leukocyte production of tissue factor activity: A link between complement and coagulation. J Clin Invest 1979;63(1):147-50.

43.   Rothberger H, Zimmerman TS, Spiegelberg HL, Vaughan JH. Leukocyte procoagulant activity: Enhancement of production in vitro by IgG and antigen-antibody complexes. J Clin Invest 1977;59(3):549-57.

44.   Grabowski EF, Zuckerman DB, Nemerson Y. The functional expression of tissue factor by fibroblasts and endothelial cells under flow conditions. Blood 1993;81(12):3265-70.

45.   Mackman N. Regulation of the tissue factor gene. FASEB Journal 1995;9(10):883-89.

46.   Taubman MB, Marmur JD, Rosenfield CL, Guha A, Nichtberger S, Nemerson Y. Agonist-mediated tissue factor expression in cultured vascular smooth muscle cells. Role of Ca2+ mobilization and protein kinase C activation. J Clin Invest 1993;91(2):547-52.

47.   Schecter AD, Fallon JT, Thiruvikraman SV, et al. Delayed surface expression of active tissue factor in human arterial smooth muscle cells determined by a novel in situ activity assay. Circulation 1995;92:I-804.

48.   Taby O, Rosenfield CL, Bogdanov V, Nemerson Y, Taubman MB. Cloning of the rat tissue factor cDNA and promoter: Identification of a serum-response region. Thromb Haemost 1996;76(5):697-702.

49.   Maynard JR, Heckman CA, Pitlick FA, Nemerson Y. Association of tissue factor activity with the surface of cultured cells. J Clin Invest 1975;55(4):814-24.

50.   Bach R, Rifkin DB. Expression of tissue factor procoagulant activity: Regulation by cytosolic calcium. Proc Natl Acad Sci USA 1990;87(18):6995-99.

51.   Carson SD. Manifestation of cryptic fibroblast tissue factor occurs at detergent concentrations which dissolve the plasma membrane. Blood Coagul Fibrinolysis 1996;7(3):303-13.

52.   Drake TA, Ruf W, Morrissey JH, Edgington TS. Functional tissue factor is entirely cell surface expressed on lipopolysaccharide-stimulated human blood monocytes and a

constitutively tissue factor-producing neoplastic cell line. J Cell Biol 1989;109(1):389-95.

53.   Le DT, Rapaport SI, Rao LV. Relations between factor VIIa binding and expression of factor VIIa/tissue factor catalytic activity on cell surfaces. J Biol Chem 1992;267(22):15447-54.

54.   Mulder AB, Smit JW, Bom VJ, et al. Association of smooth muscle cell tissue factor with caveolae. Blood 1996;88(4):1306-13.

55.   Sevinsky RJ, Rao MVL, Ruf W. Ligand-induced protease receptor translocation into caveolae: A mechanism for regulating cell surface proteolysis of the tissue factor-dependent coagulation pathway. J Cell Biol 1996;133:293-304.

56.   Dvorak HF, Van DeWater L, Bitzer AM, et al. Procoagulant activity associated with plasma membrane vesicles shed by cultured tumor cells. Cancer Res 1983;43(9):4434-42.

57.   Broze GJ, Jr. Tissue factor pathway inhibitor. Thromb Haemost 1995;74(1):90-93.

58.   Dunwiddie C, Thornberry NA, Bull HG, et al. Antistasin, a leech-derived inhibitor of factor Xa. Kinetic analysis of enzyme inhibition and identification of the reactive site. J Biol Chem 1989;264(28):16694-99.

59.   Waxman L, Smith DE, Arcuri KE, Vlasuk GP. Tick anticoagulant peptide (TAP) is a novel inhibitor of blood coagulation factor Xa. Science 1990;248(4955):593-96.

FIBRINOGEN: RISK FACTOR OR RISK MARKER?

Edzard Ernst and Wolfgang Koenig

Introduction

Our knowledge of "accepted" risk factors has become compelling. Its application to clinical practice has started to result in a considerable reduction of cardiovascular mortality and morbidity. Yet our understanding of cardiovascular risk factors is still incomplete. Only about 30% of all cardiovascular events can be "explained" on the basis of "accepted" risk factors [1]. Additional risk factors are therefore likely to exist, and fibrinogen is a prime candidate [2]. This review is aimed at summarizing data linking fibrinogen with cardiovascular risk.

Epidemiological Evidence

PROSPECTIVE STUDIES

In the Northwick Park Heart Study 1,510 individuals were tested for a range of clotting factors, including fibrinogen. At the 4-year follow-up, 49 individuals had died, 27 from cardiovascular diseases [3]. A significant association between cardiovascular deaths and fibrinogen existed, which was independent of other risk factors. At the 10-year follow-up [4], 109 individuals had suffered a first coronary event. An association between fibrinogen and ischemic heart disease (IHD) was demonstrated, which was again independent of conventional risk factors. Approximately half of all the incident coronary events occurred in the upper tertile of fibrinogen. This study recently reported 16-20 years of follow-up data in women [5]. The average fibrinogen level of those who had died of IHD during follow-up (n=19) was not significantly different from that of survivors (n=621): 3.38 versus 3.31 g/l.

About 2,000 men were recruited for the Speedwell Study [6]. Baseline fibrinogen was positively associated with prevalent IHD. When the study was expanded into the Caerphilly and Speedwell Studies it involved more than 4,700 men [7]. Its baseline data revealed a significant association of smoking with fibrinogen. The prospective evaluation of the Caerphilly and Speedwell Studies with an average follow up of 5.1 and 3.2 years respectively, included a total of 251 major coronary events [8]. Fibrinogen was implicated as an independent risk factor for IHD. Its predictive power was stronger than that of conventional coronary risk factors like total cholesterol, blood pressure, or body mass index.

A. M. Gotto, Jr. et al. (eds.), Multiple Risk Factors in Cardiovascular Disease, 75–84.
© 1998 Kluwer Academic Publishers and Fondazione Giovanni Lorenzini. Printed in the Netherlands.

Data on the ten-year follow-up of the same cohort [9] including 603 events confirmed these earlier results. After controlling for the major cardiovascular risk factors, the relative odds of IHD in the top compared to the bottom quintile were 2.2 (95% CI; 1.6-3.1). The finding that low fibrinogen characterizes patients at low risk for IHD events in the presence of elevated cholesterol, as reported in two recent studies [10,11] and withdrawn later by one of them [12], could not be confirmed in this much larger cohort.

In the Gothenburg Study, fibrinogen risk factors were recorded for a random sample of 792 men, all of them born in 1913 [13]. After a follow-up period of 13.5 years, there were 92 cases of myocardial infarction, 37 strokes, and 60 noncardiovascular deaths. Univariate analyses identified smoking, cholesterol, and fibrinogen as risk factors for myocardial infarction, while blood pressure and fibrinogen were risk factors for stroke. In a multivariate analysis the association between fibrinogen and cardiovascular events weakened, but was still statistically significant for stroke. When the study was extended to a 21-year follow-up, 119 myocardial infarctions, 81 strokes, and 333 other deaths had occurred [14]. Stroke and total mortality were significantly associated with fibrinogen. From the same area [15], it was shown recently that fibrinogen was not only strongly associated with the incidence of IHD, but also with total mortality. The adjusted relative risk for total mortality in the top tertile compared to the bottom tertile was 3.8 (95% CI; 1.01-14.4) compared to 5.4 (95% CI; 1.4-20.0) for IHD.

In a relatively small prospective study (Leigh study), 297 men, initially free of IHD, were recruited from one general practice [16]. After a mean follow-up period of 7.3 years, 40 cases of myocardial infarction had occurred, and fibrinogen was positively correlated with its incidence. In hypertensive patients, the incidence was six times higher when fibrinogen levels exceeded 3.5 g/l compared to the subpopulation with values below this threshold. Multivariate analyses showed that the predictive power of all variables, in descending order were: fibrinogen, age, systolic blood pressure, total cholesterol, obesity, number of cigarettes smoked per day, and very low density lipoproteins (VLDL).

The tenth biannual examination of the Framingham Study analyzed the interrelation of fibrinogen with smoking [17]. During a 14-year follow-up period, the risk of cardiovascular disease in men and women increased as a function of initial fibrinogen levels. The age-adjusted incidence in male smokers with high fibrinogen levels was doubled compared to a low fibrinogen subgroup. Fibrinogen was demonstrated to be a risk factor for coronary heart disease independent of smoking or other accepted risk factors [18]. In women, the magnitude of the fibrinogen-mediated risk declined with age. Fibrinogen was also a risk factor for stroke in men, but not in women. The relative impact of fibrinogen was comparable to those of blood pressure, obesity, smoking, and diabetes. A more recent analysis of the Framingham data [19] revealed that, in men, the fibrinogen risk ratio was greatest for stroke and smallest for peripheral vascular disease. For women, the risk ratio was greatest for coronary heart disease.

The PROCAM study [20] examined 1,674 men without a history of myocardial infarction or stroke. Fifteen cardiovascular events were observed during 2 years of follow up. Ten of these fell into the high fibrinogen tertile. When this study was extended to 2,116 men, followed for 6 years, 82 coronary events had occurred. The incidence of coronary events in the upper tertile of fibrinogen was 2.4-fold higher than in the lower tertile [10]. The combination of high fibrinogen and elevated LDL levels lead to an increase of coronary risk by factor 6.1. However, this finding had to be withdrawn later on [12].

The GRIPS Study [21], is a prospective cohort study of 5,239 men initially free of cardiovascular disease. One hundred and seven myocardial infarctions had occurred after 5 years of follow-up. Fibrinogen was a strong predictor in an univariate model. Its average level (± SD) was 3.6 ± 0.8 g/l in the non-event and 4.2 ± 1.0 g/l in the event group. Using a multivariate regression model, which accounted for LDL-cholesterol, measured directly, the relationship weakened, yet remained statistically significant. In the final model, the rank order of predictors was as follows: LDL cholesterol, familial disposition, Lp (a), HDL cholesterol, fibrinogen, age, smoking, glucose, and blood pressure.

When these prospective epidemiological studies were submitted to a formal meta-analysis, it was shown that the overall odds ratio for fibrinogen was 2.3 (95% CI; 1.9-2.8) [22], when the upper tertile of its distribution at baseline was compared to its bottom tertile.

CROSS-SECTIONAL STUDIES

In the Scottish Heart Health Study [23], the age-standardized odds ratios for myocardial infarction were 2.99 (95% CI; 1.97-3.53) for men and 2.45 (95% CI; 1.34-4.83) for women, when the top quartiles of fibrinogen distributions were compared with the bottom quartiles. Similar results were seen with angina pectoris. The FINRISK study [24] related hemostatic factors in 2,365 subjects to prevalent IHD (88 men and 44 women). Men and women with IHD had significantly higher plasma fibrinogen than those without. Similar findings were obtained in the ARIC study [25].

A study of 3,571 elderly Japanese male survivors within the Honolulu Heart Program evaluated the association of fibrinogen levels with coronary heart disease [26]. Fibrinogen was strongly associated with current cigarette smoking. The highest IHD prevalence (34%) was noted in current and ex-smokers who were also in the highest fibrinogen quintile.

An association between fibrinogen and subclinical atherosclerotic disease was reported from the ARIC Study [27]. Three hundred eighty-five subjects with asymptomatic atherosclerosis of the carotid artery were identified by high-resolution transcutaneous ultrasound. Controls matched for field center, race, sex, and age had to be free of atherosclerotic vessel wall thickening. Mean values were 3.16 g/L for cases and 2.87 g/L for controls (mean difference 0.29 g/L [95% CI, 0.18-0.38 g/L]). Unadjusted odds ratio for carotid atherosclerosis associated with one standard deviation (0.67 g/L) increase in fibrinogen was 1.6 (p < 0.001), after adjustment for cholesterol, blood pressure, smoking, and body mass index it decreased slightly, but remained significant (p=0.01).

In the Rotterdam Elderly Study [28] the associations between moderate or severe stenosis of the right carotid artery and conventional risk factors as well as hemostatic parameters were studied in more than 11,000 people. In 954 persons ultrasonic duplex examinations of the right internal carotid artery were done. Subjects with moderate-to-severe carotid artery disease had, compared with participants without stenosis, higher mean fibrinogen levels (difference 0.24 g/L; 95% CI, 0.04-0.45) after adjusting for age, sex, and body mass index.

The association between fibrinogen levels and the presence and extent of plaques over three different arterial sites was assessed in 652 men, aged 40-60 years. An odds ratio of 1.6 and 1.4, respectively, was obtained when the upper fibrinogen tertiles were compared to the lower [29]. Most recently, the associations between various coagulation factors and measures of subclinical disease were examined in 5,024 persons older than 65 years within the Cardiovascular Health Study (CHS) [30]. Fibrinogen was significantly associated with carotid artery stenosis, internal (but not common) carotid artery wall thickness, and ankle-arm blood pressure measurements.

In the MONICA Project fibrinogen was increased in male and female smokers [31]. In another center [32] plasma viscosity (strongly influenced by fibrinogen) was raised in males with hypercholesterolemia, untreated hypertension, or in smokers, as well as in females with hypercholesterolemia or obesity. In a later cross-sectional survey from the Augsburg MONICA study, positive associations for fibrinogen were reported with body weight, waist-to-hip ratio, smoking, and age, and a negative association with alcohol consumption [33].

In the Scottish Heart Health Study 8,824 men and women were examined. Women had higher fibrinogen levels than men [34]. Fibrinogen was positively associated with age, smoking, cholesterol, and body mass index and negatively linked to alcohol consumption. Female menopause also coincided with higher fibrinogen levels. A Danish study [35] of 439 men aged 51, showed positive associations of fibrinogen with low social class, psychological variables, smoking, physical inactivity, low HDL cholesterol, low physical fitness and high LDL cholesterol.

The largest (n=15,803) epidemiological study to include fibrinogen is the ARIC Study [36], showed fibrinogen to be 22 mg/dl higher in blacks compared to whites. It also confirmed higher values in women than in men. Fibrinogen was furthermore increased with age, smoking, body size, diabetes, fasting serum insulin, LDL, Lp (a), leukocyte count, and menopause. It was decreased with ethanol intake, exercise, HDL, and postmenopausal female hormone use.

Clinical Evidence

It has long been appreciated that an acute myocardial infarction leads to transient hyperfibrinogenemia (review [37]). Fibrinogen increases progressively with the severity and extent of coronary atherosclerosis [38-41]. This could be interpreted in terms of an acute phase response following tissue necrosis. Yet fibrinogen (or plasma viscosity) remains elevated for years following an infarction [42].

In a prospective study, 1,716 men were observed for two years who, six months before, had suffered a myocardial infarction [43]. During this period, 126 had suffered a second ischemic event. Fibrinogen was significantly elevated in this subgroup. Statistically significant differences in fibrinogen also existed between patients who survived and those who died. The relative odds for death showed an approximately linear relationship with fibrinogen levels.

In 1,755 men from the Diet and Reinfarction Trial (DART) who had recovered from an acute myocardial infarction, increased fibrinogen levels (measured 6 months after the acute event) were predictive of a recurrent infarction within 2 years of follow-up. Smoking cessation following the infarct was associated with a lower mortality compared to continued smoking and this effect appeared to be mediated by fibrinogen levels. However, smoking habit accounted for only part of the prognostic effect of fibrinogen [44].

In the ECAT-Angina Pectoris Study 3,043 patients, angiographically diagnosed to suffer from IHD, were followed for 2 years. The incidence of myocardial infarction was positively and significantly associated with baseline fibrinogen [11]. C-reactive protein (CRP) was also measured and was found to be directly and independently predictive of coronary events Interestingly, the predictive power of fibrinogen persisted after controlling for CRP, but not vice versa. Similarly, in 323 patients with stable angina followed for 60 months, fibrinogen represented an independent predictor for sudden death [45]. Recently 3,092 IHD male patients were followed for 3.2 years on average [46]. In this time span 204 men died, 111 (54%) of IHD. Their baseline fibrinogen had been 29.4 mg/dl higher than that of survivors. An increase of one SD (75 mg/dl) of fibrinogen was found to increase risk of IHD and total mortality by 29% and 31%, respectively. The longest follow-up (9 years) thus far being reported comes from a clinical cohort study of 209 IHD patients [47]. All underwent clinical assessment, angiography, and blood tests for hemostatic variables at baseline. At the end of follow-up, 58 patients (28%) had suffered a major cardiac event the risk of which was positively related to fibrinogen (risk ratio per SD increase 1.29, 95% CI; 0.99-1.68).

The involvement of increased levels of fibrinogen in the process of restenosis has recently been studied in 107 consecutive patients undergoing coronary angioplasty [48]. Fibrinogen measured within 6 months of follow-up was significantly increased in all patients with restenosis, based on four different definitions. Patients with a fibrinogen concentration > 3.5 g/L at follow-up had higher restenosis rates than patients with lower concentrations ranging between 55%-74% versus 22%-37%. This is supported by the observation, that plasma levels of interleukin-6, a strong trigger of the hepatic fibrinogen synthesis, was also able to predict restenosis post-percutaneous transluminal coronary angioplasty (PTCA) in patients with unstable angina [49].

Fibrinogen levels increase after an acute stroke [50]. As in the case of IHD, this has been attributed to an acute phase reaction subsequent to tissue necrosis. However, plasma viscosity is significantly increased in transient ischemic attack (TIA) patients, suggesting that fibrinogen levels are elevated before a relevant amount of necrosis occurs [51,52]. In a population-based case-control study, 105 patients with a TIA or minor stroke were compared to 352 age- and sex-matched subjects. Plasma fibrinogen levels were found to be significantly different in patients compared with controls, and the population attributable risk was 26% [53].

In a prospective study of stroke survivors, fibrinogen was significantly higher in patients who suffered a second cardiovascular event during the two years after the initial stroke. The effect was independent of concomitant risk factors [54]. These results are in accordance with data showing that patients with a progression of carotid artery lesions had significantly higher fibrinogen levels compared to those with nonprogressing lesions in the angiogram [55].

In peripheral arterial occlusive disease (PAOD) fibrinogen is significantly increased [56,57]. In a large cross-sectional study fibrinogen had a stronger impact on the risk of disease than conventional risk factors [58]. A large-scale study [59] demonstrated that fibrinogen is independently associated with peripheral arterial narrowing and in another study [60], fibrinogen and D-dimer (the main degradation product of cross-linked fibrin) were positively correlated with the severity of peripheral atherosclerosis. In an 11-year follow-up study of the general population it was shown that fibrinogen predicted to a certain extent the development of intermittent claudication [61]. In claudicants, fibrinogen is sometimes elevated in the absence of gross angiographic narrowing of the arteries, a finding that lead to the concept of "rheologic claudication" [57]. Longitudinal data from the Edinburgh Artery Study [62] in 1,592 men and women aged 55-74 years and followed for 5 years showed a 20% increase in the relative risk of cardiovascular events for an increase of one standard deviation of fibrinogen (0.60 g/L). There were 272 fatal and nonfatal events during the observation period. Longitudinal data in PAOD patients also showed that high fibrinogen was a predictor for reocclusion of femoro-popliteal vein grafts [63]. When 1,011 patients with PAOD were followed for 18 months, 246 of them had a major cardiovascular event [64]. In male patients (84%), ankle/arm pressure index below 0.8 and elevated fibrinogen and blood pressure were the most important predictors for secondary events.

Collectively these findings suggest that fibrinogen is elevated in overt atherosclerotic disease which might be interpreted in terms of a hematological stress syndrome [57]. Longitudinal data identify fibrinogen as a valuable prognostic indicator. Suggesting that it also represents a risk factor for cardiovascular disease and its sequelae.

Comment

The term "risk factor" by definition implies the causal involvement of a given variable in the disease process. "Risk marker" or "risk indicator" describe an association between a variable and disease with no implication of causality. In the case of fibrinogen, such a distinction is difficult to make [65]. There is abundant evidence from large observational studies that document a strong, direct, and independent relationship to various manifest or subclinical cardiovascular diseases (see above). In addition, multiple pathophysiological pathways make a direct involvement of fibrinogen in both the early and advanced stages of atherosclerosis plausible. Yet, fibrinogen may still be merely a marker of an underlying low-grade inflammation in atherosclerotic disease. Intervention studies investigating the effect of lowering of fibrinogen on cardiovascular endpoints should shed more light on this issue. However, in the absence of oral drugs that selectively act on fibrinogen levels such trials are not easy to interpret.

A link between fibrinogen and atherothrombogenesis is likely and plausible. Epidemiological studies indicate that a plasma fibrinogen level in excess of around 3.0 g/L is a powerful, independent risk factor for brain, and/or heart infarction. Increased fibrinogen is also a risk factor for the sequelae of cardiovascular disease. Future research of atherothrombotic diseases should attempt to conclusively answer the question whether fibrinogen is a risk factor or a risk marker. At present the data seems to favor the former hypothesis.

References

1.   Heller RF, Chinn S, Tunstall-Pedoe HD, Rose G. How well can we predict coronary heart disease? BMJ 1984;288:410-11.
2.   Ernst E. Plasma fibrinogen - an independent cardiovascular risk factor. J Int Med 1990;227: 365-72.
3.   Meade TW, North WRS, Chakrabarti R, et al. Hemostatic function and cardiovascular death: Early results of a prospective study. Lancet 1980;1:1050-53.
4.   Meade TW, Mellows W, Brozovic M, et al. Hemostatic function and ischemic heart disease: Principal results of the Northwick Park Heart Study. Lancet 1986;2:533-37.
5.   Meade TW, Cooper JA, Chakrabari R, Miller GJ, Stirling Y, Howarth DJ. Fibrinolytic activity and clotting factors in ischemic heart disease in women. BMJ 1996;312:1581.
6.   Baker LA, Eastham R, Elwood PC, et al. Hemostatic factors associated with ischemic heart disease in men aged 45 to 64 years. The Speedwell collaborative surveys. Br Heart J 1982;47: 490-94.
7.   Yarnell JWG, Sweetnam PM, Rogers S, et al. Some long-term effects of smoking on the hemostatic system: a report from the Caerphilly and Speedwell collaborative surveys. J Clin Pathol 1987;40:909-13.
8.   Yarnell JWG, Baker JA, Sweetnam PM, et al. Fibrinogen, viscosity, and white blood cell count are major risk factors for ischemic heart disease. Circulation 1991;83:836-44.
9.   Sweetnam RM, Thomas HF, Yarnell JWG, Beswick AD, Baker IA, Elwood PC. Fibrinogen, viscosity and the 10-year incidence of ischemic heart disease. The Caerphilly and Speedwell Studies. Eur Heart J 1996;17:1814-20.
10. Heinrich J, Balleisen L, Schulte H, Assmann G, Van De Loo J. Fibrinogen and factor VII in the prediction of coronary risk. Arterioscler Thromb 1994;14:54-59.
11. Thompson SG, Kienast J, Pyke SDM, Haverkate T, Van De Loo JCW. Hemostatic factors and the risk of myocardial infarction or sudden death in patients with angina pectoris. N Eng J Med 1995;332:635-41.
12. Heinrich J, Balleisen L, Schulte H, Assmann G, Van de Loo JCW. Fibrinogen and factor VII in the prediction of coronary risk. Results from the PROCAM Study in healthy men (Correction). Arterioscler Thromb 1994;14:1392.
13. Wilhelmsen L, Svärdsudd K, Korsan-Bengtsen K, et al. Fibrinogen as a risk factor for stroke and myocardial infarction. N Eng J Med 1984;311:501-5.
14. Eriksson H, Korsan-Bengtsen E, Welin L, et al. 21-year follow-up of CVD and total mortality among men born in 1913. In: Ernst E, Koenig W, Lowe GDO, Meade TW, editors. Fibrinogen, a "new" cardiovascular risk factor. Oxford: Blackwell, 1992: 115-20.
15. Rosengren A, Wilhelmsen L. Fibrinogen, coronary heart disease and mortality from all causes in smokers and nonsmokers. The Study of Men Born in 1933. J Intern Med 1996;239:499-507.
16. Stone MC, Thorp JM. Plasma fibrinogen - a major coronary risk factor. J R Coll Gen Prac 1985;35:565-69.

17.   Kannel WB, D'Agnostino RB, Belanger AJ. Fibrinogen, cigarette smoking, and risk of cardiovascular disease: Insights from the Framingham Study. Am Heart J 1987; 113:1006-10.

18.   Kannel WB, Wolf PA, Castelli WP, D'Agostino RB. Fibrinogen and risk of cardiovascular disease. J Am Med Assoc 1987;258:1183-86.

19.   Kannel WB. Fibrinogen - a major cardiovascular risk factor. In: Ernst E, Koenig W, Lowe GDO, Meade TW, editors. Fibrinogen, a "new" cardiovascular risk factor. Oxford: Blackwell, 1992:101-9.

20.   Balleisen L, Schulte H, Balleisen L, Assmann G, Van De Loo J. Coagulation factors and the progress of coronary heart disease. Lancet 1987;1:461.

21.   Cremer P, Nagel D, Labrot B, et al. Lipoprotein Lp (a) as a predictor of myocardial infarction in comparison to fibrinogen, LDL cholesterol and other risk factors. Europ J Clin Invest 1994; 24:444-53.

22.   Ernst E, Resch KL. Fibrinogen as a cardiovascular risk factor: A meta- analysis and review of the literature. Ann Int Med 1993;118:956-63.

23.   Lee AJ, Lowe GDO, Woodward M, Tunstall-Pedoe H. Fibrinogen in relation to personal history of prevalent hypertension, diabetes, stroke, intermittent claudication, coronary heart disease, and family history: The Scottish Heart Study. Br Heart J 1993;69:338-42.

24.   Salomaa V, Rasi, Pekkanen J, et al. Hemostatic factors and prevalent coronary heart disease; the FINRISK hemostatic study. Eur Heart J 1994;15:1293-99.

25.   Folsom AR, Wu KK, Shahar E, Davis CE. Association of hemostatic variables with prevalent cardiovascular disease and asymptomatic carotid artery atherosclerosis. Arterioscler Thromb 1993;13:1829-36.

26.   Sharp DS, Abbott RD, Burchfield CM, et al. Plasma fibrinogen and coronary heart disease in elderly Japanese-American men. Arterioscler Thromb Vasc Biol, 1996;16: 262-68.

27.   Wu KK, Folsom AR, Heiss G, Davis CE, Conlan MG, Barnes R. Association of coagulation factors and inhibitors with carotid artery atherosclerosis. Early results of the ARIC study. Ann Epidemiol 1992;2:471-80.

28.   Bots ML, Breslau PJ, Briet E et al. Cardiovascular determinants of carotid artery disease: The Rotterdam Elderly Study. Hypertension 1992;19:717-20.

29.   Levenson J, Giral P, Razavian M, Gariepy J, Simon A. Fibrinogen and silent atherosclerosis in subjects with cardiovascular risk factors. Arterioscler Thromb Vasc Biol 1995;15:1263-68.

30.   Tracy RP, Bovill EG, Yanez D, et al. Fibrinogen and factor VIII, but not factor VII, are associated with measures of subclinical cardiovascular disease in the elderly. Results from the Cardiovascular Health Study. Arterioscler Thromb Vasc Biol 1995; 15:1269-79

31.   Lowe GDO, Smith WCS, Tunstall-Pedoe HD, et al. Cardiovascular risk and haemorheology - results from the Scottish Heart Health Study and the MONICA-Project, Glasgow. Clin Hemorheol 1988;8:507-15.

32.   Ernst E, Koenig W, Matrai A, Keil U. Plasma viscosity and hemoglobin in the presence of cardiovascular risk factors. Clin Hemorheol 1988;8:507-15.

33.   Krobot K, Hense HW, Cremer P, Eberle E, Keil U. Determinants of plasma fibrinogen: Relation to body weight, waist-to-hip ratio, smoking, alcohol, age, and sex: Results from the Second MONICA Augsburg Survey 1989-1990. Arterioscler Thromb 1992;12:780-87.

34.   Lee AJ, Smith WCS, Lowe GDO, Turnstall-Pedow H. Plasma fibrinogen and coronary risk factors: The Scottish Health Study. J Clin Epidem 1990;43:913-19.

35.   Möller L, Kristensen TS. Plasma fibrinogen and ischemic heart disease risk factors. Arterioscl Thromb 1991;11:344-50.

36.   Folsom A, Wu KK, Davis CE, Conlan MG, Sorlie PD, Szklo M. Population correlates of

plasma fibrinogen and factor VII, putative cardiovascular risk factors. Atherosclerosis 1991; 91:199-205.

37. Dormandy J, Ernst E, Matrai A, Flute P. Hemorheological changes following acute myocardial infarction. Am Heart J 1982;104:1364-67.

38. Kruskal JB, Patrick CB, Commerford J, Franks JJ, Kirsch RE. Fibrin and fibrinogen-related antigens in patients with stable and unstable coronary artery disease. N Eng J Med 1987;317: 1361-65.

39. Lowe GDO, Drummond MM, Lorimer AR, et al. Relation between extent of coronary artery disease and blood viscosity. BMJ 1980;1:673-4.

40. Handa K, Kiono S, Saku K. Plasma fibrinogen levels as an independent indicator of severity of coronary atherosclerosis. Atherosclerosis 1989;77:209-13.

41. Broadhurst P, Kelleher C, Hughes L, Imeson JD, Raftery EB. Fibrinogen, factor VII clotting activity and coronary artery disease severity. Atherosclerosis 1990;85:169-73.

42. Ernst E, Resch KL, Krauth U, Paulsen HF. Does blood rheology revert to normal after myocardial infarction? Brit Heart J 1990;64:248-50.

43. Martin JF, Bath PMW, Burr ML. Influence of platelet size on outcome after myocardial infarction. Lancet 1992;338:1409-11.

44. Burr ML, Holliday RM, Fehily AM, Whitehead PJ. Hematological prognostic indices after myocardial infarction: Evidence from the diet and reinfarction trial (DART). Eur Heart J 1992; 13:166-70.

45. Benchimol D, Dartigues JF, Benchimol H, et al. Predictive value of hemostatic factors for sudden death in patients with stable angina pectoris. Am J Cardiol 1995;76:241-44.

46. Benderly M, Graff E, Reicher-Reiss H, Behar S, Brunner D, Goldbourt U. Fibrinogen is a predictor of mortality in coronary heart disease patients. Arterioscler Thromb Vasc Biol 1996; 16:351-56.

47. Thompson SG, Fechtrup C, Squire E, et al. Antithrombin III and fibrinogen as predictors of cardiac events in patients with angina pectoris. Arterioscler Thromb Vasc Biol 1996;16:357-62.

48. Montalescot G, Ankri A, Vicaut E, Drobinski G, Grosgogeat Y, Thomas D. Fibrinogen after coronary angioplasty as a risk factor for restenosis. Circulation 1995;92:31-38.

49. Liuzzo G, Buffon A, Vitelli A, et al. Plasma levels of interleukin-6 predict restenosis following coronary angioplasty in patients with unstable angina. Circulation 1996; 94:I-330.

50. Eisenbert S. Blood viscosity and fibrinogen concentration following cerebral infarction. Circulation 1966;(Suppl.2)33/34:10-14.

51. Ernst E, Matrai A, Marshall M. Blood rheology in patients with transient ischemic attacks. Stroke 1988;19:634-36.

52. Coull BM, Beamer N, de Garmo P, et al. Chronic hyperviscosity in subjects with acute stroke, transient ischemic attack, and risk factors for stroke. Stroke 1991;22: 162-68.

53. Qizilbash N, Jones L, Warlow C, Mann J. Fibrinogen and lipid concentrations as risk factors for transient ischemic attacks and minor ischemic strokes. BMJ 1991;303: 605-9.

54. Resch KL, Ernst E, Matrai A, Paulsen HF. Fibrinogen and viscosity, risk factors for stroke survivors. Ann Int Med 1992;177:371-75.

55. Grotta JC. Prediction of carotid stenosis progression by lipid and hematologic measurements. Neurology 1989;39:1325-31.

56. Stuart J, George AJ, Davies AJ, Aukland A, Hurlow RA. Hematological stress syndrome in atherosclerosis. J Clin Pathol 1981;34:464-67.

57. Dormandy JA, Hoare E, Colley J, Arrowsmith DE, Dormandy TL. Clinical haemodynamic,

rheological and biochemal findings in 126 patients with intermittent claudication. BMJ 1973; 4:576-81.

58.   Leng GC, Lee AJ, Fowkes FGR, Lowe GDO, Housley E. The relationship between cigarette smoking and cardiovascular risk factors in peripheral arterial disease compared with ischemic heart disease. Eur Heart J 1995;16:1542-48.

59.   Lowe GDO, Fowkes FGR, Dawes J, Donnan PT, Lennie SE, Housley E. Blood viscosity, fibrinogen, and activation of coagulation and leukecytes in peripheral arterial disease and the normal population in the Edinburgh Artery Study. Circulation 1993;87:1915-20.

60.   Lassila R, Peltonen S, Lepäntalo M, Saarinen O, Kauhanen P, Manninen V. Severity of peripheral atherosclerosis is associated with fibrinogen and degradation of cross-linked fibrin. Arterioscler Thromb 1993;13:1738-42.

61.   Bainton D, Sweetnam P, Baker I, Elwood P. Peripheral vascular disease: consequence for survival and association with risk factors in the Speedwell prospective heart disease study. Br Heart J 1994;72:128-32.

62.   Lowe GDO, Lee AJ, Rumley A, Price JF, Fowkes GR. Blood viscosity and risk of cardiovascular events: The Edinburgh Artery Study. Br J Haematol 1997;96:168-73.

63.   Wiseman S, Kenehington G, Dain R. Influence of smoking and plasma factors on patency of femoro-poplitean vein grafts. BMJ 1989;299:643-46.

64.   Violi F, Criqui M, Longoni A, Castiglioni C. Relation between risk factors and cardiovascular complications in patients with peripheral vascular disease. Results from the ADEP study. Atherosclerosis 1996;120:25-35.

65.   Koenig W. Establishing causality: The case of fibrinogen. In: Ernst E, Koenig W, Lowe GDO, Meade TW, editors. Fibrinogen, a "new" cardiovascular risk factor. Oxford: Blackwell, 1992: 96-100.

PAI-1 AND THE RISK OF CARDIOVASCULAR DISEASE

Irène Juhan-Vague and Marie Christine Alessi

Introduction

Among the list of coronary risk factors, it has recently been proposed that impairment of the fibrinolytic system detected in plasma, due to increased plasminogen activator inhibitor -1 (PAI-1) level, could predict complications of atherosclerosis.

This could account for the properties of the fibrinolytic system [1]. Inactive plasminogen is converted into active plasmin by plasminogen activators, t-PA and uPA. Beside its contribution to the degradation of fibrin, plasmin plays a great part in vessel wall remodelling through activation of metalloproteinases and growth factors and degradation of the extracellular matrix.

The fibrinolytic system is regulated by a balance between activators and inhibitors, PAI-1 which inhibits t-PA and u-PA, being the main inhibitor of plasminogen activation. An increased PAI-1 concentration induces a decreased plasmin formation and leads to an accumulation of fibrin [2-4] and change in the vessel wall remodelling [5-7]. Besides its antiprotease activity, PAI-1 also participates in the cellular adhesion and migration processes. By the mere fact that it binds to vitronectin in the same part of the molecule as the vitronectin receptor or uPA receptor, it mediates the release of cells from their substrate [8,9].

All of these properties indicate that PAI-1 can be involved in the risk of developing atherothrombosis.

Clinical and Epidemiological Studies

PAI-1 and other fibrinolytic variables have been investigated in plasma in many clinical studies. The main variables studied (PAI-1 activity and antigen and t-PA antigen, which represent mainly inactive t-PA/PAI-1 complexes), are strongly positively correlated between each other and negatively correlated with resulting fibrinolytic activity. In other words, an increased PAI-1 or t-PA antigen concentration corresponds to a decreased circulating fibrinolytic activity.

Case/control studies have shown an increased plasma PAI-1 concentration in patients with coronary heart disease, or other forms of atherosclerosis, and in patients with obesity or noninsulin dependent diabetes [10-12]. PAI-1 expression is also increased in the

A. M. Gotto, Jr. et al. (eds.), Multiple Risk Factors in Cardiovascular Disease, 85–92.

atherosclerotic lesions [13-15].

Fibrinolytic variables have been assayed in prospective epidemiological studies and results are in favor of a role of these parameters as predictor of coronary events. The predictive capacity of fibrinolytic variables has been demonstrated in longitudinal studies [16] including healthy subjects such as in the Northwick Park Heart Study [17] or the Physicians' Health Study [18], or including patients with coronary heart disease [19-26]. However discrepant results have been reported in the literature, which could be attributed to the choice of controlled confounding variables, fibrinolytic parameters being strongly related to other coronary risk markers.

To illustrate the predictive capacity of PAI-1, some recent results of the ECAT Angina Pectoris study [27] are described. A large group of angina patients were followed for 2 years in this multicentric European study. t-PA antigen, fibrinogen, C reactive protein, and von Willebrand factor were considered as risk factors for myocardial infarction, after adjustment for many parameters (body mass index [BMI], blood pressure, cholesterol, triglyceride, smoking, drug used, previous myocardial infarction, diabetes, extent of coronary artery disease, and left ventricular ejection fraction). PAI-1 was predictive of events only before these adjustments [26].

The relative risk of coronary events according to the distribution of PAI activity, PAI-1 antigen, and t-PA antigen before adjustments was calculated. The risk increased almost 5-fold from the bottom to the top quintile of t-PA antigen, 3-fold for PAI-1 antigen, and 2-fold for PAI-1 activity. In order to understand in which context PAI-1 or t-PA antigen are predictive of events, we performed adjustments with different clusters of variables which are known to be related to fibrinolytic parameters, mainly insulin resistance [28-37], and inflammation [38,39]. Another cluster was added, related to endothelial cell damage, represented by von Willebrand factors which is, like PAI-1 and t-PA, produced by endothelial cells. After adjustment for insulin resistance parameters (BMI, triglyceride, high density lipoprtotein [HDL] cholesterol), PAI-1 activity, and PAI-1 antigen were no longer considered as risk factors. Whereas adjustment for inflammation markers (fibrinogen, C reactive protein) or endothelial cell marker had no effect at all on PAI-1 predictive capacity. The results were different with t-PA antigen; the 3 different adjustments affected its prognostic value to the same extent and, when the adjustments were combined, the predictive capacity of t-PA antigen disappeared.

Taking these results from angina patients into consideration, plasma PAI-1 levels seem to be mainly related to insulin resistance whereas t-PA antigen is influenced by 3 phenomena: insulin resistance, inflammation, and endothelial cell damage. Therefore PAI-1 is a risk marker in the context of the insulin resistance syndrome and t-PA antigen is a marker of a combination of pathological pathways.

PAI-1 and Insulin Resistance

Insulin resistance also called plurimetabolic syndrome, is a largely distributed abnormality [40,41]. It is considered as predisposing to the development of atherosclerosis [42-45] and includes a cluster of variables such as obesity, with a repartition of the fat in the central part of the body (usually quantified by the waist-to-hip ratio), high blood pressure, glucose intolerance, and, among the biological abnormalities, fasting hyperinsulinemia, abnormalities of the lipid profile with elevated triglyceride, and decreased HDL cholesterol. Increased PAI-1 and increased t-PA antigen levels must be added to the cluster of atherogenic abnormalities of this syndrome [28-37]. PAI-1 or t-PA antigen levels are very strongly correlated with all of the variables included in the metabolic syndrome and modulations of insulin resistance (by hypocaloric diet with weight loss, physical training, or oral antidiabetic drugs) induce parallel changes in PAI-1 and t-PA antigen levels [46-51].

The mechanisms involved in PAI-1 production in the context of insulin resistance are beginning to be better understood. A production of PAI-1 by adipose tissue has attracted much attention recently. Folsom et al. [51] have shown that the reduction in PAI-1 antigen levels after weight loss was more related to the degree of weight loss than to triglyceride or insulin changes. It was also underlined that PAI-1 antigen levels were not increased in type II diabetic patients without obesity [35]. Moreover plasma levels of adipsin a serine protease mainly produced by adipocytes were independently and positively associated with those of PAI-1 [52].

Data on PAI-1 expression by adipose tissue were first provided in rodents [53-57]. We have recently investigated PAI-1 production by human adipose tissue and its different cellular fractions [58]. As the relative degree of android (central) adiposity is better correlated with the risk of coronary heart disease than the absolute degree of fatness [59-60] and as the waist-to-hip ratio or direct measurement of visceral fat are strongly correlated with insulin resistance and plasma PAI-1 levels [31-33,61,62], we were interested in studying the capacity to produce PAI-1 of human adipose tissue from different territories. PAI-1 protein detected by immunolocalization was present at the stromal and adipocyte level whatever the territories tested (omental, mammary, gluteal). In subcutaneous tissue, where only stromal vascular cells expressed a detectable amount of PAI-1 mRNA in the basal state, adipocyte fractions were able to express PAI-1 mRNA under incubation. No effect was observed on PAI-1 antigen production by the adipocyte fraction in the presence of TNFα, whereas TGFβ induced a significantly increased PAI-1. Interestingly omental tissue explants produced significantly more PAI-1 antigen than subcutaneous tissue from the same individual. These results suggest that adipose tissue, in particular visceral tissue accumulation, participates in the elevated PAI-1 levels observed in insulin resistant patients [58]. The nature of the cells responsible for PAI-1 production in adipose tissue, as well as the mechanisms related to the insulin resistance involved, are so far an open field of investigation.

PAI-1 and Genetic Polymorphisms

Different polymorphisms on the PAI-1 gene have recently been described [63-65] and a contribution of genetic variation to plasma PAI-1 levels has been proposed [63,64,66-68]. An insertion-deletion on the promoter, 675 4G/5G [63,64] has been extensively studied and it was shown that subjects homozygous for the 4G allele presented higher plasma PAI-1 levels than the others. This relationship has principally been shown in patients with previous myocardial infarction [63-65,69]. A stronger association between triglyceride levels and plasma PAI-1 activity has been observed in diabetic patients homozygous for the 4G allele than in those homozygous for the 5G allele [67,69]. It has been proposed that the candidate site in the promoter could have a sequence involved in the binding of a transcriptional factor, whose level could be influenced by very low density lipoproteins (VLDL) [68]. However in the large population of the ECTIM Study, a case-control study of myocardial infarction, no significant difference in the relationships between PAI-1 levels and triglyceride among the genotype classes was noted [66]. Interestingly the prevalence of the 4G allele was significantly higher in a group of 100 patients aged 35-45 years with myocardial infarction than in controls [68]. However this relation was not confirmed in the ECTIM study of patients aged 25-64 years [66] and in the Physicians' Health Study [70].

To illustrate the relative contribution of both the insulin resistance syndrome and polymorphisms of the PAI-1 gene to plasma levels of PAI-1 in a healthy population, we have recently performed a family study involving 228 healthy nuclear families from the Stanislas cohort of Nancy (France) [71]. A gender difference was observed with fathers exhibiting higher PAI-1 levels than mothers and children. PAI-1 was as expected strongly correlated with insulin resistance variables, such as BMI, waist-to-hip circumference ratio, and insulin. They explained 48% and 28% of the variability of PAI-1 in fathers and mothers respectively, whereas the 4G/5G polymorphism, in univariate and multivariate analysis, explained less than 5%; the effect being smaller in fathers than in mothers. Therefore in a healthy population, plasma PAI-1 levels are primarily determined by the insulin resistance syndrome, the genetic effect being weak. The influence of a gene-environment interaction needs to be further investigated

Conclusion

It has been shown that PAI-1 is a risk factor of cardiovascular disease in the context of insulin resistance and it is produced in this context by adipose tissue, especially by fat from omentum. It could therefore be proposed that PAI-1 is a link between insulin resistance, obesity, and cardiovascular disease. The causal contribution of the impairment of fibrinolysis to vascular disease development has to be more extensively documented. Evaluation of a protective effect of the specific modulation of PAI-1 [72] opens up a promising field of interest.

References

1.   Collen D, Lijnen HR. Basic and clinical aspects of fibrinolysis and thrombolysis. Blood 1991;78:3114-24.
2.   Reilly CF, Fujita T, Hutzelmann JE, Mayer EJ, Shebuski RJ. Plasminogen activator inhibitor 1 suppresses endogenous fibrinolysis in a canine model of pulmonary embolism. Circulation 1991;84:287-92.
3.   Vaughan DE, Declerck PJ, Van Houtte E, De Mol M, Collen D. Reactivated recombinant plasminogen activator inhibitor 1 (rPAI-1) effectively prevents thrombolysis in vivo.

Thromb Haemostas 1992;68:60-63.

4. Biemond BJ, Levi M, Coronel R, Janse MJ, Ten Cate JW, Pannekoek H. Thrombolysis and reocclusion in experimental jugular vein and coronary artery thrombosis. Effect of a plasminogen activator inhibitor type 1 neutralizing monoclonal antibody. Circulation 1995; 91:1175-81.

5. Erickson LA, Fici GJ, Lund JE, Boyle TP, Polites HG, Marotti KR. Development of venous occlusions in mice transgenic for the PAI-1 gene. Nature 1990;346:74-76.

6. Carmeliet P, Bouche A, Schoonjans L, et al. Physiological consequences of loss of plasminogen activator gene function in mice. Nature 1994;368:419-24.

7. Carmeliet P, Bouche A, De Clercq C, et al. Biological effects of disruption of the tissue-type plasminogen activator, urokinase type plasminogen activator and plasminogen activator inhibitor-1 genes in mice. Ann NY Acad Sci 1995;748:367-82.

8. Stefansson S, Lawrence DA. The serpin PAI-1 inhibits cell migration by blocking integrin avb3 binding to vitronectin. Nature 1996;323:441-43.

9. Deng G, Curriden SA, Wang S, Rosenberg S, Loskutoff DJ. Is plasminogen activator inhibitor 1 the molecular switch that governs urokinase receptor-mediated cell adhesion and release? J Cell Biol 1996;134:1563-71.

10. Juhan-Vague I, Alessi MC. Plasminogen activator inhibitor 1 and atherothrombosis. Thromb Haemostas 1993;70:138-43.

11. Prinz MH, Hirsh J. A critical review of the relationship between impaired fibrinolysis and myocardial infarction. Amer Heart J 1991;122:545-51.

12. Rocha E, Paramo JA. The relationship between impaired fibrinolysis and coronary heart disease. A role for PAI-1. Fibrinolysis 1994;8:294-303.

13. Schneiderman J, Sawdey MS, Keeton MR, et al. Increased type 1 plasminogen activator inhibitor gene expression in atherosclerotic human arteries. Proc Natl Acad Sci USA 1992; 89:6998-7002.

14. Chomiki N, Henry M, Alessi MC, Anfosso F, Juhan-Vague I. Plasminogen activator inhibitor 1 expression in human liver and healthy or atherosclerotic vessel walls. Thromb Haemostas 1994;72:44-53.

15. Lupu F, Bergonzelli GE, Heim DA, et al. Localization and production of plasminogen activator inhibitor-1 in human healthy and atherosclerotic arteries. Arterioscler Thromb 1993;13:1090-1100.

16. Juhan-Vague I, Alessi MC. Fibrinolysis and risk of coronary artery disease. Fibrinolysis 1996;10:127-36.

17. Meade TW, Ruddock V, Stirling Y, Chakrabarti T, Miller GJ. Fibrinolytic activity, clotting factors and long-term incidence of ischaemic heart disease in the Northwick Park Heart Study. Lancet 1993;342:1076-79

18. Ridker PM, Vaughan DE, Stampfer MJ, Manson JE, Hennekens CH. Endogenous tissue type plasminogen activator and risk of myocardial infarction. Lancet 1993;341:1165-68.

19. Jansson JH, Nilsson TK, Olofsson BO. Tissue plasminogen activator and other risk factors as predictors of cardiovascular events in patients with severe angina pectoris. Eur Heart J 1991;12:157-61.

20. Jansson JH, Olofsson BO, Nilsson TK. Predictive value of tissue plasminogen activator mass concentration on long-term mortality in patients with coronary artery disease. A 7 year follow up. Circulation 1993;88:2030-34.

21. Hamsten A, De Faire U, Walldius G, et al. Plasminogen activator inhibitor in plasma: Risk factor for recurrent myocardial infarction. Lancet 1987;II:3-9.

22.   Gram J, Jespersen J, Kluft C, Rijken DC. On the usefulness of fibrinolysis variables in the characterization of a risk group for myocardial infarction. Acta Med Scand 1987;221:149-53.

23.   Cortellaro M, Cofrancesco E, Boschetti C, et al., for the PLAT Group. Increased fibrin turnover and high PAI-1 activity as predictors of ischemic events in atherosclerotic patients: A case-control study. Arterioscler Thromb 1993;13:1412-17.

24.   Cimmiello C. Tissue type plasminogen activator and risk of myocardial infarction. Lancet 1993;342:48-49.

25.   Munkvad S, Gram J, Jespersen J. A depression of active tissue plasminogen activator in plasma characterizes patients with unstable angina pectoris who develop myocardial infarction. Eur Heart J 1990;11:525-28.

26.   Thompson SG, Kienast J, Pyke SDM, Haverkate F, van de Loo JCW. Hemostatic factors and the risk of myocardial infarction or sudden death in patients with angina pectoris. N Engl J Med 1995;332:635-41.

27.   Juhan-Vague I, Pyke SDM, Alessi MC, Jespersen J, Haverkate F, Thompson SG. Fibrinolytic factors and the risk of myocardial infarction or sudden death in patients with angina pectoris. Circulation 1996;94:2057-63.

28.   Juhan-Vague I, Alessi MC, Vague P. Increased plasma plasminogen activator inhibitor 1 levels. A possible link between insulin resistance and atherothrombosis. Diabetologia 1991; 34:457-62.

29.   Juhan-Vague I, Thompson SG, Jespersen J. Involvement of the hemostatic system in the insulin resistance syndrome. A study of 1500 patients with angina pectoris. Arterioscler Thromb 1993;13:1865-73.

30.   Potter van Loon BJ, Kluft C, Radder JK, Blankenstein MA, Meinders AE. The cardiovascular risk factor plasminogen activator inhibitor type 1 is related to insulin resistance. Metabolism 1993;42:945-49.

31.   Eliasson M, Evrin PE, Lundblad D. Fibrinogen and fibrinolytic variables in relation to anthropometry, lipids and blood pressure. The Northern Sweden MONICA Study. J Clin Epidemiol 1994;47:513-24.

32.   Vague P, Juhan-Vague I, Chabert V, Alessi MC, Atlan C. Fat distribution and plasminogen activator inhibitor activity in non diabetic obese women. Metabolism 1989;38:913-15.

33.   Landin K, Stigendal L, Eriksson E, et al. Abdominal obesity is associated with an impaired fibrinolytic activity and elevated plasminogen activator inhibitor-1. Metabolism 1990;39: 1044-48.

34.   Schneider DJ, Sobel BE. Augmentation of synthesis of plasminogen activator inhibitor type 1 by insulin and insulin-like growth factor type 1: Implications for vascular disease by hyperinsulinemic states. Proc Nat Acad Sci USA 1991;88:9959-63.

35.   Mc Gill JB, Schneider DJ, Arfken CL, Lucore CL, Sobel BE. Factors responsible for impaired fibrinolysis in obese subjects and NIDDM patients. Diabetes 1994;43:104-9.

36.   Hamsten A, Karpe F, Bavenholm P, Silveira A. Interactions amongst insulin, lipoproteins and haemostatic function relevant to coronary heart disease. J Int Med 1994;236:75-88.

37.   Nagi DK, Hendra TJ, Ryle AJ, et al. The relationships of concentrations of insulin, intact proinsulin and 32-33 split proinsulin with cardiovascular risk factors in type 2 (non insulin dependent) diabetic subjects. Diabetologia 1990;33:532-37.

38.   Juhan-Vague I, Alessi MC, Joly P, et al. Plasma plasminogen activator inhibitor 1 in angina pectoris. Influence of plasma insulin and acute-phase response. Arteriosclerosis 1989;9:362-67.

39.   Haverkate F, Thompson SG, Duckert F. Haemostasis factors in angina pectoris: Relation to gender, age and acute-phase reaction. Thromb Haemostas 1995;73:561-67.
40.   Reaven GO. Banting lecture 1988. Role of insulin resistance in human disease. Diabetes 1988;37:1595-607.
41.   Zimmet P. The epidemiology of diabetes mellitus and related conditions. In: Alberti KGMM, Krall CP, editors. The Diabetes Annual 6. Amsterdam: Elsevier, 1991: 1-19.
42.   Ferrannini E, Haffner SM, Mitchell BD, Stern MP. Hyperinsulinemia. The key feature of a cardiovascular and metabolic syndrome. Diabetologia 1991;34:416-22.
43.   Eschwege E, Richard JL, Thibult N, et al. Coronary heart disease mortality in relation with diabetes, blood glucose and plasma insulin levels. The Paris Prospective Study, ten years later. Horm Metab Res 1985;15:41-46.
44.   Pyörälä K, Savolainen E, Kaukola S, Haapakoski J. Plasma insulin as coronary heart disease risk factor: Relationship to other risk factors and predictive value during 9-year follow-up of the Helsinki Policemen Study population. Acta Med Scand 1985;701(Suppl.):38-52.
45.   Desprès JP, Lamarche B, Mauriège P, et al. Hyperinsulinemia as an independent risk factor for ischemic heart disease. N Eng J Med 1996;334:952-57.
46.   Sundell IB, Dahlgren S, Ranby M, Lundin E, Stenling R, Nilsson TK. Reduction of elevated plasminogen activator inhibitor levels during modest weight loss. Fibrinolysis 1989;3:51-53.
47.   Vague P, Juhan-Vague I, Alessi MC, Badier C, Valadier J. Metformin decreases the high plasminogen activator inhibition capacity, plasma insulin and triglyceride levels in non diabetic obese subjects. Thromb Haemostas 1987;57:326-28.
48.   Landin K, Tengborn L, Smith U. Treating insulin resistance in hypertension with Metformin reduces both blood pressure and metabolic risk factors. J Int Med 1991;229:181-87.
49.   Estelles A, Aznar J, Tormo G, Sapena P, Tormo V, Espana F. Influence of a rehabilitation sports program on the fibrinolytic activity of patients after myocardial infarction. Thromb Res 1989;55:203-12.
50.   Gris JC, Schved JF, Aguilar-Martinez P, Arnaud A, Sanchez N. Impact of physical training on plasminogen activator inhibitor activity in sedentary men. Fibrinolysis 1990;4:97-98.
51.   Folsom AR, Qamhieh HT, Wing RR, et al. Impact of weight loss on plasminogen activator inhibitor (PAI-1) factor VII, and other hemostatic factors in moderately over weight adults. Arterioscler Thromb 1993;13:162-69.
52.   Alessi MC, Parrot G, Guenoun E, Scelles V, Vague P, Juhan-Vague I. Relation between plasma PAI activity and Adipsin levels. Thromb Haemostas 1995;74:1200-1202.
53.   Sawdey S, Loskutoff DJ. Regulation of murine type 1 plasminogen activity inhibitor (PAI-1) gene expression in vivo. Tissue specificity and induction by lipopolysaccharide, tumor necrosis factor a and transforming growth factor b. J Clin Invest 1991;8:1346-53.
54.   Samad F, Yamamoto K, Loskutoff DJ. Distribution and regulation of plasminogen activator inhibitor 1 in murine adipose tissue in vivo. J Clin Invest 1996;97:37-46.
55.   Lundgren CH, Brown SL, Nordt TD, Sobel BE, Fujii S. Elaboration of type 1 plasminogen activator inhibitor from adipocytes. A potential pathogenetic link between obesity and cardiovascular disease. Circulation 1996;93:106-10.
56.   Samad F, Loskutoff DJ. Tissue distribution and regulation of plasminogen activator inhibitor-1 in obese mice. Mol Med 1996;2:568-82.
57.   Shimomura I, Funahashi T, Takahashi M, et al. Enhanced expression of PAI-1 in visceral fat: Possible contributor to vascular disease in obesity. Nature Medicine 1996;2:800-803.
58.   Alessi MC, Peiretti F, Morange P, Henry M, Nalbone G, Juhan-Vague I. Production of plasminogen activator inhibitor 1 by human adipose tissue. Possible link between visceral

fat accumulation and vascular disease. Diabetes 1997; in press.

59.   Björntorp P. "Portal" adipose tissue as a generator of risk factors for cardiovascular disease
       and diabetes. Arteriosclerosis 1990;10:493-96.

60.   Larsson B, Svärdsud DK, Welin L, Wilhelmsen L, Björntorp P, Tibbin G. Abdominal
       adipose tissue distribution, obesity and risk of cardiovascular disease and death : 13 year
       follow-up of participants in the study of men born in 1913. Br Med J 1984;288:1401-04.

61.   Sundell IB, Nilsson TK, Ranby M, Hallmans G, Hellsten G. Fibrinolytic variables are related
       to age, sex, blood pressure, and body build measurements : A cross-sectional study in
       Norsjö, Sweden. J Clin Epidemiol 1989:42:719-23.

62.   Cigolini M, Targher G, Bergamo Andreis IA, Tonoli M, Agostino G, De Sandre G. Visceral
       fat accumulation and its relation to plasma hemostatic factors in healthy men. Arterioscler
       Thromb Vasc Biol 1996;16:368-74.

63.   Dawson S, Hamsten A, Wiman B, Henney A, Humphries S. Genetic variation at the
       plasminogen activator inhibitor-1 locus is associated with altered levels of plasma
       plasminogen activator inhibitor-1 activity. Arterioscler Thromb 1991;11:183-90

64.   Dawson SJ, Wiman B, Hamsten A, Green F, Hamphries S, Henney AM. The two allele
       sequences of a common polymorphism in the promoter of the plasminogen activator
       inhibitor 1 (PAI-1) gene respond differently to interleukin 1 in HepG2 cells. J Biol Chem
       1993;268:10739-45.

65.   Henry M, Chomiki N, Scarabin PY, et al. Five frequent polymorphisms of plasminogen
       activator inhibitor 1 gene : Lack of association between genotypes, PAI activity and
       triglycerides levels in a healthy population. Arterioscler Thromb Vasc Biol 1997; in press.

66.   Ye S, Green FR, Scarabin PY, et al. The 4G/5G genetic polymorphism in the promoter of
       the plasminogen activator inhibitor-1 (PAI-1) associated with differences in plasma PAI-1
       activity but not with risk of myocardial infarction in the ECTIM study. Thromb Haemostas
       1995;74:837-41.

67.   Panahloo A, Mohamed-Ali V, Lane A, Green F, Humphries SE, Yudkin JS. Determinants
       of plasminogen activator 1 activity in treated NIDDM and its relation to a polymorphism in
       the plasminogen activator inhibitor 1 gene. Diabetes 1995;44:37-42.

68.   Eriksson P, Kallin B, van't Hooft, Bavenholm P, Hamsten A. Allele-specific increase in
       basal transcription of the plasminogen-activator inhibitor 1 gene is associated with
       myocardial infarction. Proc Natl Acad Sci USA 1995;92:1851-55.

69.   Mansfield MW, Strickland MH, Grant PJ. Environmental and genetic factors in relation to
       elevated circulating levels of plasminogen activator inhibitor 1 in Caucasian patients with
       non insulin dependent diabetes mellitus. Thromb Haemostas 1995;74:842-48.

70.   Ridker PM, Hennekens CH, Lindpaintner K, Stampfer MJ, Miletich JP. Arterial and venous
       thrombosis is not associated with the 4G/5G polymorphism in the promoter of the
       plasminogen activator inhibitor gene in a large cohort of US men. Circulation 1997;95:59-
       62.

71.   Henry M, Tregouët DA, Alessi MC, et al. Family study of metabolic and genetic
       determinants of PAI-1 activity and PAI-1 antigen plasma concentrations. The Stanislas
       cohort study. Thromb Haemostas XVIth ISTH Congress, Florence 1997, Abstract.

72.   Charlton PA, Faint RW, Bent F, et al. A series of low molecular weight inhibitors of
       plasminogen activator inhibitor (PAI-1) increase fibrinolysis and protect against thrombus
       formation in the rat. Abstract. Thromb Haemostas 1995;73:1005.

PLASMA HOMOCYST(E)INE [H(E)] AND ARTERIAL OCCLUSIVE DISEASES: GENE-
NUTRIENT INTERACTIONS

M. Rene Malinow

Interest in the association between plasma homocyst(e)ine[1] and vascular diseases has increased substantially. Table 1 shows the number of reports in the last 30 years listed in Medline under "homocysteine/blood." The data indicate that the annual rate of publications was initially 1.4 and it raised to 62 in the last five years, i.e. about a 44-fold increase within the span covered by the literature search. Such an accelerated growth probably reflects the potential clinical importance of homocyst(e)inemia in vascular occlusive diseases and the usual decrease of homocyst(e)ine levels brought about by inexpensive vitamin therapy. The availability of methods for accurately measuring plasma homocyst(e)ine and the more recent emphasis on genes regulating the expression of enzymes involved in the methionine/homocysteine metabolism, may also have contributed to such growth in publications [see reviews in 1-6]. This presentation will be necessarily selective in view of the large number of reports dealing with the subject. Thus, the association of elevated homocyst(e)ine to idiopathic venous thrombosis and pulmonary embolism [7-9] will not be considered. Moreover, in order to comply with time restraints, potentially involved mechanisms at the cellular level and results obtained postmethionine loading test, a procedure that may unmask abnormalities in the metabolism of methionine/homocysteine [10] will not be discussed, except as noted. Previous publications by the author will be quoted freely here.

---

[1] Plasma/serum homocyst(e)ine is the sum of the thiol-containing amino acid homocysteine and the homocysteinyl moiety of the disulfides homocysteine and cysteine-homocysteine, whether free or bound to proteins. *Homocyst(e)inemia* relates to the amount of homocyst(e)ine in blood, plasma, or serum; *hyperhomocyst(e)inemia* indicates above-normal concentrations of homocyst(e)ine (i.e. about > 16 μmol/L). Moderate, intermediate, and severe hyperhomocyst(e)inemia refer to concentrations between 16 and 30, between 31 and 100, and > 100 μmol/L, respectively. Thus, homocystinuria is also called severe hyperhomocyst(e)inemia [1].

A. M. Gotto, Jr. et al. (eds.), Multiple Risk Factors in Cardiovascular Disease, 93–104.
© 1998 *Kluwer Academic Publishers and Fondazione Giovanni Lorenzini. Printed in the Netherlands.*

Table 1. Number of Publications on "Homocyst(e)ine/Blood" in Medline

Dates	Publications (N)	Rate/Year
1966-79	19	1.4
1980-85	27	4.5
1986-91	92	15.3
1992-96	310	62.0

Homocystinuria

Homocystinuria, a rare genetic autosomal recessive disorder with defective activity of cystathionine β synthase, an enzyme which requires pyridoxal phosphate as cofactor in the transsulfuration of homocysteine to cysteine [11], brought initial attention to the potential association of homocyst(e)ine and cardiovascular disease. Thus, affected subjects may show neurologic, ocular, skeletal, and vascular abnormalities that could result in early death secondary to myocardial infarction, stroke, or pulmonary embolism [11]. In a number of these patients, intake of large doses of vitamin B_6 decreased the severity of symptoms and may have prolonged life [11]. Biochemical findings in blood, and postmortem studies in homocystinuric children, supported McCully's proposal of the "homocysteine hypothesis for arteriosclerosis" [12]. Subsequent observations demonstrated the frequent occurrence of moderately elevated levels of plasma homocyst(e)ine in adults with clinically apparent atherosclerosis, but not showing other abnormalities observed in homocystinuria.

Homocyst(e)inemia in Coronary Artery Disease (CAD)

Wilcken and Wilcken [13] described increased concentrations of cysteine-homocysteine disulfide after methionine loading in CAD patients. Murphy-Chutorian et al. [14] and Clarke et al. [15] also reported increased homocysteine species postmethionine-loading in similar patients. Kang et al. [16] found increased basal concentrations of homocyst(e)ine in CAD subjects.

Several colleagues and I measured basal homocyst(e)ine in 405 consecutive patients attending an internist's office [17]. The age of men and women with CAD was 64.5 ± 9.6 (SD) and 70.1 ± 8.2 years, respectively, compared with 56.6 ± 11.3 and 62.4 ± 11.5 years in the controls. The patients with CAD had higher homocyst(e)ine concentrations than the control subjects, i.e. 13.07 ± 4.32 versus 11.21 ± 3.71 μmol/L in men (P = 0.02), and 12.97 ± 7.39 versus 10.15 ± 4.99 μmol/L in women (P = 0.03, in-ln-transformed values with age as covariate). About 20% of male coronary patients had homocyst(e)ine concentrations exceeding the 95th percentile distribution of the control subjects. In another study [18], the presence of CAD was established by coronary angiography in 175 men (age 50 ± 7 years) and contrasted their homocyst(e)ine levels with those in 255 control subjects (age 49 ± 6 years) clinically free of CAD. Concentrations were greater in the CAD subjects than in controls, i.e. 13.66 ± 6.44 versus 10.93 ± 4.92 µmol/L respectively, (P = 0.001). Stepwise discriminant analysis on cases versus controls was performed with models including usual risk factors for atherosclerosis. Smoking, high-density lipoprotein cholesterol, hypertension, homocyst(e)ine, and diabetes were associated (P = 0.05) in descending order with the presence of CAD in the first model. In a second model, apolipoproteins B and A-I were used and homocyst(e)ine remained associated with the presence of CAD. These data suggested that homocyst(e)ine could be considered an independent risk factor for atherosclerosis [19].

Homocyst(e)inemia in Cerebrovascular Disease

High concentrations of homocyst(e)ine have been observed in patients with cerebrovascular disease [15,20-22]. As previously reported [23], 41 patients with acute strokes and 27 patients with transient ischemic attacks had higher mean concentrations of homocyst(e)ine i.e. 15.78 ± 5.40 (P<10^{-4}) and 14.76 ± 6 (P<10^{-2}) µmol/L, respectively, than 31 controls (10.68 ± 3.20 µmol/L). About one-third of the patients had homocyst(e)ine concentrations higher than arbitrarily defined control levels. No relation between homocyst(e)ine concentration and other recognized stroke risk factors or stroke type were detected; however, concentrations of serum uric acid and plasma homocyst(e)ine were positively correlated [23].

In 142 survivors of stroke, mean homocyst(e)ine concentrations were greater than in 66 controls, and hyperhomocyst(e)inemia was present in 40% of the stroke patients and in 6% of the controls [24]. The homocyst(e)ine concentrations were increased in patients with lacunar, hemorrhagic, or embolic strokes. Plasma homocyst(e)ine showed no significant association with the presence of hypertension, smoking, or hypercholesterolemia or with the concentration of blood glucose, glycohemoglobin, or plasma fibrinogen. About 40% of the homocyst(e)ine variance could be predicted by the values of blood folate, plasma pyridoxal 5'-phosphate, and serum creatinine. Thus, hyperhomocyst(e)inemia seemed to be partly related to renal function and to the concentration of cofactors involved in the metabolism of homocysteine [24].

Homocyst(e)inemia in Peripheral Arterial Disease

Boers et al. [20], Clarke et al. [15] and Mansoor et al. [25] found high concentrations of plasma homocyst(e)ine in subjects with peripheral arterial occlusive disease. In a study of 47 patients with carotid arterial involvement (n = 35) or ileofemoral lesions (n = 32), most patients had both arterial territories involved. Plasma homocyst(e)ine was elevated in these patients, i.e. 16.16 ± 6.94 µmol/L in cases versus 10.10 ± 2.16 µmol/L in controls (P = 0.05) [26].

Seventy-eight patients with intermittent claudication were selected from an epidemiological survey of all middle-aged men (n = 15,253; age 45-69 years) in Linkoping County, Sweden [27]. As controls, 98 randomly selected, age-matched men were included.

Concentration of homocyst(e)ine was significantly higher in the affected subjects than in controls (16.74 ± 5.45 versus 13.80 ± 3.21 µmol/L; P = 0.0002). Twenty-three percent of the patients had homocyst(e)ine concentrations above the 95th percentile of the controls. The homocyst(e)ine levels were independent of other risk factors for peripheral atherosclerotic disease, but increased homocyst(e)ine was observed mainly in subjects with low concentrations of serum folate. The authors concluded that folic acid supplementation could be appropriate in the treatment of these patients [27].

Homocyst(e)ine and Genetic Factors

The importance of genetic factors in the control of homocyst(e)inemia in patients without homocystinuria, was demonstrated in several studies. Families of 71 hyperhomo- cyst(e)inemic CAD patients were selected on the basis of availability of relatives. In 20 families (28%), the proband had homocyst(e)ine concentrations greater than the 90th percentile of controls. Familial segregation of homocyst(e)ine levels was observed in 10 of these kindred, i.e. in 14% of the probands, suggesting the likelihood of familial hyperhomocyst(e)inemia, terms then introduced in the literature [19]. A significant correlation was found between the homocyst(e)ine levels of off-springs and probands (r = 0.248; P = 0.002). Moreover, significant correlation (r = 0.264; P = 0.041) between spouses, suggested that environmental factor may also have been involved [19].

To further test familial segregation, homocyst(e)ine was measured in plasma samples from 37 men and women with early familial coronary heart disease, and from 48 controls matched for age and sex [28]. The subjects were selected to include 13 male sibling pairs with CAD as well as 13 male sibling pairs and 13 spouse pairs as controls (all age-matched). The mean homocyst(e)ine concentrations were significantly higher in CAD patients, both in men (14.31 versus 11.09 µmol/L; P = 0.02) and women (9.51 versus 7.40 µmol/L; P = 0.02). A strong familial correlation of plasma homocyst(e)ine was observed among all 26 male sibling pairs (r = 0.52; P < 0.01) and was present separately in subjects with CAD as well as in control siblings. The data suggested that hyperhomocyst(e)inemia was an inherited abnormality that might explain certain cases of early familial CAD. Moreover, Wu et al. [29] found concordant high homocyst(e)inemia in at least 12% of 85 families with two or more siblings affected by early CAD, a prevalence similar to the one indicated above in previous observations. Furthermore, genetic control of homocyst(e)inemia was suggested in observations on mono-[30] and dizogotic twins [30,31], in which the paired correlation of homocyst(e)ine was significantly higher in monozygotic twins than in dizogotic twins. Finally, Tonstad et al. [32] assessed the predictive value of homocyst(e)ine levels in children from families experiencing premature cardiovascular disease. Homocyst(e)ine was higher in children whose father, grandfather, or uncle died at age ≤ 55 years of myocardial infarction or sudden cardiac arrest than in control children.

Plasma Homocyst(e)ine and Graded Risk for Myocardial Infarction

Kang et al. published histograms of homocyst(e)ine concentrations in CAD and control subjects, demonstrating a displacement to the right in the values of CAD patients [16]. These observations suggested that the risk of CAD was continuous across the concentration of homocyst(e)inc. Similar results were reported in a prospective study of 21,826 subjects from Tromso, Norway: serum homocyst(e)ine was a risk factor for CAD with no threshold effect [33]. Collaborators and I conducted a study on 420 survivors of myocardial infarction (cases) and 486 controls from northern France and Northern Ireland [34]. The age-adjusted rate of myocardial infarction in the upper quintile of homocyst(e)ine levels, i.e. homocyst(e)ine levels ≥ 17.2 $\mu mol/L$, compared with the lowest quintile (< 9.8 $\mu mol/L$) was 3.4 fold higher in Northern Ireland ($P < 10^{-3}$), and 5.2 fold higher in northern France ($P < 10^{-4}$). Additional adjustment for body mass index, alcohol intake, cigarette smoking, systolic blood pressure, and certain lipid parameters, maintained the statistical significance only in the subjects from northern France. Figure 1 shows the age-adjusted, odds ratios in subjects in northern France. The data suggested that there was a graded risk of myocardial infarction across the entire distribution of homocyst(e)ine levels. Moreover, a recent report has extended these findings. Basal and postmethionine load homocyst(e)ine levels were determined in 131 cases with severe CAD documented by angiography and in 189 controls [35]. The homocyst(e)ine data suggested that fasting, postload, and the increase after methionine loading had a positive association with the risk of severe CAD. The association existed over a wide range of homocyst(e)ine levels without showing a threshold below which there was no increased risk. A similar lack of threshold effect in the association of homocyst(e)ine and CAD was also observed by Robinson et al. [36]. Thus, the findings reported by different authors suggest that treatment of homocyst(e)inemia probably should not be limited only to hyperhomocyst(e)inemic individuals. However, which individuals would be treated remains to be established.

The Interrelationship Between Plasma Homocyst(e)ine and Folic Acid Supplementation; Modulation Effects of Methylenetetrahydrofolate Reductase (MTHFR) Gene Polymorphism

High concentration of homocyst(e)ine has been reported in subjects with low levels of folate [37,38] and of vitamins B_{12} [38,39], and B_6 [36]. Robinson et al. considered the latter case to be a common and independent reversible risk for CAD [36]. The effects of B-vitamins supplementation in reducing homocyst(e)ine levels, given as single or multiple agents, has been documented following the oral use of folic acid (0.6-15 mg/d) [40-42], vitamin B_{12} (parenteral) in patients with pernicious anemia [43], and vitamin B_6 (20-250 mg/d) in subjects with abnormal post methionine loading tests [44,45]. However, the following discussion will be focused on folic acid and MTHFR gene polymorphism.

The enzyme MTHFR catalyzes the reduction of 5,10-methylenetetrahydrofolate to 5-methyltetrahydrofolate, the most common form of circulating folic acid. This active form of folate transfers a methyl group to cobalamin. Thereby, methionine synthase catalyzes the transfer of a methyl group for the transmethylation of homocysteine to methionine [11]. Kang et al. [46,47] reported the presence of a common homozygous thermolabile form of MTHFR in 5% of white controls and in 17% of CAD patients. The DNA mutation responsible for the heat labile variant has been identified as a C- to T-mutation at nucleotide 677, which substitutes a valine for alanine at position 114 of the MTHFR protein [48,49]. The frequency of the homozygous form (T677T) of this polymorphism was 12% in French Canadians and 12% to 15% in populations of European, Middle Eastern, and Japanese origin [50]. The frequency of homozygotes for the T677 allele in 60 Dutch patients with arterial occlusive diseases was 15%, compared with 5.2% in 111 control subjects [51]. Also, Gallagher et al. also observed a higher frequency of the T/T homozygotes in CAD patients than in controls (i.e. 17% and 7%, respectively) [52]. In a current study [53], homocyst(e)ine was higher in subjects homozygous for the T677 allele, and T/T homozygotes were more prevalent in CAD patients than in non-CAD subjects (12.1% versus 7.8%, respectively). However, such differences in homozygous prevalence between CAD cases and control subjects, were not confirmed by several investigators [54-59]. Whether these disparities are due to differences in genetic pools or other undetermined factors needs further study.

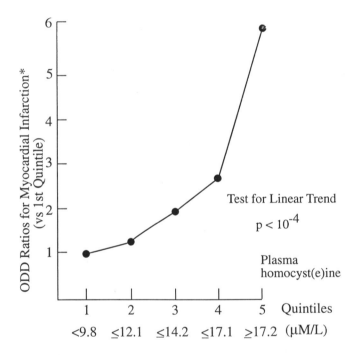

*Adjusted for age, BMI, alcohol intake, cigarette smoking

Figure 1. Odd ratios for subjects with previous myocardial infarction versus controls in northern France. Adapted from Malinow et al. [34].

Collaborators and I aimed to identify factors responsible for interindividual heterogeneity in responsiveness to folate supplementation. It was hypothesized that allelic variations in the C677T gene for MTHFR as well as baseline homocyst(e)ine and vitamin levels may contribute to such heterogeneity. To test this hypothesis, the effects of a three-week daily supplement of either 1 or 2 mg of folic acid on plasma homocyst(e)ine levels were examined in subjects with or without CAD who were homozygous, heterozygous, or null for the C677T mutation in the MTHFR gene. The modulation effects of multivitamins use and baseline homocyst(e)ine and plasma vitamin levels on responsiveness to folic acid supplementation in these subjects also were tested [53].

The study involved 140 subjects which were diagnosed more than three months previously with a history of acute myocardial infarction, angina pectoris documented by a cardiologist, percutaneous transarterial coronary angioplasty, or coronary bypass graft surgery (cases). Control subjects had no history of CAD (n = 102). Case and control subjects reported having no history of stroke, intermittent claudication, or peripheral arterial revascularization. Decreases of homocyst(e)ine were essentially similar after the intake of 1 or 2 mg/d of folic acid regardless of sex, age, CAD status, body mass index, smoking, or plasma creatinine concentration. Nonusers of multivitamins had higher basal levels of homocyst(e)ine and lower levels of B-vitamins, but the decrease of homocyst(e)inemia in response to folic acid supplementation was greater than in users of multivitamins. Folate levels increased approximately to the same levels in all subjects, suggesting similar folate absorption in users and nonusers of multivitamins [53].

The influence of MTHFR genotype on the response to folic acid supplementation is shown in Figure 2.

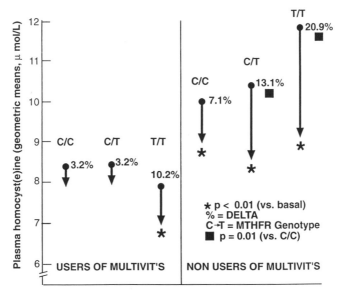

Figure 2. Decreases in plasma homocyst(e)ine following three-week daily intake of folic acid supplementation as function of MTHFR C677T genotype. Adapted from Malinow et al. [53].

Users of multivitamins with C/C and C/T genotypes had a blunted response to folic acid supplementation whereas nonusers of multivitamins responded to folic acid supplementation regardless of MTHFR genotype. However, the therapeutic response was more marked in the T/T homozygotes. An observation by Guttormsen et al. [60] also suggested the T/T homozygotes are very sensitive to folic acid supplementation: in 21 of 37 subjects with homocyst(e)ine > 20 μmol/L, homocyst(e)inemia was normalized with a small intake of folic acid (0.2 mg/d).

The negative correlation between levels of homocyst(e)ine and folate, and the influence of MTHFR genotype on these correlations is shown in Figure 3. The slopes of the regression equations are almost identical in C/C and C/T subjects. However, subjects with T/T MTHFR genotype are more susceptible to show higher levels of homocyst(e)ine at lower folate levels than the other genotypes.

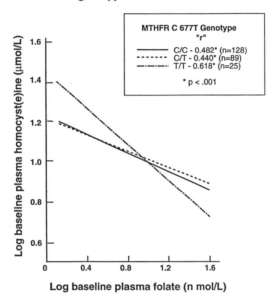

Figure 3. Log baseline homocyst(e)ine versus log baseline folate levels. Regression equations: C/C, y=1.210-0.199 x; C/T, y=1.222-0.212; T/T, y=1.42g-0.359x. Adapted from Malinow et al. [53].

Conclusion

Levels of homocyst(e)ine are frequently elevated in patients with coronary, cerebral and peripheral arterial occlusive diseases. Folate status is an important determinant of homocyst(e)ine levels, which are modulated by MTHFR genotypes. Further research is necessary to delineate those interactions. Daily intake of folic acid (2.5 mg) and vitamins B_6 (20 mg)and B_{12} (0.4 mg) has been proposed to test the hypothesis that reducing levels of homocyst(e)ine will decrease the incidence of brain infarction [61]. Whether vitamin supplementation will affect the evolution of atherosclerosis, must await the results of prospective placebo-controlled, randomized, clinical trials.

Acknowledgments

This work is supported in part by grant RR00163-34 from the National Institutes of Health.

References

1. Kang SS, Wong PWK, Malinow MR. Hyperhomocyst(e)inemia as a risk factor for occlusive vascular disease. Ann Rev Nutr 1992;12:259-78.
2. Duell PB, Malinow MR. Homocyst(e)ine:An important risk factor for atherosclerotic vascular disease. Curr Opin Lipid 1997;8:28-34.
3. Malinow MR. Hyperhomocyst(e)inemia. A common and easily reversible risk factor for atherosclerosis. Circulation 1990;81:2004-6.
4. Malinow MR. Homocyst(e)ine and arterial occlusive diseases. J Intern Med 1994;236:603-17.
5. Malinow MR. Plasma homocyst(e)ine and arterial occlusive diseases: A mini-review. Clin Chem 1994;41:173-76.
6. Mayer EL, Jacobsen DW, Robinson K. Homocysteine and coronary atherosclerosis. J Am Coll Cardiol 1996;27:517-27.
7. den Heijer M, Koster T, Blom HJ, et al. Hyperhomocysteinemia as a risk factor for deep-vein thrombosis. N Engl J Med 1996;334:759-62.
8. Ridker PM, Hennekens CH, Lindpainter K, Stampfer MJ, Eisenberg PR, Miletich JP. Mutation in the gene coding for coagulation factor V and the risk of myocardial infarction, stroke, and venous thrombosis in apparently healthy men. N Engl J Med 1995;332:912-17.
9. Ridker PM, Hennekens CH, Selhub J, Miletich JP, Malinow MR, Stampfer MJ. Interrelation of hyperhomocyst(e)inemia, factor V Leiden, and risk of future venous thromboembolism. Circulation 1997;95:1777-82.
10. Bostom AG, Jacques PF, Nadeau MR, Williams RR, Ellison RC, Selhub J. Post-methionine load hyperhomocysteinemia in persons with normal fasting total plasma homocysteine: Initial results from the NHLBI family heart study. Atherosclerosis 1995;116:147-51.
11. Mudd SH, Levy HL. Disorders in transsulfuration. In: Scriver CR, Beaudet AL, Sly WS, Valle D, editors. The metabolic basis of inherited disease, 6th ed. McGraw-Hill: New York, 1989: 693-734.
12. McCully KS. Vascular pathology of homocysteinemia: Implications for the pathogensis of arteriosclerosis. Am J Pathol 1969;56:111-28.
13. Wilcken DEL, Wilcken B. The pathogenesis of coronary artery disease. A possible role for methionine metabolism. J Clin Invest 1976;57:1079-82.
14. Murphy-Chutorian DR, Wexman MP, Grieco AJ, et al. Methionine intolerance: A possible risk factor for coronary artery disease. J Am Coll Card 1985;6:725-30.
15. Clarke R, Daly L, Robinson K, et al. Hyperhomocysteinemia: An independent risk factor for vascular disease. N Engl J Med 1991;324:1149-55.
16. Kang SS, Wong PWK, Cook HY, Norusis M, Messer JV. Protein-bound homocyst(e)ine. A possible risk factor for coronary heart disease. J Clin Invest 1986;77:1482-86.
17. Malinow MR, Sexton G, Averbuch M, Grossman M, Wilson DL, Upson B. Homocyst(e)inemia in daily practice: Levels in coronary heart disease. Coron Art Dis 1990;

1:215-20.

18.   Genest JJ, McNamara JR, Salem DN, Wilson PWF, Schaefer EJ, Malinow MR. Plasma homocyst(e)ine levels in men with premature coronary artery disease. J Am Coll Card 1990; 16:1114-18.

19.   Genest JJ, McNamara MT, Upson B, et al. Prevalence of familial hyperhomocyst(e)inemia in men with premature coronary artery disease. Arterioscler Thromb 1991;11:1129-36.

20.   Boers GHJ, Smals AGH, Trijbels FJM, et al. Heterozygosity for homocystinuria in premature peripheral and cerebral occlusive arterial disease. N Engl J Med 1985;313:709-15.

21.   Brattstrom LE, Hardebo JE, Hultberg BL. Moderate homocysteinemia—a possible risk factor for arteriosclerotic cerebrovascular disease. Stroke 1984;14:1012-16.

22.   Araki A, Sako Y, Fukushima Y, Matsumoto M, Asada T, Kita T. Plasma sulfhydryl-containing amino acids in patients with cerebral infarction and in hypertensive subjects. Atherosclerosis 1989;79:139-46.

23.   Coull BM, Malinow MR, Beamer N, Sexton G, Nordt F, deGarmo P. Elevated plasma homocyst(e)ine in acute stroke and TIA: A possible independent risk factor for stroke. Stroke 1990;21:572-76.

24.   Brattstrom L, Lindgren A, Israelsson B, Malinow MR, Norrving B, Upson B. Hyperhomocysteinaemia in stroke—prevalence, cause, and relationships to type of stroke and stroke risk factors. Eur J Clin Invest 1992;22:214-21.

25.   Mansoor MA, Bergmark C, Svardal AM, Lonning PE, Ueland PM. Redox status and protein binding of plasma homocysteine and other aminothiols in patients with early-onset peripheral vascular disease. Arterioscler Thromb Vasc Biol 1995;15:232-40.

26.   Malinow MR, Kang SS, Taylor LM, et al. Prevalence of hyperhomocyst(e)inemia in patients with peripheral arterial occlusive disease. Circulation 1989;79:1180-88.

27.   Molgaard J, Malinow MR, Lassvik C, Holm AC, Upson B, Olsson AG. Hyperhomocyst(e)inemia: An independent risk factor for intermittent claudication. J Intern Med 1992;231:273-80.

28.   Williams, RR, Malinow MR, Hunt SC, et al. Hyperhomocyst(e)inemia in Utah siblings with early coronary disease. Coron Art Dis 1990;1:681-85.

29.   Wu LL, Wu J, Hunt SC, James BC, et al. Plasma homocyst(e)ine as a risk factor for early familial coronary artery disease. Clin Chem 1994;40:552-61.

30.   Reed T, Malinow MR, Christian JC, Upson B. Estimates of heritability of plasma homocyst(e)ine levels in aging adult male twins. Clin Genet 1991;39:425-28.

31.   Berg K, Malinow MR, Kierulf P, Upson B. Population variation and genetics of plasma homocyst(e)ine level. Clin Genet 1991;41:315-21.

32.   Tonstad S, Refsum H, Sivertsen M, Christophersen B, Ose L, Ueland PM. Relation of total homocysteine and lipid levels in children to premature cardiovascular death in male relatives. Pediatr Res 1996;40:47-52.

33.   Arnesen E, Refsum H, Bonaa KH, Ueland PM, Forde OH, Nordrehaug JE. Serum total homocysteine and coronary heart disease. Int J Epidemiol 1995;24:704-9.

34.   Malinow MR, Ducimetiere P, Luc G, et al. Plasma homocyst(e)ine levels and graded risk for myocardial infarction: Findings in two populations at contrasting risk for coronary heart disease. Atherosclerosis 1996;126:27-34.

35.   Verhoef P, Kok FJ, Kruyssen D, et al. Plasma total homocyst(e)ine, B vitamins, and risk of coronary atherosclerosis. Arterioscler Thromb Vasc Biol 1997;17:989-95.

36.   Robinson K, Mayer EL, Miller DP, et al. Hyperhomocysteinemia and low pyridoxal phosphate. Circulation 1995;92:2825-30.

37.   Kang SS, Wong PWK, Norusis M. Homocyst(e)inemia due to folate deficiency. Metabolism 1987;36:458-62.

38.   Ueland PM, Refsum H, Stabler SP, Malinow MR, Andersson A, Allen RH. Total homocysteine in plasma or serum. Methods and clinical application. Clin Chem 1993;39: 1764-79.

39.   Lindenbaum J, Rosenberg IH, Wilson PWF, Stabler SP, Allen RH. Prevalence of cobalamin deficiency in the Framingham elderly population. Am J Clin Nutr 1994;60:2-11.

40.   Ubbink JB, van der Merwe A, Vermaak WJH, et al. Hyperhomocysteinemia and the response to vitamin supplementation. Clin Invest 1993;71:993-98.

41.   Brattstrom LE, Israelsson B, Jeppsson J-O, Hultberg BL. Folic acid—an innocuous means to reduce plasma homocysteine. Scand J Clin Lab Invest 1988;48:215-21.

42.   Bostom AG, Shemin D, Lapane KL, et al. High dose B-vitamin treatment of hyperhomocysteinemia in dialysis patients. Kidney Int 1996;49:147-52.

43.   Lindenbaum J, Helaton EB, Savage DG, et al. Neuropsychiatric disorders caused by cobalamin deficiency in the absence of anemia or macrocytosis. N Engl J Med 1988;318: 1720-28.

44.   Ubbink JB, van der Merwe A, Delport R, et al. The effect of a subnormal vitamin B6 status on homocysteine metabolism. J Clin Invest 1996;98:177-84.

45.   van den Berg M, Franken DG, Boers GH, et al. Combined vitamin B6 plus folic acid therapy in young patients with arteriosclerosis and hyperhomocysteinemia. J Vasc Surg 1994;20:933-40.

46.   Kang SS, Passen EI, Ruggie N, Wong PWK, Sora J. Thermolabile defect of methylenetetrahydrofolate reductase in coronary artery disease. Circulation 1993;88:1463-69

47.   Kang SS, Wong PWK, Susmano A, Sora J, Norusis M, Ruggie N. Thermolabile methylenetetrahydrofolate reductase: An inherited risk factor for coronary artery disease. Am J Hum Genet 1991;48:536-45.

48.   Goyette P, Sumner JS, Milos R, et al. Human methylenetetrahydrofolate reductase: Isolation of DNA, mapping and mutation identification. Nat Genet 1994;7:195-200.

49.   Frosst P, Blom HJ, Milos R, et al. A candidate genetic risk factor for vascular disease: A common mutation in methylenetetrahydrofolate reductase. Nat Genet 1995;10:111-3.

50.   Motulsky AG. Nutritional ecogenetics: Homocysteine-related arteriosclerotic vascular disease, neural tube defects, and folic acid. Am J Hum Genet 1996;58:17-20.

51.   Kluijmans LAJ, Lambert PWJ, van den Heuvel WJ, et al. Molecular genetic analysis in mild hyperhomocysteinemia: A common mutation in the methylenetetrahydrofolate reductase gene is a genetic risk factor for cardiovascular disease. Am J Hum Genet 1996;58:35-41.

52.   Gallagher PM, Meleady R, Shields DC, et al. Homocysteine and risk of premature coronary heart disease. Circulation 1996;94:2154-58.

53.   Malinow MR, Nieto FJ, Kruger WD, et al. The effects of folic acid supplementation on plasma total homocysteine are modulated by multivitamin use and methylenetetrahydrofolate reductase genotypes. Arterioscler Thromb Vasc Biol 1997;17:in press.

54.   Wilcken DEL, Wang ZL, Sim AS, McCredie RM. Distribution of healthy and coronary populations of the methylenetetrahydrofolate reductase (MTHFR) $C_{677}T$ mutation. Arterioscler Thromb Vasc Biol 1996;16:878-82.

55.   Schmitz C, Lindpaintner K, Verhoef P, Gaziano JM, Buring J. Genetic polymorphism of methylenetetrahydrofolate reductase and myocardial infarction: A case-control study. Circulation 1996;94:1812-14.

56.   Deloughery TG, Evans A, Sadeghi A, et al. Common mutation in methylenetetrahydrofolate

reductase: Correlation with homocysteine metabolism and late-onset vascular disease. Circulation 1996:94:3074-78.

57. van Bockxmeer FM, Mamotte CDS, Vasikaran SD, Taylor RR. Methylenetetrahydrofolate reductase gene and coronary artery disease. Circulation 1997;95:21-23.

58. Brugada R, Marian AJ. A common mutation in methylenetetrahydrofolate reductase gene is not a major risk of coronary artery disease or myocardial infarction. Atherosclerosis 1997;128: 107-12.

59. Christensen B, Frosst P, Lussier-Cacan S, et al. Correlation of a common mutation in the methylenetetrahydrofolate reductase gene with plasma homocysteine in patients with premature coronary artery disease. Arterioscler Thromb Vasc Biol 1997;17:569-73.

60. Guttormsen AB, Ueland PM, Nesthus I, et al. Determinants and vitamin responsiveness of intermediate hyperhomocysteinemia. J Clin Invest 1996;98:2174-83.

61. Howard VJ, Chambless LE, Malinow MR, Lefkowitz D, Toole JF. Results of a homocyst(e)ine lowering pilot study in acute stroke patients. Stroke 1997;28:234.

THE ROLE OF SOCIAL AND PSYCHOEMOTIONAL FACTORS IN THE DEVELOPMENT OF CARDIOVASCULAR DISEASE: THE EXPERIENCE IN EASTERN EUROPEAN COUNTRIES

Eugene I. Chazov

The socio-economic state of society and the associated level of psychoemotional tension and "stress" currently do not play a significant role in the assessment of factors which determine cardiovascular morbidity and mortality. It is difficult to determine their role in the formation of cardiovascular morbidity and mortality, while at the same time taking into account the presence of various risk factors in the observed population groups (smoking, lipid metabolism abnormalities, high level of arterial blood pressure, etc.).

Nevertheless, clinical studies as well as experimental data convincingly prove the significance of "stress" and psychoemotional tension in the formation of heart and vessel disease. For example, our experimental studies demonstrated that chronic neurotization of animals and stresses of different character cause alteration of neurotransmitters' content (adrenaline, noradrenalin, serotonin) in the hypothalamus and adrenal and, depending on their basal content, cause elevation of arterial blood pressure.

But life has conducted the best experiment. Between 1990 and 1995, particularly 1992-1993, a rapid leap in mortality from cardiovascular diseases took place in the majority of Eastern European countries [1-2]. Cardiovascular disease in Russia increased from 617 deaths per 100,000 in 1990 to 790 deaths per 100,000 in 1995. In Byelorussia, cardiovascular mortality increased from 542.1 to 640.1 per 100,000 during the same time period; in Ukraine, from 641.5 to 875.0; in the Republic of Moldova, from 435.1 to 559.3; and in Armenia, from 333.8 to 357.8 deaths. A similar situation was observed in Bulgaria, where cardiovascular mortality increased from 158.6 to 174.2 per 100,000 during 1990-1993, and in Rumania, where deaths from cardiovascular disease increased from 148.2 to 170.7 per 100,000.

The question arises as to what has caused such a radical leap. A simple analysis indicates that life in these countries has been characterized recently by many complex political and economic transformations which have led to economic crises, lack of trust in the society, political and social opposition, poverty, and spiritual deterioration.

In Russia, for example, the 1995 annual income of 25% of the population was lower than subsistence minimum. Satisfaction with life has decreased from 40% in 1991 to 16% in 1995. According to official statistics the difference in the annual income of the 10% most well-provided for segment of the population and the 10% most poorly provided for segment was 13.5-fold. In Russia the gross national product has declined by 50% during 1989-1994.

A. M. Gotto, Jr. et al. (eds.), Multiple Risk Factors in Cardiovascular Disease, 105–107.

By way of comparison, during 1930-1935, the years of the Great Depression in the United States, the American gross national product declined by 30%. The correlation between the level of the gross national product and the health of the nation is well known [2].

How do such socio-economic and political transformations influence the health of the nation, specifically cardiovascular morbidity and mortality? To determine this, we have carried out studies in randomized groups of population from the same region of Moscow. Between 1985 and 1995, there was a 1.7-fold increase in the frequency of ischemic heart disease cases and a significant increase in arterial blood pressure levels in the general population [2]. At the same time though, the level of plasma cholesterol has decreased as well as the index of bodyweight. This suggests that lipid metabolism disturbances did not play a significant role in this situation. However, it should be noted that from 1991 to 1995 sales of foodstuffs such as butter, meat, chocolate, and other cholesterol-rich products have decreased by 21% and that the average nutritional value of the Russian diet represented 2,293 Kcal.

One explanation for the changes in the levels of heart disease and blood pressure may be that the levels of psychoemotional tension as well as "stress" have radically increased. Studies carried out by the Research Center for Preventive Medicine in 3,000 male and female Moscow residents have demonstrated rapid growth in psychoemotional tension (according to the L. Reeder et al. scale). L. Reeder's scale introduced in 1969 is based on the questionnaire which estimates the degree of tension. In 1989 the level of stress in the studied population group was 1.40, according to the above-mentioned scale, and has rapidly risen during the complicated economical and political situation in 1992 [2]. During this period the stress level increased to 1.59. The most distinct changes were detected in people over forty years old, as well as those individuals with elevated arterial blood pressure. It is well known that the lability of the central mechanisms of vascular regulation is a characteristic feature of these two groups.

Levels of vitality and depression were also studied. Material and spiritual instability, high levels of unemployment (which according to official statistics accounts for 8.2% of the active population), concerns for individual safety and high levels of crime, uncertainty, and destruction of traditional values have led to a considerable loss of vitality [3]. This parameter for the past four years has increased from 9.96 to 12.33. It should be noted that in those countries of Eastern Europe where the political and economic situation was stable or improved, the death rate from cardiovascular diseases has declined. For example, in the Republic of Chekhia, the death rate from cardiovascular disease has decreased from 145.7 deaths per 100,000 in 1990 to 120.9 per 100,000 in 1993 and in Poland, the rate has fallen from 157.4 per 100,000 in 1990 to 142.4 per 100,000 in 1993.

While analyzing the state of cardiovascular morbidity and mortality, the quality of health care delivery, prevention, and patient monitoring in particular should be taken in account, although assessment of the data obtained in regions with different levels of health care delivery demonstrated an insignificant influence on the mortality rate. The key factor affecting cardiovascular morbidity and mortality is played by socio-economics and the resultant levels of psychoemotional tension and "stress."

References

1. The Demographic Yearbook of Russia. Statistical Yearbook. Goscomstat of Russia. Moscow, Russia. 1995.
2. Gundarov A. Why are people dying in Russia, how can we survive? (Facts and arguments). Media Sphere Publishing House: Moscow, 1995: 1,7,9,13,41,45.
3. Towards healthy Russia. The State Research Center for Preventive Medicine. Moscow. 1994: 37-38.

D.A. Wood on behalf of the EUROASPIRE Study Group[1]

Introduction

Coronary heart disease (CHD) mortality is increasing in a number of central and eastern European countries, remains unchanged in other parts of Europe, and in some countries has declined significantly over recent decades [1]. CHD remains the leading cause of mortality in men over 45 years old and in women over 65 years old throughout Europe. In addition, CHD causes substantial morbidity and premature disability and is a major burden on the cardiological, medical, and social services of all European countries.

In the Joint European Societies recommendations on the prevention of CHD in clinical practice, published in the *European Heart Journal* in 1994, preventive strategies were reviewed [2]. A comprehensive CHD prevention policy must include three components:

1. A population strategy: for altering, in the entire population, those lifestyle and environmental factors, and their social and economic determinants, that are the underlying causes of the mass occurrence of CHD;
2. A high risk strategy: identification of high risk individuals, and action to reduce their risk factor levels; and
3. Secondary prevention: prevention of recurrent CHD events and progression of the disease in patients with clinically established CHD.

In Europe the number of patients with established CHD is large and the number of healthy individuals at high risk of developing the disease is huge. Therefore, it is useful to define priorities for CHD prevention in clinical practice and these are set out in Table 1. The highest priority is given to patients with clinically established CHD, or other atherosclerotic vascular disease, and secondly to asymptomatic subjects with particularly high risk factors levels, or with a cluster of several risk factors which puts them at high risk. The closest relatives of patients with early onset CHD and other individuals follow as priorities for

---

[1]G. Ambrosio (Italy), P. Amouyel (France), D. De Bacquer (Belgium), G. De Backer (Belgium), J. Deckers (The Netherlands), I. Graham (Ireland), F. Gutzwiller (Switzerland), U. Keil (Germany), E. Östör (Hungary), K. Pyörälä (Finland), S. Sans (Spain), J. Simon (Czech Republic), J. Turk (Slovenia)

A. M. Gotto, Jr. et al. (eds.), Multiple Risk Factors in Cardiovascular Disease, 109–117.

action.

Table 1. Joint European Societies[+] Priorities of Coronary Heart Disease Prevention in Clinical Practice

---

1.   Patients with established CHD or other atherosclerotic vascular disease;
2.   Asymptomatic subjects with particularly high risk (subjects with severe hypercholesterolemia or other forms of dyslipidemia, diabetes or hypertension, and subjects with a cluster of several risk factors);
3.   Close relatives of patients with early-onset CHD or other atherosclerotic vascular disease and asymptomatic subjects with particularly high risk;
4.   Other individuals met in connection with ordinary clinical practice.

[+] European Societies of Cardiology, Atherosclerosis, and Hypertension (ESC, EAS, ESH)

As secondary prevention was made the highest priority, the ESC decided to define the current status of preventive action in patients with CHD in Europe and thus ascertain the potential for secondary prevention. In the United Kingdom, a survey assessing risk factor recording and management as part of the ordinary care of CHD patients—ASPIRE (Action on Secondary Prevention through Intervention to Reduce Events)—was carried out in 1994-1995 at the initiative of the British Cardiac Society [3]. The ASPIRE survey laid the foundation for EUROASPIRE (European Action on Secondary Prevention through Intervention to Reduce Events) which was conducted in nine European countries: Czech Republic, Finland, France, Germany, Hungary, Italy, The Netherlands, Slovenia, and Spain in 1995-1996 [4].

AIMS OF EUROASPIRE

The specific aims of EUROASPIRE were:
1.   To determine whether the major high risk factors for CHD (cigarette smoking, obesity, blood pressure, cholesterol, diabetes, and family history of CHD) and their management are identified and recorded in patients medical records;
2.   To interview patients at least six months after hospitalization for a coronary event (coronary artery bypass grafting [CABG], percutaneous transluminal coronary angioplasty [PTCA], acute myocardial infarction [MI] or acute myocardial ischemia without infarction) and measure the modifiable risk factors (current smoking habit, obesity, blood pressure, and plasma lipids) and describe their management in terms of lifestyle (smoking, diet, and exercise) and drug therapy; and
3.   To determine whether family members (first-degree blood relatives) have been screened, where appropriate, for CHD risk factors.

STUDY POPULATION AND METHODS

Within each country one geographical arca was selected and all hospitals serving that population identified. The area included at least one hospital offering interventional cardiology and cardiac surgery, and one or more acute hospitals receiving patients with acute MI and ischemia. A sample of hospitals (or all hospitals) was taken so that any patient presenting within the area with acute symptoms of CHD, or requiring revascularization in the form of angioplasty or coronary artery surgery, had an approximately equal chance of being included in the patient sample.

Within each hospital, consecutive male or female patients ($\leq$ 70 years) were identified retrospectively from the following diagnostic groups: CABG, PTCA, acute MI (ICD-9 410) and acute myocardial ischemia without evidence of infarction (ICD-9 411, 413). Data collection was conducted in two stages: 1) a retrospective review of hospital medical records; and 2) an interview and examination of the patients at least 6 months or more after the hospital admission.

As the results from the United Kingdom survey have already been published this report covers the results from the other nine European countries.

RESULTS

Four thousand eight hundred sixty-three patients' records were reviewed of which 1,201 (25%) were women. Patient interviews were conducted on 3,569 (73%) of the patients and after allowing for deaths and losses to follow up, the adjusted overall response rate to interview was 85%.

At the time of the hospital admission, the prevalence of risk factors recorded in medical records was as follows:
- 34% of patients were smoking cigarettes;
- 18% were obese with a body mass index > 30 kg/m^2;
- 58% had raised blood pressure (SBP $\geq$ 140 mmHg and/or DBP $\geq$ 90 mmHg and/or on antihypertensive medication);
- 71% had a raised plasma cholesterol (total cholesterol $\geq$ 5.5 mmol/l and/or on lipid lowering medication); and
- 22% had diabetes mellitus.

At the follow-up interview the prevalence of current smoking (validated by a breath carbon monoxide concentration greater than 10 ppm), raised blood pressure, and raised plasma cholesterol by European center are shown in Figures 1-3. Overall, 21% of men and 14% of women were smoking cigarettes at interview; the prevalence for all patients was 19%. Fifty-three percent had raised blood pressure and in 7.5% this was severe. In patients using blood pressure lowering drugs (and here all drugs that lower blood pressure are included) only half had reached the therapeutic target of a systolic blood pressure less than 140 mmHg. Forty-four percent of patients had a raised plasma cholesterol and in 14% this was severe. Of the minority (36%) on lipid lowering medication, 13% had a total cholesterol less than 4.5 mmol/l, 52% less than 5.5 mmol/l, and 83% less than 6.5 mmol/l.

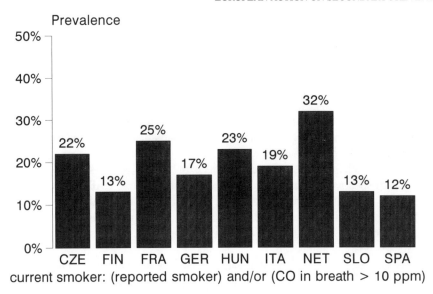

Figure 1. Prevalence of current smoking by European center. Current smoker: (reported smoker) and/or (CO in breath > 10 ppm).

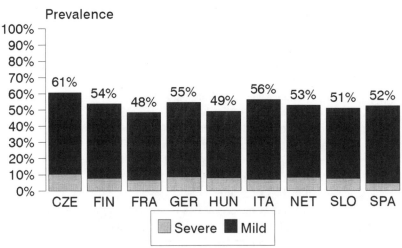

mild hypertension: (140 mmHg ≤ SBP < 180 mmHg) and/or (90 mmHg ≤ DBP < 105 mmHg)
severe hypertension: (SBP ≥ 180 mmHg) and/or (DBP ≥ 105 mmHg)

Figure 2. Prevalence of raised blood pressure by European center. Raised blood pressure: moderate 140 mmHg ≤ SBP < 180 mmHg and/or 90 mmHg ≤ DBP < 105 mmHg; severe SBP ≥ 180 mmHg and/or DBP ≥ 105 mmHg.

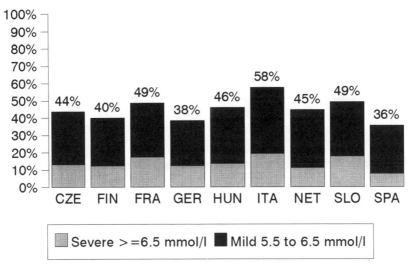

Figure 3. Prevalence of raised plasma cholesterol by European center. Raised plasma cholesterol: moderate 5.5 mmol/l < total cholesterol, 6.5 mmol/l; severe total cholesterol > 6.5 mmol/l.

The prevalence of reported medication at interview by European centers is given in Table 2 for those classes of drugs which have been shown in single trials or meta-analysis to reduce total mortality.

21% of patients had received advice to have first-degree blood relatives screened for coronary risk factors.

Discussion

This nine-country European survey demonstrates a high prevalence of modifiable coronary risk factors in patients with established heart disease, a result consistent with the UK ASPIRE survey. A real clinical potential therefore exists for specialist and general practitioners to further reduce CHD morbidity and mortality and also to improve life expectancy.

Although current cigarette smoking had fallen from the time of hospitalization, almost one-fifth of the patients were smoking cigarettes at follow up. The background prevalence of smoking in each country partly explains the threefold difference in smoking prevalence between centers, and also the substantially lower exposure to cigarettes in women compared to men in most countries. Smokers who continue the habit following unstable angina or MI have up to a fivefold greater all cause mortality and fatal reinfarction compared with those who stop smoking, and this excess risk is likely to apply to patients who continue to smoke following revascularization [5]. Long-term follow up shows the benefits of giving up smoking in patients with acute ischemic syndromes. Personal advice and encouragement to stop smoking given by a physician during a single routine consultation is effective, particularly in CHD patients.

Table 2. Reported Medication at Interview by European Center

	Anti-platelets	Beta-Blockers	ACE Inhibitors	Lipid Lowering	Anti-coagulants
CZE	85%	65%	28%	29%	4%
FIN	82%	78%	17%	39%	7%
FRA	82%	56%	34%	42%	6%
GER	83%	44%	31%	35%	6%
HUN	72%	58%	46%	22%	14%
ITA	86%	49%	32%	25%	3%
NET	78%	47%	27%	8%	12%
SLO	80%	52%	31%	30%	6%
SPA	84%	35%	18%	30%	7%
Total	81%	54%	29%	32%	7%

With increasing obesity all cause mortality increases, largely due to an increase in cardiovascular mortality [6]. Obesity adversely influences other risk factors, including blood pressure, plasma low density lipoprotein (LDL) cholesterol, high density lipoprotein (HDL) cholesterol, triglycerides, and glucose tolerance. As about a quarter of all patients were obese at interview there is potential to reduce the prevalence of obesity and associated risk factors. For CHD patients who are overweight, the lipid lowering diet (reduction in total dietary intake of fat to 30% or less of total energy intake, the intake of saturated fat to no more than one-third of total fat intake, and the intake of cholesterol to less than 300 mg per day) needs to be modified with regard to calorie restriction, and a suitable regular exercise program.

While the relative benefit from blood pressure lowering is the same in those with and without previous myocardial infarction, the absolute benefit is greater in those with established CHD because they are at higher absolute risk. Overall, about half of the patients had raised blood pressure at the time of interview, and 7.5% were severely hypertensive. In those patients receiving blood pressure lowering drugs one-half still had raised blood pressure with a systolic blood pressure > 140 mmHg. Guidelines on the treatment of hypertension in patients with established CHD maintain that blood pressure should be consistently below 140 over 90 mmHg [7].

An even larger proportion of patients had raised blood cholesterol requiring treatment with diet and, where appropriate, drug therapy. The EAS recommendations published prior to this survey had advised that total cholesterol should be reduced to below 5.2 mmol/l in coronary patients [8]. Since the joint ESC/EAS/ESH recommendations were published, the Scandinavian Simvastatin Survival Study (4S) and the Cholesterol and Recurrent Event Study (CARE) have been reported. In 4S, patients with CHD (MI or angina pectoris) with an average total cholesterol of 6.7 mmol/l (> 5.5 mmol/l but < 8.0 mmol/l) on diet and simvastatin had a significantly lower coronary morbidity and mortality and improved survival compared to patients receiving placebo [9]. The results of CARE which tested pravastatin in MI patients with an average total cholesterol of 5.4 mmol/l (< 6.2 mmol/l) on diet confirmed those of 4S in relation to CHD morbidity and mortality, and showed that CHD patients with cholesterol below 5.5 mmol/l also benefit from statin therapy [10]. In CARE the reduction in CHD events was related to the baseline level of LDL cholesterol, and the lower the value the smaller the reduction, if any, in risk. In the lowest quintile of baseline LDL cholesterol distribution (less than 3.3 mmol/l), there was no evidence of benefit with pravastatin. These major trial results will certainly influence existing professional recommendations on lipid lowering, both in terms of the level at which to start treatment and the therapeutic target. Almost one-half of the patients in the EUROASPIRE survey had at interview a total cholesterol > 5.5 mmol/l (the lower limit for cholesterol inclusion criteria for 4S) and one-half of those patients who were receiving lipid lowering drugs still had a cholesterol level > 5.5 mmol/l. So there is considerable potential in CHD patients, through a combination of diet and drug therapy, to reduce the risk of recurrent CHD.

Diabetes substantially increases the risk of recurrent CHD and one-fifth of patients reported a medical diagnosis of diabetes at interview [11]. Diabetes is a particularly strong risk factor in women and markedly diminishes the relative protection of female gender in relation to CHD. Noninsulin dependent (type 2) diabetes, which accounts for the vast majority of diabetic patients in this survey, is associated with profound abnormalities in other cardiovascular risk factors, namely elevated plasma triglycerides and low plasma HDL cholesterol levels, increased prevalence of hypertension, central obesity, and hyperinsulinemia. Although there is no direct trial evidence that good metabolic control of diabetes will decrease the risk of subsequent CHD, this does not preclude the active management of associated risk factors and, in particular, blood pressure and lipid levels.

The use of prophylactic drug therapies [12-15] in CHD patients shows, with one exception, a striking variation between European centers. Aspirin is the exception, with the vast majority of patients reporting that they took this drug (or another antiplatelet agent). All centers used aspirin to a similar extent with the exception of Hungary where only three quarters of patients were taking this form of drug therapy, but this was counterbalanced by a higher use of anticoagulants in that country. In contrast the reported use of beta-blockers shows over a twofold difference between centers despite convincing evidence from controlled trials that early and late beta-blockade postinfarction reduces CHD mortality and improves survival. ACE inhibitors are the next most commonly prescribed group of drugs and there was also considerable variation in reported use by European center, although not as great as seen for beta-blockers. The evidence for ACE inhibitors in those with symptoms or signs of heart failure in the context of myocardial infarction, or with chronic left ventricular systolic dysfunction is more recent than for beta-blockade, but the variation between centers is still surprisingly large. While only a minority of patients are taking anticoagulants, the evidence for this class of drugs is similar to that of other prophylactic drugs in terms of survival, but the widespread use of aspirin, the need for regular monitoring and the risk of significant side effects has all resulted in a more conservative approach to anticoagulant prescribing in the context of CHD.

The variation in use of prophylactic drug therapies between centers is particularly interesting given a common evidence base from randomized controlled trials which has been interpreted differently in clinical practice across Europe. The factors which influence prescribing behavior require investigation as patient management depends not only on evidence from trials, but on how these trials are interpreted and implemented in clinical practice.

About half of the patients had a family history of CHD affecting one or more first-degree blood relatives. Yet two-thirds of patients in this survey said that their family members had not been advised to be screened for coronary risk factors, and this proportion was almost the same for those who had a family history of premature (less than 65 years) CHD. Screening is particularly important in those with a family history of premature CHD, as this group will embrace those with familial hypercholesterolemia, or other forms of inherited dyslipidemia, which deserves specialist investigation and management.

This European survey has shown a high prevalence of modifiable risk factors in CHD patients and therefore real potential to further reduce CHD morbidity and mortality and improve patients chances of survival. If the joint ESC/EAS/ESH recommendations on prevention of CHD in clinical practice were adopted by every cardiologist and physician responsible for cardiac patients then this potential could be achieved in the majority who are able to comply. The clinical return of such vigorous secondary prevention policy is a lower requirement for revascularization procedures, fewer hospitalizations, and lower CHD morbidity and mortality. For the patients this is perceived in terms of a better quality of life and a longer life expectancy.

Acknowledgments

The EUROASPIRE survey was undertaken as part of the initiatives of the Joint ESC/EAS/ESH Implementation Group on Coronary Prevention (Chairman: Professor D A Wood). The EUROASPIRE study group is grateful to all the hospitals at which the study was conducted, their administrative staff, physicians, nurses, and other personnel, as well as to the patients themselves. The EUROASPIRE study was supported by an educational grant made to the European Society of Cardiology by Merck, Sharp and Dohme.

References

1.   Sans S, Kasteloot H, Kromhout D on behalf of the Task Force. The burden of cardiovascular diseases mortality in Europe. Task Force of the European Society of Cardiology on Cardiovascular Mortality and Morbidity Statistics in Europe. Eur Heart J 1997;18:1231-48.

2.   Pyörälä K, De Backer G, Graham I, Poole-Wilson PA, Wood DA, on behalf of the Task Force. Prevention of coronary heart disease in clinical practice. Recommendations of the Task Force of the European Society of Cardiology, European Atherosclerosis Society and European Society of Hypertension. Eur Heart J 1994;15:1300-1331.

3.   Bowker TJ, Clayton TC, Ingham JE, et al. A British Cardiac Society Survey of the Potential for Secondary Prevention of Coronary Diseases - "ASPIRE". Heart 1996;75:334-42.

4.   EUROASPIRE Study Group. EUROASPIRE: A European Society of Cardiology survey of secondary prevention of coronary heart disease: Principal results. Eur Heart J 1997;18(10): 1569-82.

5.   Daly LE, Mulcahy R, Graham IM, Hickey N. Long term effect on mortality of stopping smoking after unstable angina and myocardial infarction. BMJ 1983;287:324-26.

6.   Larsson B. Obesity and body fat distribution as predictors of coronary heart disease. In: Marmot M, Elliot P, editors. Coronary heart disease epidemiology. From aetiology to public health. Oxford: Oxford University Press, 1922:233-41.

7.   The Fifth Report of the Joint National Committee on Detection, Evaluation and Treatment of High Blood Pressure (JNCV). Arch Int Med 1993;153:154-83.

8.   Prevention of coronary heart disease: Scientific background and new guidelines. Recommendations of the European Atherosclerosis Society. Prepared by the International Task Force for Prevention of Coronary Heart Disease. Nutr Metab Cardiovasc Dis 1992;2: 113-56.

9.   Scandinavian Simvastatin Survival Study Group. Randomized trial of cholesterol lowering in 444 patients with coronary heart disease: The Scandinavian Simvastatin Survival Study (4S). Lancet 1994;344:1383-89.

10. Sacks FM, Pfeffer MA, Lemvel Am, et al. The effect of pravastatin on coronary events after myocardial infarction in patients with average cholesterol levels. N Engl J Med 1996;335: 1001-9.

11. Pyörälä K, Laakso M, Uusitupa M. Diabetes and atherosclerosis: An epidemiological view. Diabetes/Metab Rev 1987;3:463-524.

12. Antiplatelet Trialists' Collaboration. Collaborative overview of randomized trials of antiplatelet therapy. I. Prevention of death, myocardial infarction and stroke by prolonged antiplatelet therapy in various categories of patients. BMJ 1994;308:82-105.

13. Yusuf S, Peto R, Lewis J, Collins R, Sleight P. Beta-blockade during and after myocardial infarction: An overview of the randomized trials. Prog Cardiovasc Dis 1985;27:335-71.

14. Lonn EM, Yusuf S, Jha P, et al. Emerging role of angiotensin converting enzyme inhibitors in cardiac and vascular protection. Circulation 1994;90:2056-69.

15. Smith P, Arnesen H, Holme T. The effect of warfarin on mortality and reinfarction after myocardial infarction. N Engl J Med 1990;323:147-52.

CARDIOVASCULAR RISK FACTORS IN NORMOTENSIVE AND HYPERTENSIVE EGYPTIANS: PRELIMINARY RESULTS, EGYPTIAN NATIONAL HYPERTENSION PROJECT (NHP)

M. Mohsen Ibrahim, for the NHP Investigative Team

Introduction

Following eradication of many infectious and parasitic diseases and the sharp decline in infant mortality rate, cardiovascular disease constitutes now the main cause of morbidity and mortality in many third world countries [1,2]. Death secondary to cardiovascular causes have increased more than threefold and they are now responsible for more than 40% of deaths in Egyptians in comparison to reports of 12.4 % two decades earlier [3]. A number of demographic, social, and environmental factors might also contribute to this change in health profile. These include rapid urbanization, inadequate shelter and crowding, increased consumption of junk food, more sedentary life style, and other social stress [4]. It is not known whether these social and demographic changes are associated with higher prevalence rates of the established cardiovascular risk factors such as hypertension, dyslipidemia, obesity, diabetes, and cigarette smoking. Recent data from the Egyptian National Hypertension Project (NHP), the first cross-sectional national survey in a developing country showed that hypertension is very common in Egyptians and constitutes a major health problem [5]. On the other hand, clustering of cardiovascular risk factors has been shown in studies from Western countries to occur in hypertensive patients [6]. It is not known whether this increased cardiovascular risk profile is present in hypertensives living in developing countries with possibly different life styles, dietary habits, and demographic characteristics. Also it is not known whether borderline elevations, or high normal levels of blood pressure are associated with increased prevalence of risk factors. The present study is based upon preliminary data collected during the Egyptian NHP Survey and has three main objectives: first, to identify the prevalence of a number of important cardiovascular risk factors in normotensive and hypertensive Egyptians; secondly, to find the relationship between minimal elevations of blood pressure in the high normal range and the prevalence of risk factors; and finally, to examine the effect of demographic characteristics on risk factor prevalence.

Methods

Data were collected during the Egyptian NHP Survey. The details of the methodology were

119

A. M. Gotto, Jr. et al. (eds.), Multiple Risk Factors in Cardiovascular Disease, 119–129.
© 1998 Kluwer Academic Publishers and Fondazione Giovanni Lorenzini. Printed in the Netherlands.

discussed in previous communications [7,8]. Briefly, the survey was conducted during the period 1991-1994. The sample design was a multistage probability sample of clusters of households in geographically defined areas. The 26 governorates of Egypt were stratified into five strata and governorates were subjectively selected. Twenty-one sampling locations were selected in six Egyptian governorates that represent all Egyptian geographic regions and socioeconomic groups. Field survey consisted of two phases for each governorate. In Phase I, the whole sample in the survey site was interviewed by the data collection staff, filling questionnaire forms that address the demographic variables, socioeconomic characteristics, dietary habits, smoking, parity, and education. Blood pressure was measured four times according to a standardized protocol using a regular mercury sphygmomanometer. Pressure was recorded to the closest 2 mmHg after 5 minutes rest in the sitting position using an appropriate cuff size. Phase II followed Phase I by 1-2 weeks where all hypertensives, i.e. those whose average systolic blood pressure (SBP) $\geq$ 140 mmHg, and/or average diastolic blood pressure (DBP) $\geq$ 90 mmHg, or those receiving antihypertensive medications, were reevaluated together with gender-matched normotensives in specialized local centers for detailed clinical and laboratory investigations. The latter included fundus examination, standard 12-lead electrocardiograms, echocardiographic studies, urine and blood tests, 12-hour urine collection for creatinine, and electrolyte estimation. Blood pressure was measured twice following the same protocol. Weight, height, and waist and hip circumferences were measured. Blood samples were collected after 12 hours of fasting for blood sugar and serum lipids, samples were processed locally, frozen at -30° C and then transported to Cairo for batch analysis. Samples (10 ml blood) were taken in the field free of hemolysis, collected in clean dry tubes with rubber stopper. At the central biochemical laboratory in Cairo, all frozen samples were thawed and then analyzed by a semiautomated autoanalyzer. Twelve cuvettes were run in one tray batch measurement. The first three cuvettes were left for blank, high standard, and low standard; the rest of the 9 cuvettes were used for sample analysis. Reagent (0.7 ml) (according to test performed) was added and put in the analyzer to incubate, mix, and read the results within 3 minutes.

Quality control was done on 5 % of the sample by repeating the analysis by the same operator and on 5% by a different operator in a control-certified laboratory. Calibration was done daily and in each run.

Based upon the average of six arterial pressure (AP) readings measured on two separate occasions, individuals in the sample were classified into the groups: normotensives (NT): average AP readings less than 130/85 mmHg; high normal (HN): AP readings between 130-139/85-89 mmHg; and hypertensives (HT): average AP equal to or greater than 140/90 mmHg.

A total number of 2,313 individuals had detailed clinical and laboratory evaluations. The prevalence of the following risk factors were examined in 1,733 individuals who were not receiving medications: body mass index (BMI: body weight in kg/height in m^2), waist/hip ratio, fasting and 2-hour postprandial blood glucose, current cigarette smoking, total serum cholesterol, high density lipoprotein (HDL) cholesterol, triglycerides, and low density lipoprotein (LDL) cholesterol.

HEIGHT AND WEIGHT

Height was measured to the nearest 0.5 cm. Standard weight was taken in light clothing without shoes using a beam balance to the nearest 0.1 kg.

WAIST AND HIP

Waist girth was measured from the horizontal plane across the minimum girth between the lowest lateral portion of the rib cage and iliac crest. Hip girth was measured at the level of maximal protrusion of the gluteal muscles.

BLOOD SAMPLES

These were obtained between 9:00 and 10:00 A.M. from the antecubital vein after 12 hours of fasting with the subject in the sitting position. Total cholesterol, triglycerides, and HDL cholesterol were measured directly while LDL cholesterol was computed. A second blood sample was collected after ingestion of 75 gm of glucose for blood sugar estimation.

CRITERIA OF THE DIAGNOSIS OF RISK FACTORS

Hypercholesterolemia was considered if serum cholesterol were greater than or equal to 240 mg/dl, low HDL-cholesterol if less than 35 mg/dl, increased LDL-cholesterol if equal to or more than 160 mg/dl. Also noted were serum triglycerides more than 200 mg/dl, obesity by a BMI > 30 kg/m^2, central obesity in presence of waist/hip ratio > 0.85, diabetes mellitus by a fasting blood sugar (FBS) $\geq$ 140 mg/dl, impaired glucose tolerance by a postprandial (75 g of oral glucose) between 140 and 200 mg/dl.

Results

POPULATION CHARACTERISTICS

Table 1 shows the baseline characteristics of the population studied. Hypertensives were one decade older than normotensives, and with higher prevalence in males and lower rates of education. There were no important differences in rural-urban distributions.

PREVALENCE OF CARDIOVASCULAR RISK FACTORS

Table 2 shows the prevalence of risk factors in the three groups. All risk factors with the exception of cigarette smoking and low HDL-cholesterol were more prevalent in hypertensives in comparison to normotensives. Individuals with high normal blood pressure levels have increased prevalence of the majority of risk factors similar to patients with established hypertension. Increased waist/hip ratio and impaired glucose tolerance were less common in this intermediate group and prevalence of obesity was close to normotensive rates.

Table 1. Baseline Characteristics

	NT	HN	HT
N	668	322	743
Age (mean ± SD)	43.4 (12)	48.9 (13)	54.7 (13)
Gender (M/F)	40.3/59.7	46.3/53.7	48.9/51.1
SBP (mmHg)	114.5 (9)	132.4 (6)	153.9 (17)
DBP (mmHg)	72.5 (7)	81.3 (7)	89.4 (11)
Heart Rate (b/m)	79 (11)	82 (12)	84 (13)
Urban/Rural	69.6/30.4	64.3/35.7	65.6/34.4
Low Education (%)*	25.8	13.1	35.1

*Illiterate or just reads and writes

Table 2. Prevalence of CV Factors

	NT	HN	HT
Hypercholesterolemia	8.6	12.4	15.6
Hypertriglyceridemia	10.6	16.8	17.4
Low HDL-C	25.2	25.6	26.4
Increased LDL-C	15.3	23.9	25.4
Obesity	25.3	27.3	35.1
Increased W/H Ratio	23.2	12.6	34.8
Diabetes Mellitus	4.9	8.3	10.8
Impaired Glucose Tolerance	19.6	9.8	46.7
Cigarette Smoking	19.5	22.0	18.2

AGE DISTRIBUTION

Figures 1 to 4 shows the prevalence of some selected risk factors in different age decades in normotensives, high normal, and hypertensive individuals. There was a trend for higher prevalence rates with aging in the risk factors studied. Hypercholesterolemia, hypertriglyceridemia, and obesity were more prevalent in hypertensives in all age groups compared to normotensives. Individuals of high normal blood pressure were similar to hypertensives in older age decades regarding rates of hypercholesterolemia. Prevalence of diabetes mellitus was similar in old age in the three groups (Figure 3) while it was more common in young and middle aged hypertensives.

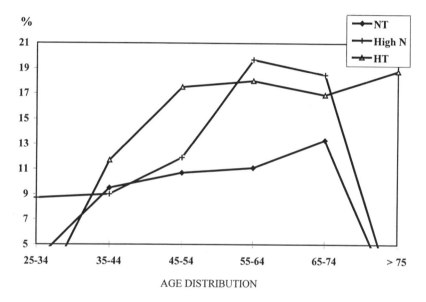

Figure 1. Prevalence of hypercholesterolemia in normotensives (NT), high normal (high N) and hypertensive individuals at different age decades.

GENDER DISTRIBUTION

Table 3 shows the influence of gender on the prevalence of risk factors in the three groups. Hypercholesterolemia, obesity, diabetes mellitus were more prevalent in females than males in all groups, while the reverse was true for hypertriglyceridemia and increased waist to hip ratio. Cigarette smoking was very rare in Egyptian females.

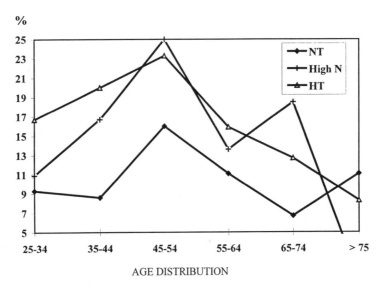

Figure 2. Prevalence of hypertriglyceridemia in normotensives, high normal, and hypertensive individuals at different age decades.

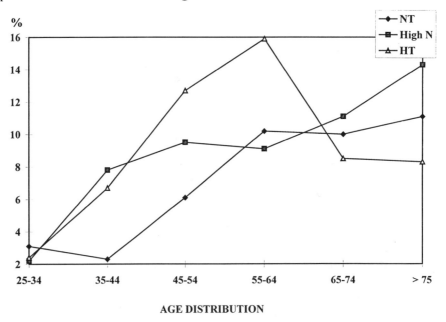

Figure 3. Prevalence of diabetes mellitus in normotensives, high normal, and hypertensive individuals at different age decades.

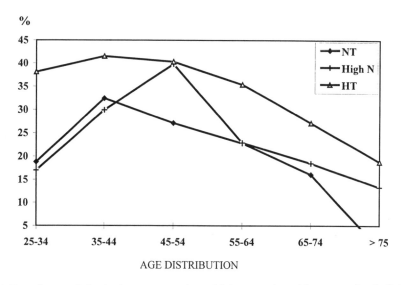

Figure 4. Prevalence of obesity in normotensives, high normal, and hypertensive individuals at different age decades.

Table 3. Prevalence of CV Risk Factors by Gender

	Males			Females		
	NT	HN	HT	NT	HN	HT
Hypercholesterolemia	7.3	8.6	14.2	9.4	18.9	16.9
Hypertriglyceridemia	11.6	19.2	21.6	9.7	14.6	14.3
Low HDL-C	31.6	36.2	31.8	20.7	18.7	20.3
Obesity	14.9	13.7	25.3	32.3	39.8	44.1
Increased W/H Ratio	26.2	15.2	43.1	20.8	10.3	27.9
Diabetes Mellitus	3.1	6.7	9.7	6.1	9.8	11.9
Impaired Glucose Tolerance	2.2	4.4	5.6	3.0	1.9	5.6
Cigarette Smoking	46.1	43.9	35.8	1.5	1.8	1.8

Table 4 compares the prevalence of risk factors in individuals surveyed, classified as young and old.

Table 4. Prevalence of CV Risk Factors by Age

	Young (< 45y)			Old (≥ 45y)		
	NT	HN	HT	NT	HN	HT
Hypercholesterolemia	7.0	8.9	8.6	10.8	14.7	17.6
Hypertriglyceridemia	8.6	14.5	20.2	13.0	18.3	17.1
Obesity	26.5	25.0	41.0	23.5	28.7	33.4
Diabetes Mellitus	2.6	5.7	5.5	8.2	9.9	12.3
Cigarette Smoking	18.1	21.6	16.5	21.5	22.3	18.7
Low HDL-C	23.3	23.6	24.0	27.7	25.4	26.6
Impaired Glucose Tolerance	38.5	7.7	30.8	16.5	10.1	49.4
Increased W/H Ratio	30.9	10.9	17.8	18.2	13.6	45.9

URBAN-RURAL RESIDENCE

Table 5 shows the influence of urban-rural residence on the prevalence of risk factors. In all groups, in general, risk factors were more prevalent in urban compared to rural areas.

Table 5. Prevalence of CV Risk Factors by Residence

	Urban			Rural		
	NT	HN	HT	NT	HN	HT
Hypercholesterolemia	8.7	14.8	18.6	8.2	8.0	9.8
Hypertriglyceridemia	11.2	20.7	19.2	8.8	9.8	15.1
Obesity	31.0	33.7	45.5	11.8	14.3	14.9
Diabetes Mellitus	5.7	10.4	11.8	3.1	4.5	9.0
Cigarette Smoking	20.9	24.9	21.4	16.3	17.1	11.9
Low HDL-C	26.5	32.2	28.9	22.1	16.7	20.3
Impaired Glucose Tolerance	20.8	9.1	45.5	13.3	13.3	53.3
Increased W/H Ratio	24.8	12.0	35.2	20.1	13.6	33.9

Rates of obesity were almost threefold greater in urban than rural areas for the three groups studied.

SERUM LIPID LEVELS, BLOOD SUGAR, AND BODY MASS INDEX

Levels of fasting serum cholesterol, triglycerides, HDL-cholesterol, LDL-cholesterol, blood sugar, and BMI are seen in Table 6. Lipid levels, blood sugar, and BMI were higher in hypertensive and high normal groups compared to normotensive individuals.

Table 6. Serum Lipids, Sugar, BMI, and W/H Ratio

	NT	HN	HT
Cholesterol (mg/dl)	183 (40)	192 (45)	197 (43)
Triglycerides (mg/dl)	129 (69)	145 (75)	155 (83)
HDL-C (mg/dl)	42 (10)	42 (11)	42 (10)
LDL-C (mg/dl)	116 (36)	120 (39)	123 (39)
FBS (mg/dl)	96 (40)	100 (37)	107 (50)
BMI (kg/m^2)	27.6 (6)	28.4 (6)	29.3 (7)
W/H Ratio	0.87 (0.08)	0.89 (0.08)	0.91 (0.08)

Discussion

The results of this cross-sectional survey showed that cardiovascular risk factors were common in urban Egyptians, and with the exception of cigarette smoking they were more prevalent in hypertensives compared to normotensive individuals. Also, the prevalence of risk factors was influenced by gender, age, and urban versus rural residence. The clustering of cardiovascular risk factors in hypertensive patients was previously reported in studies from Western countries [6,9]. The present survey showed that the same pattern was present in developing countries with different demographic, environmental, and dietary habits. Framingham data [6] showed that lipid abnormalities and glucose intolerance were associated with hypertension more often than chance would predict and that this clustering was not entirely attributable to obesity. However, the role of obesity should not be underestimated particularly when looking to differences in risk profiles between urban and rural Egyptians where obesity was almost three times more prevalent in urban areas. All cardiovascular risk factors were more prevalent in urban than rural Egyptians (Table 5) both in normotensives and hypertensives. A positive correlation was reported between the prevalence of obesity and other cardiovascular risk factors [10,11]. A metabolic link in terms of insulin resistance was described between noninsulin dependent diabetes mellitus, obesity, hypertension, and dyslipidemia [12]. Insulin resistance also characterizes the aging process [12]. Aging was associated with increasing prevalence of risk factors and hypertension [5]. The older age in our hypertensive patients might explain some of the differences in risk profile between normotensives and hypertensives, however, the higher prevalence rates of risk factors in hypertensives were present in all age groups in comparison to normotensives (Figures 1-4). This together with the double prevalence rates of diabetes mellitus and impaired glucose tolerance imply that aging was not the only factor responsible for the very high rates in hypertensives. An important finding in this study was the increased prevalence of risk factors in individuals with high normal blood pressure approaching rates similar to those in patients with established hypertension. This clustering of risk factors in individuals with minimal elevations of blood pressure has practical implications. The higher morbidity and mortality rates associated with mild hypertension [13,14] is not only due to elevation of blood pressure, but also secondary to the associated risk factors. It seems that the trend in increased risk is blood pressure related with no clear definition between hypertensives and normotensives, i.e. the lower the blood pressure, the lesser the associated cardiovascular risk factors. Hypertensive patients, even those with mild elevations of blood pressure should be routinely screened for the presence of other risk factors. This might limit the need to pharmacologic therapy in patients with mild hypertension and low cardiovascular risk profile. Risk factors other than hypertension strongly condition the degree of hazard imposed by blood pressure level. There are suggestions that some patients with mild hypertension have cardiovascular risk low enough that they can safely be spared antihypertensive drug treatment [15,16]. On the other hand, aggressive treatment of hypertension might be needed in patients with mild elevations and associated risk factors.

The gender differences in cardiovascular risk profile factors in our survey was reported in studies from Western countries [17]. Obesity was very common in Egyptian women specially the hypertensive group (44.1 %, Table 4), and this was associated with higher prevalence rates of hypercholesterolemia and diabetes mellitus. Hypertriglyceridemia, low HDL-cholesterol and increase in waist/hip ratio were less common in women compared to men. Cigarette smoking was very rare in Egyptian women both normotensive and hypertensive. On the other hand, smoking was more common in normotensive than hypertensive men (46.1 % versus 35.8 %).

The present study has a number of special features. First, it is one of the few studies examining the prevalence of cardiovascular risk factors in a developing country that followed rigorous quality controlled measures, including a relatively large sample representing all geographic regions, socioeconomic groups over a wide age spectrum. Secondly, effect of antihypertensive medications on risk profile was eliminated by including only individuals not receiving medications. Thirdly, the large number of blood pressure measurements (six) over two occasions in an epidemiologic survey could reliably classify individuals in the three groups studied. Fourthly, the identification of a high normal group as a special entity with increased cardiovascular risk was an original finding and needs further investigation.

References

1. Dodu SRA. Emergency of cardiovascular disease in developing countries. Cardiology 1988; 75:56-64.
2. Murray CJL, Lopez AD. Global and regional cause of death pattern in 1990. Bull WHO 1994; 72:447-80.
3. The Central Agency for Public Mobilization and Statistics (CAPMAS). The annual health report of the year 1990. Cairo, Egypt:CAPMAS;1990.
4. Omran AR. The epidemiological transition - a theory of the epidemiology of population change. Milbank Memorial Fund Q 1971;4:509-38.
5. Ibrahim MM, Rizk H, Appel LJ, et al. Hypertension, Prevalence, Awareness, Treatment and Control in Egypt. Hypertension 1995;26:886-90.
6. Kannel W. Blood pressure as a cardiovascular risk factor: Prevention and treatment. JAMA 1996;275:1571-76.
7. Ashour Z, Ibrahim MM, Appel LJ, Ibrahim AS, Whelton PK, for the Investigative Team. The Egyptian National Hypertension Project (NHP). Design and Rationale. Hypertension 1995;26: 880-85.
8. Ibrahim MM. The Egyptian National Hypertension Project (NHP): Preliminary results. J Human Hypertension 1996;10:539-41.
9. Defranzo RA, Ferrannini E. Insulin resistance: A multifacted syndrome responsible for NIDDM, obesity, hypertension, dyslipidemia and other atherosclerotic cardiovascular disease. Diabetes Care 1991;14:173-94.
10. Modan M, Afkin H, Almay S. Hyperinsulinemia: A link between hypertension, obesity and glucose intolerance. J Clin Invest 1985;75:809-17.
11. Folsom AR, Kaye SA, Sellers TA, et al. Body fat distribution and 5 year risk of death in older women. JAMA 1993;269:483-87.
12. DeFronzo RA. Insulin resistance: the metabolic link between noninsulin-dependent diabetes mellitus, obesity, hypertension, dyslipidemia and atherosclerotic cardiovascular disease. Current Opinion in Cardiology 1990;5:586-93.
13. Relmon AS. Mild hypertension: No more benign neglect. N Engl J Med 1980;302:293-94.
14. Moser M, Gifford RW. Why less severe degrees of hypertension should be treated. J Hypertens 1985;3:437-47.
15. Freis ED. Should mild hypertension be treated? N Engl J Med 1982;307:306-9.
16. McAlister NH. Should we treat mild hypertension? JAMA 1983;249:379-82.
17. Wenger NK. Hypertension and other cardiovascular risk factors in women. Am J Hypertens 1995;8:945-95.

LIPID DEPOSITION AND OXIDATION IN THE EVOLUTION OF THE ATHEROSCLEROTIC LESION: LESSONS LEARNED FROM HYPERCHOLESTEROLEMIC ANIMAL MODELS

Michael E. Rosenfeld

Introduction

A focus of this symposium is the potential of multifactorial approaches to managing simultaneous risk factors for prevention of atherosclerosis. In keeping with this theme, this chapter discusses how hyperlipidemia-induced increases in the deposition of lipid within the artery wall, coupled with oxidative processes occurring within the artery may play important causative roles in the pathogenesis of atherosclerosis. The data suggest that combined hypolipidemic and antioxidant therapy may be most effective in the prevention of atherosclerosis in many high risk individuals.

As we do not yet have adequate quantitative measures of oxidative activity within the artery wall, it is still currently unknown whether excessive oxidative activity could be considered as a positive risk factor for cardiovascular disease. Readily accessible markers of oxidation in the plasma have not definitively established oxidative processes as risk factors. For example, because there are reports of both positive and negative associations, it is still controversial as to whether plasma lipid peroxides, the susceptibility of plasma lipoproteins to *in vitro* oxidation, or high titers of autoantibodies which recognize oxidized low density lipoprotein (LDL), can be used as markers of the severity of cardiovascular disease [1-15]. Furthermore, to date, there have been very few clinical studies of the long-term effects of combined hypolipidemic and antioxidant therapy [16-19] and none that have attempted this intervention in high risk younger adults [20].

In contrast to the lack of clinical data, recent studies of hypercholesterolemic rabbits, monkeys, and genetically engineered mice have shown that the deposition of lipid in the artery wall is accompanied by formation of oxidation products [21-23] and that both occur at each stage in the evolution of atherosclerotic lesions from fatty streaks to advanced plaques [21]. Additional studies have demonstrated that a variety of different antioxidants are inhibitory of atherosclerotic lesion initiation and progression in these same animal models [22, 24-35]. Based on the experimental data, the simultaneous administration of hypolipidemic agents and both fat- and water-soluble antioxidants to younger, high risk individuals may be warranted and could prove to be a more effective treatment for preventing both the initiation and progression of atherosclerotic lesions than hypolipidemic agents alone.

A. M. Gotto, Jr. et al. (eds.), Multiple Risk Factors in Cardiovascular Disease, 131–140.

The Potential Role of Lipid Deposition and Oxidation in the Initiation of the Atherogenic Process

The trapping and retention of lipoproteins within the extracellular matrix of arteries at lesion prone sites is the first measurable event in the atherogenic process. The seminal studies of Scwenke and Carew [36,37] elegantly demonstrated that within days of initiating hypercholesterolemia in rabbits, there was a specific increase in the concentration of LDL particles that accumulated at sites within the aorta that are known to later develop atherosclerotic lesions. These studies clearly showed that the increase in the concentration of LDL at these sites was not due to an increase in endothelial permeability, but was due to the retention or trapping of the particles within the artery wall. We subsequently showed that this process continues in young rabbits already exhibiting very early fatty streaks [38]. Using electron microscopic autoradiography and LDL particles labeled with a nondegradable, radioiodinated probe, we observed that a significant percentage of the particles were associated with the extracellular matrix (Figure 1). Additional high resolution, freeze-fracture, electron microscopic studies have further demonstrated the presence of aggregates of lipoproteins within the extracellular matrix of the artery [39].

Trapping of lipoproteins within the extracellular matrix increases the retention time within the artery wall allowing the particles to undergo either a spontaneous or cell-mediated oxidative modification. Numerous *in vitro* studies have attempted to elucidate the mechanism(s) by which lipoproteins become oxidized and several excellent reviews of these studies have recently been published [40-44]. But, it is still unclear how and to what extent lipoproteins become oxidized *in vivo*.

Following the development of antibodies which specifically recognize epitopes characteristic of oxidized LDL, we and others demonstrated the presence of these oxidation products within developing atherosclerotic lesions [21,23,45-47]. Our studies showed that there was extensive oxidation product associated primarily with macrophages at all stages in the atherogenic process in rabbits [21]. Similar observations have recently been made in early lesions in the apoE-deficient mouse [23].

It is currently thought that the presence of oxidized lipoprotein particles within the matrix induces a chronic inflammatory response. Oxidized LDL activates endothelial cells *in vitro* to express leukocyte specific adhesion molecules and secrete potent leukocyte chemotactic proteins [48-50]. Furthermore, oxidized LDL is itself a chemoattractant for both monocytes and lymphocytes [51,52]. Once situated within the body of the artery, monocytes mature into tissue macrophages which rapidly become transformed into lipid engorged foam cells. This transformation into foam cells is likely a result of the maturation dependent expression of a family of scavenger receptors which enable the cells to perform their normal function of removing toxic debris from their surroundings [53]. Thus, the presence of lipid oxidation products within the intima appears to be the prerequisite for the formation of the early fatty streak which is composed largely of macrophage-derived foam cells [54]. The essential role of oxidation processes in the induction of the fatty streak is strongly supported by all of the experimental studies showing a reduction in fatty streaks in antioxidant treated rabbits, monkeys, and mice [22,24-35]. In addition, several studies of the effects of chronic probucol treatment have demonstrated a significant reduction in the number of macrophage-derived foam cells in the lesions as a result of the antioxidant therapy [34,55,56].

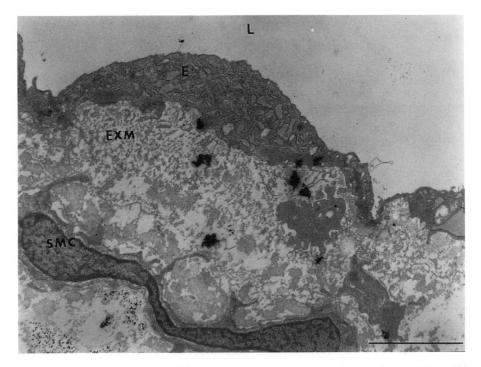

Figure 1. Trapping of LDL in the extracellular matrix in the aorta of a WHHL rabbit. Young, WHHL rabbits were injected with a bolus of autologous LDL that was labeled with the non-degradable iodinated probe, ^{125}I-tyramine-cellobiose-LDL. After 48 hours, the animals were sacrificed and the arteries were dissected out and processed for electron microscopic autoradiography. This figure demonstrates the localization of silver grains (black squiggles) representative of the distribution of LDL particles in the extracellular matrix of an early fatty streak in the aorta of a 4 month old WHHL rabbit. Bar = 1 uM. EXM = extracellular matrix, EC = endothelial cell, L – lumen, SMC = smooth muscle cells.

The Potential Role of Lipid Deposition and Oxidation in the Transition of the Fatty Streak to an Atheroma

The hallmarks of the transition from an early lesion to a more advanced plaque are the formation of an atheromatous necrotic core and a fibrous cap [57]. Currently it is believed that the lipid component of the necrotic core is derived from the coalescence of cellular lipid released following the apoptotic and/or necrotic death of macrophage-derived foam cells coupled with the continuous direct deposition and aggregation of lipoprotein particles [58].

As noted previously, we showed that macrophage-derived foam cells situated throughout the lesion and at all stages of lesion development contain oxidation products. We also observed immunoreactive oxidation products associated with extracellular lipids within the necrotic core [21]. Evidence suggests that accumulation of these oxidation products may be the ultimate cause of the death of foam cells. For example, *in vitro* studies have shown that accumulation of excess oxidized LDL can be cytotoxic to cells [59].

Fragmentation of cellular DNA can occur during a pro-oxidant-induced apoptotic or necrotic cell death. We have observed that macrophages which contain oxidation products and are situated adjacent to a developing necrotic core in rabbit lesions exhibit a significant amount of DNA fragmentation (Figure 2). Furthermore, in preliminary studies we have observed that macrophage-derived foam cells isolated from atherosclerotic lesions in rabbits contain a much higher content of oxidized lipids and exhibit a higher degree of DNA fragmentation than macrophages isolated simultaneously from other tissues in the same animals. We have also observed that chronic treatment of hypercholesterolemic rabbits with probucol reduces the number of cells containing fragmented DNA in lesions throughout the aorta (data not shown).

The formation of the fibrous cap involves smooth muscle cell migration, proliferation, and connective tissue synthesis. It is still unclear as to what role lipid deposition and oxidation play in stimulating this smooth muscle cell behavior. However, recent studies have shown that oxidized LDL (and in particular the lysophosphatidylcholine derived from oxidized LDL) are mitogenic for both smooth muscle cells and macrophages [60-62]. It is now thought that the particles induce proliferation by directly activating signal transduction pathways involving mitogen-activated protein kinases [62].

The Potential Role of Lipid Deposition and Oxidation in Plaque Destablization

Advanced atherosclerotic lesions do not compromise blood flow in an artery unless there is a failure of the artery to undergo compensatory remodeling and/or the plaque ruptures causing the formation of an occlusive thrombus. Compensatory remodeling is a process whereby the medial layer of the artery enlarges in an attempt to maintain normal lumen size [63]. It is currently unknown precisely how the media enlarges, but accumulating evidence suggests that the process may involve expansion of the internal elastic lamina and chronic dilation [64]. The deposition and oxidation of lipid may play a role in inhibiting this compensatory remodeling. We have observed that in stenotic lesions in the carotid arteries of apoE-deficient mice there is a strong positive correlation between the degree of stenosis and thinning of the underlying media. We have also observed a high degree of adventitial inflammation in these stenotic arteries. Upon close inspection of the lesions, we further observed that the vast majority of these stenotic lesions also had accumulations of cholesterol clefts and lipid engorged smooth muscle cells situated along the internal elastic lamina and within the media. The thickness of the media was significantly reduced primarily where there were deposits of cholesterol clefts along the internal elastic lamina. Palinski et al. [23] have demonstrated the presence of oxidation products associated with these cholesterol clefts in atherosclerotic lesions in the apoE-deficient mouse. Thus, it is likely

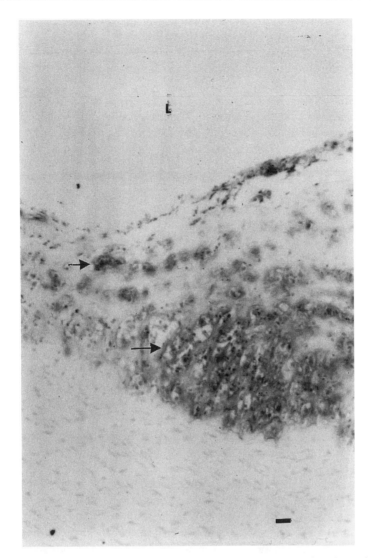

Figure 2. DNA fragmentation in foam cells in an atherosclerotic lesion from the aorta of a WHHL rabbit. Sections of aorta were incubated in the presence of biotin-labeled UTP and terminal deoxynucleotide transferase (TDT) followed by avidin-labeled alkaline phosphatase. The color reaction for alkaline phosphatase activity (arrows) is representative of those cells containing fragmented DNA and where the biotin-labeled UTP was incorporated into the DNA during repair by TDT. This figure shows the large number of macrophages situated within the lateral margin, adjacent to a developing necrotic core, of an atherosclerotic lesion in the thoracic aorta of a 12-month-old WHHL rabbit. Bar = 10 uM. L = lumen

that this lipid deposition and oxidation both attracts inflammatory cells into the adventitia and may compromise the capacity of the media to dilate by contributing to the apoptotic and/or necrotic death of medial smooth muscle cells. The death of smooth muscle cells could account for the observed thinning of the media in areas containing extracellular lipid deposits.

The rupture of plaques with formation of occlusive thrombi are the underlying cause of clinical events such as unstable angina and myocardial infarction. Recent studies of autopsy material from individuals dying of myocardial infarction have demonstrated that the plaques which rupture are generally not more than 50% stenotic, are rich in lipid and inflammatory cells, and most frequently rupture along the lateral margins where the fibrous cap is the thinnest. In most cases, the thinning of the fibrous cap occurs over the areas of the lesion which are most enriched with inflammatory cells and deposits of extracellular lipid, for example where the necrotic core encroaches on the fibrous cap [65]. Again, these areas also appear to contain the largest concentrations of cells exhibiting fragmented DNA (Figure 2) [66] and suggests that lipid accumulation and oxidation may be responsible for the death of cells in areas where plaques rupture. Thus, the thinning of the fibrous cap may be a response to the toxic effects of lipid deposition and analogous to what may induce the thinning of the media and the failure of compensatory remodeling in the apoE-deficient mouse.

Finally, inflammatory activation of macrophages by oxidized lipids leading to an increase in the expression and secretion of pro-apoptotic cytokines and proteolytic enzymes may be another mechanism by which the structural integrity of the plaque becomes compromised. Recent studies have demonstrated the expression of biologically active metalloproteinases by macrophages within the lateral margins of advanced plaques [67].

In summary, it is now clear from numerous animal studies that under conditions of chronic hyperlipidemia, lipid deposition within the artery wall is a continuous process occurring at all stages in the development of atherosclerotic lesions. Furthermore, the evidence is now quite compelling that lipid deposition is accompanied by the formation of lipid-derived oxidation products. The initial formation of these oxidation products induces an inflammatory response leading to the establishment of the fatty streak. The unregulated accumulation of oxidation products can be cytotoxic and may cause foam cell death. The release of lipid from dead cells coupled with continued influx of lipoproteins contribute to the formation of the necrotic core. Excessive lipid deposition and cell death may also contribute to the loss of compensatory remodeling leading to the formation of stenotic lesions and to the destabilization and rupture of plaques. Thus, the evidence suggests that the chronic administration of the combination of hypolipidemic agents and antioxidants should be extremely effective in preventing the formation and inhibiting the progression of atherosclerotic lesions and thus, may constitute an important multifactorial approach to reducing cardiovascular disease.

References

1.   Sanderson KJ, van Rij AM, Wade CR, Sutherland WH. Lipid peroxidation of circulating low

density lipoproteins with age, smoking and in peripheral vascular disease. Atherosclerosis 1995;118:45-51.

2.   Belch JJ, Mackay IR, Hill A, Jennings P, McCollum P. Oxidative stress is present in atherosclerotic peripheral arterial disease and further increased by diabetes mellitus. Int Angiol 1995;14:385-88.

3.   Joensuu T, Salonen R, Winblad, I, Korpela H, Salonen JT. Determinants of femoral and carotid artery atherosclerosis. J Intern Med 1994;236:79-84.

4.   Plachta H, Bartnikowska E, Obara A. Lipid peroxides in blood from patients with atherosclerosis of coronary and peripheral arteries. Clin Chim Acta 1992;211:101-12.

5.   Vel'azquez E, Winocour PH, Kesteven P, Alberti KG, Laker MF. Relation of lipid peroxides to macrovascular disease in type 2 diabetes. Diabet Med 1991;8:752-58.

6.   Stringer MD, Kakkar VV. Markers of disease severity in peripheral atherosclerosis. Eur J Vasc Surg 1990;4:513-18.

7.   Maggi E, Chiesa R, Melissano G, et al. LDL oxidation in patients with severe carotid atherosclerosis. A study of in vitro and in vivo oxidation markers. Arterioscler Thromb 1994; 14:1892-99.

8.   Kanazawa T, Osanai T, Yin XZ, Yi HZ, Onodera K, Metoki H. Peroxidized low-density lipoprotein with four kinds of hydroperoxidized cholesteryl linoleate estimated in plasma of young heavy smokers. Pathobiology 1996;64:115-22.

9.   Schreier LE, Sanguinetti S, Mosso H, Lopez GI, Siri L, Wikinski RL. Low-density lipoprotein composition and oxidability in atherosclerotic cardiovascular disease. Clin Biochem 1996;29:479-87.

10.   De Rijke YB, Verwey HF, Vogelezang CJ, et al. Enhanced susceptibility of low-density lipoproteins to oxidation in coronary bypass patients with progression of atherosclerosis. Clin Chim Acta 1995;243:137-49.

11.   Andrews B, Burnand K, Paganga G, et al. Oxidisability of low density lipoproteins in patients with carotid or femoral artery atherosclerosis. Atherosclerosis 1995;112:77-84.

12.   Marchesi E, Martignoni A, Salvini M, et al. Carotid intima-media thickening and in vivo LDL oxidation in patients with essential hypertension. J Hum Hypertens 1996;10:577-82.

13.   Palinski W, Tangirala RK, Miller E, Young SG, Witztum JL. Increased autoantibody titers against epitopes of oxidized LDL in LDL receptor-deficient mice with increased atherosclerosis. Arterioscler Thromb Vasc Biol 1995;15:1569-76.

14.   Maggi E, Marchesi E, Ravetta V, Martignoni A, Finardi G, Bellomo G. Presence of autoantibodies against oxidatively modified low-density lipoprotein in essential hypertension: A biochemical signature of an enhanced in vivo low-density lipoprotein oxidation. J Hypertens 1995;13:129-38.

15.   Uusitupa MI, Niskanen L, Luoma J, et al. Autoantibodies against oxidized LDL do not predict atherosclerotic vascular disease in non-insulin-dependent diabetes mellitus. Arterioscler Thromb Vasc Biol 1996;16:1236-42.

16.   Walldius G, Regnstrom J, Nilsson J, et al. The role of lipids and antioxidative factors for development of atherosclerosis. The Probucol Quantitative Regression Swedish Trial (PQRST). Am J Cardiol 1993;71:15B-19B.

17.   Walldius G, Erikson U, Olsson AG, et-al. The effect of probucol on femoral atherosclerosis: The Probucol Quantitative Regression Swedish Trial (PQRST). Am J Cardiol 1994;74:875-83.

18.   Kritchevsky SB, Shimakawa T, Tell GS, et al. Dietary antioxidants and carotid artery wall thickness. The ARIC Study. Atherosclerosis Risk in Communities Study. Circulation 1995;92:

2142-50.

19.   Azen SP, Qian D, Mack WJ, et al. Effect of supplementary antioxidant vitamin intake on carotid arterial wall intima-media thickness in a controlled clinical trial of cholesterol lowering. Circulation 1996;94:2369-72.

20.   Steinberg D. Clinical trials of antioxidants in atherosclerosis: Are we doing the right thing? Lancet 1995;346:36-38.

21.   Rosenfeld M, Palinski W, Ylä-Herttuala S, Butler S, Witztum JL. Distribution of oxidation specific lipid-protein adducts and apolipoprotein B in atherosclerotic lesions of varying severity from WHHL rabbits. Arteriosclerosis 1990;10:336-49.

22.   Sasahara M, Raines EW, Chait A, et al. Inhibition of hypercholesterolemia-induced atherosclerosis in the nonhuman primate by probucol. I. Is the extent of atherosclerosis related to resistance of LDL to oxidation? J Clin Invest 1994;94:155-64.

23.   Palinski W, Ord VA, Plump AS, Breslow JL, Steinberg D, Witztum JL. ApoE-deficient mice are a model of lipoprotein oxidation in atherogenesis. Demonstration of oxidation-specific epitopes in lesions and high titers of autoantibodies to malondialdehyde-lysine in serum. Arterioscler Thromb 1994;14:605-16.

24.   Carew TE, Schwenke DC, Steinberg D. Antiatherogenic effect of probucol unrelated to its hypocholesterolemic effect: evidence that antioxidants in vivo can selectively inhibit low density lipoprotein degradation in macrophage-rich fatty streaks and slow the progression of atherosclerosis in the Watanabe heritable hyperlipidemic rabbit. Proc Natl Acad Sci USA 1987;84:772-79.

25.   Daugherty A, Zweifel BS, Schonfeld G. The effects of probucol on the progression of atherosclerosis in mature Watanabe heritable hyperlipidaemic rabbits. Br J Pharmacol 1991; 103:1013-18.

26.   Bjorkhem I, Henriksson-Freyschuss A, Breuer O, Diczfalusy U, Berglund L, Henriksson P. The antioxidant butylated hydroxytoluene protects against atherosclerosis. Arterioscler Thromb 1991;11:15-22.

27.   Bocan TM, Mueller SB, Brown EQ, Uhlendorf PD, Mazur MJ, Newton RS. Antiatherosclerotic effects of antioxidants are lesion-specific when evaluated in hypercholesterolemic New Zealand white rabbits. Exp Mol Pathol 1992;57:70-83.

28.   Sparrow CP, Doebber TW, Olszewski J, et al. Low density lipoprotein is protected from oxidation and the progression of atherosclerosis is slowed in cholesterol-fed rabbits by the antioxidant N,N'-diphenyl-phenylenediamine. J Clin Invest 1992;89:1885-91.

29.   Morel DW, de la Llera-Moya M, Friday KE. Treatment of cholesterol-fed rabbits with dietary vitamins E and C inhibits lipoprotein oxidation but not development of atherosclerosis. J Nutr 1994;124:2123-30.

30.   Fruebis J, Steinberg D, Dresel HA, Carew TE. A comparison of the antiatherogenic effects of probucol and of a structural analogue of probucol in low density lipoprotein receptor-deficient rabbits. J Clin Invest 1994;94:392-98.

31.   Kleinveld HA, Demacker PN, Stalenhoef AF. Comparative study on the effect of low-dose vitamin E and probucol on the susceptibility of LDL to oxidation and the progression of atherosclerosis in Watanabe heritable hyperlipidemic rabbits. Arterioscler Thromb 1994;14: 1386-91.

32.   Shaish A, Daugherty A, O'Sullivan F, Schonfeld G, Heinecke JW. Beta-carotene inhibits atherosclerosis in hypercholesterolemic rabbits. J Clin Invest 1995;96:2075-82.

33.   Fruebis J, Carew TE, Palinski W. Effect of vitamin E on atherogenesis in LDL receptor-deficient rabbits. Atherosclerosis 1995;117:217-24.

34.   Chang MY, Sasahara M, Chait A, Raines EW, Ross R. Inhibition of hypercholesterolemia-induced atherosclerosis in the nonhuman primate by probucol. II. Cellular composition and proliferation. Arterioscler Thromb Vasc Biol 1995;15:1631-40.

35.   Tangirala RK, Casanada, F, Miller E, Witztum JL, Steinberg D, Palinski W. Effect of the antioxidant N,N'-diphenyl 1,4-phenylenediamine (DPPD) on atherosclerosis in apoE-deficient mice. Arterioscler Thromb Vasc Biol 1995;15:1625-30.

36.   Schwenke DC, Carew TE. Initiation of atherosclerotic lesions in cholesterol-fed rabbits: I. Focal increases in arterial LDL concentration precede development of fatty streak lesions. Arteriosclerosis 1989;9:895-907.

37.   Schwenke DC, Carew TE. Initiation of atherosclerotic lesion in cholesterol-fed rabbits. II. Selective retention of LDL vs. selective increases in LDL permeability in susceptible sites of arteries. Arteriosclerosis 1989;9:908-18.

38.   Rosenfeld ME, Carew, TE, von Hodenberg E, Pittman RC, Ross R, Steinberg D. Autoradiographic analysis of the distribution of ^{125}I-tyramine-cellobiose-LDL in atherosclerotic lesions of the WHHL rabbit. Arteriosclerosis and Thrombosis 1992;12:985-95.

39.   Frank JS, Fogelman AM. Ultrastructure of the intima in WHHL and cholesterol-fed rabbit aortas prepared by ultra-rapid freezing and freeze-etching. J Lipid Res 1989;30:967-78.

40.   Stocker R. Lipoprotein oxidation: Mechanistic aspects, methodological approaches and clinical relevance. Curr Opin Lipidol 1994;5:422-33.

41.   Tribble DL. Lipoprotein oxidation in dyslipidemia: Insights into general mechanisms affecting lipoprotein oxidative behavior. Curr Opin Lipidol 1995;6:196-208.

42.   Rice-Evans C, Leake D, Bruckdorfer KR, Diplock AT. Practical approaches to low density lipoprotein oxidation: Whys, wherefores and pitfalls. Free Radic Res 1996;25:285-311.

43.   Jialal I, Devaraj S. Low-density lipoprotein oxidation, antioxidants, and atherosclerosis: A clinical biochemistry perspective. Clin Chem 1996;42:498-506.

44.   Esterbauer H, Schmidt R, Hayn M. Relationships among oxidation of low-density lipoprotein, antioxidant protection, and atherosclerosis. Adv Pharmacol 1997;38:425-56.

45.   Haberland ME, Fong D, Cheng L. Malondialdehyde-altered protein occurs in atheroma of Watanabe heritable hyperlipidemic rabbits. Science 1988;241:215-18.

46.   Palinski W, Rosenfeld ME, Yla-Herttuala S, et al. Low density lipoprotein undergoes oxidative modification in vivo. Proc Natl Acad Sci USA 1989;86:1372-76.

47.   Boyd HC, Gown AM, Wolfbauer G, Chait-A. Direct evidence for a protein recognized by a monoclonal antibody against oxidatively modified LDL in atherosclerotic lesions from a Watanabe heritable hyperlipidemic rabbit. Am J Pathol 1989;135:815-25.

48.   Khan BV, Parthasarathy SS, Alexander RW, Medford RM. Modified low density lipoprotein and its constituents augment cytokine-activated vascular cell adhesion molecule-1 gene expression in human vascular endothelial cells. J Clin Invest 1995;95:1262-70.

49.   Kim JA, Territo MC, Wayner E, et al. Partial characterization of leukocyte binding molecules on endothelial cells induced by minimally oxidized LDL. Arterioscler Thromb 1994;14:427-33.

50.   Cushing SD, Berliner JA, Valente AJ, et al. Minimally modified low density lipoprotein induces monocyte chemotactic protein 1 in human endothelial cells and smooth muscle cells. Proc Natl Acad Sci USA 1990;87:5134-38.

51.   Quinn MT, Parthasarathy S, Fong L, Steinberg D. Oxidatively modified low density lipoproteins: A potential role in the recruitment and retention of monocyte/macrophages during atherogenesis. Proc Natl Acad Sci USA 1987;84:2995-98.

52.   McMurray HF, Parthasarathy S, Steinberg D. Oxidatively modified low density lipoprotein is a chemoattractant for human T lymphocytes. J Clin Invest 1993;92:1004-8.

53.   Yla-Herttuala S. Expression of lipoprotein receptors and related molecules in atherosclerotic lesions. Curr Opin Lipidol 1996;7:292-97.

54.   Stary HC, Chandler AB, Glagov S, et al. A definition of initial, fatty streak, and intermediate lesions of atherosclerosis. Circulation 1994;89:2462-78.

55.   O'Brien K, Nagano Y, Gown A, Kita T, Chait A. Probucol treatment affects the cellular composition but not anti-oxidized low density lipoprotein immunoreactivity of plaques from Watanabe heritable hyperlipidemic rabbits. Arterioscler Thromb 1991;11:751-59.

56.   Braesen JH, Beisiegel U, Niendorf A. Probucol inhibits not only the progression of atherosclerotic disease, but causes a different composition of atherosclerotic lesions in WHHL-rabbits. Virchows Arch 1995;426:179-88.

57.   Stary HC, Chandler AB, Glagov S, et al. A definition of advanced types of atherosclerotic lesions and a histological classification of atherosclerosis. Arterioscler Thromb Vasc Biol 1995;15:1512-31.

58.   Guyton JR, Klemp KF. Development of the lipid-rich core in human atherosclerosis. Arterioscler Thromb Vascm Biol 1996;16:4-11.

59.   Coffey MD, Cole RA, Colles SM, Chisolm GM. In vitro cell injury by oxidized low density lipoprotein involves lipid hydroperoxide-induced formation of alkoxyl, lipid, and peroxyl radicals. J Clin Invest 1995;96:1866-73.

60.   Yui S, Sasaki T, Miyazaki A, Horiuchi S, Yamazaki M. Induction of murine macrophage growth by modified LDLs. Arterioscler Thromb 1993;13:331-37.

61.   Sakai M, Miyazaki A, Hakamata H, et al. Lysophosphatidylcholine potentiates the mitogenic activity of modified LDL for human monocyte-derived macrophages. Arterioscler Thromb Vasc Biol 1996;16:600-605.

62.   Kusuhara M, Chait A, Cader A, Berk BC. Oxidized LDL stimulates mitogen-activated protein kinases in smooth muscle cells and macrophages. Arterioscler Thromb Vasc Biol 1997;17: 141-48.

63.   Glagov S, Weisenberg E, Zarins CK, Stankunavicius R, Kolettis GJ. Compensatory enlargement of human atherosclerotic coronary arteries. N Eng J Med 1987;316:1371-74.

64.   Clarkson TB, Prichard RW, Morgan TM, Petrick GS, Klein KP. Remodeling of coronary arteries in human and nonhuman primates. JAMA 1994;271:289-94.

65.   Lendon CL, Davies MJ, Born GV, Richardson PD. Atherosclerotic plaque caps are locally weakened when macrophages density is increased. Atherosclerosis 1991;87:87-90.

66.   Mitchinson, MJ, Hardwick SJ, Bennett MR. Cell death in atherosclerotic plaques. Curr Opin Lipidol 1996;7:324-29.

67.   Libby P, Geng YJ, Aikawa M, et al. Macrophages and atherosclerotic plaque stability. Curr Opin Lipidol 1996;7:330-35.

OXIDATIVE MODIFICATION OF LDL AND ATHEROGENESIS

Daniel Steinberg

Introduction

The hypothesis that oxidative modification of low density lipoprotein (LDL) might be a critically important step in atherogenesis grew out of the recognition that cholesterol accumulation in foam cells could not be due to uptake of native LDL by way of the LDL receptor. First of all, patients who totally lack LDL receptors nevertheless develop foam cell-rich lesions much like the lesions in hypercholesterolemic subjects with normal LDL receptors [1]. Second, neither cultured monocyte/macrophages [2] nor cultured smooth muscle cells [3] can be forced to accumulate any appreciable amounts of cholesterol ester by incubation with even very high concentrations of native LDL. This led to a search for alternative forms of LDL and alternative lipoprotein receptors. Chemically acetylated LDL (AcLDL) was the first modified form demonstrated to be taken up sufficiently rapidly by monocyte/macrophages to lead to cholesterol accumulation [2]. The uptake occurred by way of a new receptor, the AcLDL receptor, quite distinct from the native LDL receptor. Unlike the native LDL receptor, the acetyl LDL receptor does not downregulate as the cell cholesterol content increases, which allows the progressive accumulation of sterol. However, there is no evidence for generation of AcLDL *in vivo*. Oxidized LDL (OxLDL) was shown to be an alternative ligand for the AcLDL receptor and to cause accumulation of cholesterol esters in monocyte/macrophages [4]. Over the past decade a large body of evidence has accumulated demonstrating that oxidation of LDL does indeed take place *in vivo* and that this process may be playing a significant role in atherogenesis, at least in animal models [5,6]. If this hypothesis is valid with respect to the human disease, it would have important implications for intervention to slow the progression of atherosclerosis. Consequently there has been intense interest in the oxidation of LDL and the factors that contribute to it.

Overview of Current Concepts of Atherogenesis

It is generally accepted that the fatty streak lesion is the earliest visible lesion of atherosclerosis and that most more advanced lesions can be traced back to the fatty streak as the progenitor lesion. Presumably, then, if we could limit the generation and rate of progression of fatty streak lesions we would reduce the number and severity of the more

141

A. M. Gotto, Jr. et al. (eds.), Multiple Risk Factors in Cardiovascular Disease, 141–147.
© 1998 *Kluwer Academic Publishers and Fondazione Giovanni Lorenzini. Printed in the Netherlands.*

advanced, clinically consequential lesions as well. The scheme in Figure 1 summarizes some of the key events believed to lead to fatty streak formation. One of the earliest responses to hypercholesterolemia is an increase in the adherence of circulating monocytes to arterial endothelial cells. This is due to an increase in the expression of adhesion molecules both on the circulating monocyte and on the endothelial cell surface [7-9]. The adherent monocytes then migrate between endothelial cells in response to chemoattractant molecules generated and released by cells of the arterial wall (including the endothelial cells themselves). In the subendothelial space the monocyte undergoes a dramatic modification of its phenotype to become a "tissue macrophage," expressing a large number of genes that are not expressed on the circulating monocyte, including the scavenger receptors involved in the uptake of AcLDL and OxLDL [10]. Presumably LDL is constantly entering the wall of the artery from the plasma compartment and returning. During its residence in the subendothelial space it may undergo some degree of oxidation. Even a very minimal degree of oxidation is enough to confer proatherogenic properties on LDL (MM-LDL), including the ability to stimulate release from endothelial cells of an important macrophage growth factor (macrophage colony stimulating factor [11]) and a potent chemoattractant for monocytes (monocyte chemoattractant protein-1 [12]). A further degree of oxidation is necessary to generate the form of LDL recognized by the scavenger receptor, now expressed on the phenotypically altered monocyte population. That presumably is the basis for the beginning of lipid accumulation leading to accumulation of foam cells.

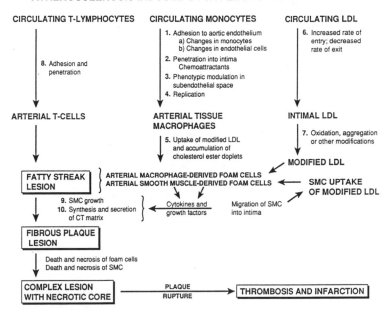

Figure 1. Schema summarizing the major features of fatty streak formation and the later evolution of the atherosclerotic plaque.

The Multiple Proatherogenic Properties of Oxidized LDL

It was recognized very early that the uptake of oxidized LDL by macrophages was due in part to the same receptor that recognizes AcLDL [4]. More recent studies have established that additional macrophage receptors are also involved in that uptake [13,14]. In any case, the first proatherogenic property described was the ability to cause cholesterol ester accumulation in cultured monocyte/macrophages [15]. It was soon found that oxidized LDL had additional proatherogenic properties, including the ability to inhibit the motility of tissue macrophages [16] and the ability to act directly as a chemoattractant for monocytes [17]. Studies of the cytotoxicity of LDL established that it only was damaging after undergoing oxidative modification [18]. OxLDL-induced damage to endothelial cells could obviously be an important proatherogenic property. Over the past six or seven years OxLDL has been shown to have many additional potentially proatherogenic properties. Just to mention a few, it can inhibit or even reverse the vasodilatation normally induced by nitric oxide [19]; it can induce the formation of autoantibodies [20,21]; and it can stimulate the release of interleukin-1 [22]. Thus, evidence from cell culture studies suggests a number of ways in which oxidized LDL might be proatherogenic but what is the evidence that is actually formed *in vivo* and that it is actually proatherogenic?

There is substantial evidence, both direct and indirect. Studies of lipoproteins extracted gently from atherosclerotic lesions (in the presence of antioxidants to prevent factitious oxidation) have demonstrated the presence of oxidatively modified LDL [23]. Antibodies raised against oxidized LDL (antibodies that do not react at all with native LDL) demonstrate the presence of epitopes of oxidized LDL in atherosclerotic lesions but not in normal arterial tissue [21]. Some investigators have reported the presence of oxidized LDL, or at least of oxidized lipids, in human plasma [24,25] but this probably represents a very small fraction of the total circulating LDL. Finally, and most important, it has been shown using several different animal models that antioxidant treatment slows the progression of early lesions, as reviewed elsewhere [6]. Inhibition has been observed with several different antioxidants (probucol, butylated hydroxytoluene, N,N-diphenylphenylenediamine, and vitamin E). Moreover, inhibition has been observed in several different animal models— (LDL receptor-deficient rabbits, cholesterol-fed rabbits, cholesterol-fed nonhuman primates, cholesterol-fed hamsters, and apoE-deficient mice).

Clinical Relevance

The positive results obtained with several different antioxidant compounds in several different animal models makes it seem reasonable to extrapolate and assume that antioxidants will indeed be effective against the human disease. That seems to be a reasonable extrapolation in view of the fact that fatty streak lesions in the animal models are very similar to those in humans. The macrophage receptors involved in the uptake of oxidized LDL are highly homologous in humans and in animals all the way back to rodents. Furthermore, the basic pathobiology of the atherogenic process seems not be radically different in humans and in animals.

On the other hand, past experience dictates caution. The pace at which lesions develop in humans is much slower than it is in the animal models and so it is quite possible that effective repair processes can occur in the course of the human disease that are not effective in the more rapidly developing lesions of experimental animals. It should also be kept in mind that in the animal models the levels of lipoproteins reached are much higher than they are in the human disease and this may lead to at least quantitative differences in response to antioxidants. Only after we have sufficiently large, double-blind clinical intervention trials with antioxidants should we conclude that the hypothesis applies in man. Until then we should not make any recommendations regarding antioxidant supplementation.

Clinical Trials

BETA-CAROTENE

When the issue of clinical trials was first under discussion [26] beta-carotene, vitamin E, and vitamin C appeared to be the most promising natural antioxidants for study. There was strong epidemiologic evidence that vitamin E intake correlated negatively with CHD risks and similar but somewhat weaker data with respect to beta-carotene and vitamin C [27-29]. When the first clinical intervention trials using beta-carotene supplementation yielded negative results [30-32] there was considerable head scratching. However, when direct tests were made of the ability of antioxidants to protect LDL against *ex vivo* oxidative modification, it became clear that vitamin E and beta-carotene were in quite different categories. Supplementation with vitamin E makes the circulating LDL much less susceptible to oxidative modification provided the dose is sufficiently high [33]. While the experimental data available are limited, it appears that a dose of somewhere above 150 international units daily is required to give substantive increases in resistance of LDL to oxidative modification [34]. Beta-carotene, on the other hand, has not been shown to be protective at all. Even with very large doses, doses that increase the plasma concentration and the LDL concentration many-fold, there is no significant increase in the resistance of the circulating LDL to *ex vivo* oxidation [33,35]. This is an unexpected finding inasmuch as the beta-carotene within LDL is progressively destroyed during oxidation of LDL, as is the vitamin E content [36]. However, it may be that the beta-carotene is degraded to compounds that have prooxidant effects or that is simply a less efficient chainbreaking antioxidant in the context of the LDL particle. The situation is made more complicated by a recent report [37] that beta-carotene supplementation can inhibit the progression of atherosclerosis in rabbits even though it is very poorly absorbed and does not confer protection against *ex vivo* oxidation of the rabbit LDL!

VITAMIN E

Vitamin E is in quite a different category, as mentioned above. Supplementation with vitamin E can increase plasma levels several-fold and can prolong the lag time of LDL in an *ex vivo* oxidation system [33,34]. Only two clinical intervention trials utilizing vitamin E have been reported. The first, the Finnish Alpha-Tocopherol-Betacarotene study [32] involved middle-aged men who had been heavy smokers for much of their lives (and presumably had, therefore, advanced atherosclerosis). The dose of vitamin E was only 50 mg per day which is insufficient to confer any important protection of circulating LDL against oxidation. No effect on either cancer or cardiovascular disease was observed. The second study, the Cambridge Heart Antioxidant Study (CHAOS) was a double-blind study in patients with coronary heart disease established by direct angiographic visualization [38]. The patients were stratified according to a number of risk factors and also according to the treatment recommended (medical, bypass surgery or angioplasty). The dose of vitamin E was 400 to 800 international units daily. After a median follow-up of slightly less than two years, there was a highly significant (p=0.005) reduction in the primary endpoint of cardiovascular death plus nonfatal myocardial infarction (47% reduction in risk). There are several additional clinical intervention studies in process, some of them using cardiovascular events as endpoints and others using carotid artery ultrasound as endpoints [29]. Until additional studies are completed it will not be possible to reach a firm conclusion on the issue.

Summary

The hypothesis that oxidation of LDL is a critical step in atherogenesis is relatively new. Still, the case is strong at the experimental level and at least one clinical intervention trial has yielded surprisingly strong positive results. However, until additional clinical trials are reported we are not in a position to make any recommendations to the general public regarding the use of antioxidant supplements.

References

1.   Goldstein JL, Hobbs HH, Brown MS. Familial hypercholesterolemia. In: Scriver CR, Beaudet AL, Sly WS, Valle D, editors. The metabolic and molecular bases of inherited disease. New York: McGraw-Hill, Inc., 1995: 1981-2030.

2.   Goldstein JL, Ho YK, Basu SK, Brown MS. Binding site on macrophages that mediates uptake and degradation of acetylated low density lipoprotein, producing massive cholesterol deposition. Proc Natl Acad Sci USA 1979;76:333-37.

3.   Weinstein DB, Carew TE, Steinberg D. Uptake and degradation of low density lipoprotein by swine arterial smooth muscle cells with inhibition of cholesterol biosynthesis. Biochim Biophys Acta 1976;424:404-21.

4.   Henriksen T, Mahoney EM, Steinberg D. Enhanced macrophage degradation of low density lipoprotein previously incubated with cultured endothelial cells: Recognition by receptors for acetylated low density lipoproteins. Proc Natl Acad Sci USA 1981;78:6499-503.

5.   Steinberg D, Parthasarathy S, Carew TE, Khoo JC, Witztum JL. Beyond cholesterol. Modifications of low-density lipoprotein that increase its atherogenicity [see comments]. N Engl J Med 1989;320:915-24.

6.   Steinberg D. Oxidative modification of LDL and atherogenesis. The 1995 Lewis A. Conner

Memorial Lecture. Circulation 1997;95:1062-71.

7.   Gerrity RG. The role of monocyte in atherogenesis. I. Transition of blood-borne monocytes into foam cells in fatty lesions. Am J Pathol 1981;103:181-90.

8.   Cybulsky MI, Gimbrone MA, Jr. Endothelial expression of a mononuclear leukocyte adhesion molecule during atherogenesis. Science 1991;251:788-91.

9.   Bath P, Gladwin A, Martin J. Human monocyte characteristics are altered in hypercholesterolemia. Atherosclerosis 1991;90:175-81.

10. Fogelman A, Haberland M, Seager J, Hokom M, Edwards P. Factors regulating the activities of the low density lipoprotein receptor and the scavenger receptor on human monocyte-macrophages. J Lipid Res 1981;22:1131-41.

11. Rajavashisth TB, Andalibi A, Territo MC, et al. Induction of endothelial cell expression of granulocyte and macrophage colony-stimulating factors by modified low-density lipoproteins. Nature 1990;344:254-57.

12. Cushing SD, Berliner JA, Valente AJ, et al. Minimally modified low density lipoprotein induces monocyte chemotactic protein 1 in human endothelial cells and smooth muscle cells. Proc Natl Acad Sci USA 1990;87:5134-38.

13. Sparrow CP, Parthasarathy S, Steinberg D. A macrophage receptor that recognizes oxidized low density lipoprotein but not acetylated low density lipoprotein. J Biol Chem 1989;264:2599-604.

14. Arai H, Kita T, Yokode M, Narumiya S, Kawai C. Multiple receptors for modified low density lipoproteins in mouse peritoneal macrophages: Different uptake mechanisms for acetylated and oxidized low density lipoproteins. Biochem Biophys Res Comms 1989;159:1375-82.

15. Henriksen T, Mahoney EM, Steinberg D. Enhanced macrophage degradation of biologically modified low density lipoprotein. Arteriosclerosis 1983;3:149-59.

16. Quinn MT, Parthasarathy S, Steinberg D. Endothelial cell-derived chemotactic activity for mouse peritoneal macrophages and the effects of modified forms of low density lipoprotein. Proc Natl Acad Sci USA 1985;82:5949-53.

17. Quinn MT, Parthasarathy S, Fong LG, Steinberg D. Oxidatively modified low density lipoproteins: A potential role in recruitment and retention of monocyte/macrophages during atherogenesis. Proc Natl Acad Sci USA 1987;84:2995-98.

18. Morel DW, Hessler JR, Chisolm GM. Low density lipoprotein cytotoxicity induced by free radical peroxidation of lipid. J Lipid Res 1983;24:1070-76.

19. Kugiyama K, Kerns SA, Morrisett JD, Roberts R, Henry PD. Impairment of endothelium-dependent arterial relaxation by lysolecithin in modified low-density lipoproteins. Nature 1990;344:160-62.

20. Palinski W, Yla-Herttuala S, Rosenfeld ME, et al. Antisera and monoclonal antibodies specific for epitopes generated during oxidative modification of low density lipoprotein. Arteriosclerosis 1990;10:325-35.

21. Palinski W, Rosenfeld ME, Yla-Herttuala S, et al. Low density lipoprotein undergoes oxidative modification in vivo. Proc Natl Acad Sci USA 1989;86:1372-76.

22. Jackson RL, Barnhart RL, Mao SJ. Probucol and its mechanisms for reducing atherosclerosis. Adv Exp Med Biol 1991;285:367-72.

23. Yla-Herttuala S, Palinski W, Rosenfeld ME, et al. Evidence for the presence of oxidatively modified low density lipoprotein in atherosclerotic lesions of rabbit and man. J Clin Invest 1989;84:1086-95.

24. Sevanian A, Hwang J, Hodis H, Cazzolato G, Avogaro P, Bittolo-Bon G. Contribution of an in vivo oxidized LDL to LDL oxidation and its association with dense LDL subpopulations.

Arterioscler Thromb Vasc Biol 1996;16:784-93.

25. Hodis HN, Kramsch DM, Avogaro P, et al. Biochemical and cytotoxic characteristics of an in vivo circulating oxidized low density lipoprotein (LDL-). J Lipid Res 1994;35:669-77.

26. Steinberg D. Antioxidants in the prevention of human atherosclerosis. Summary of the proceedings of a National Heart, Lung, and Blood Institute Workshop: September 5-6, 1991, Bethesda, Maryland. Circulation 1992;85:2337-44.

27. Stampfer MJ, Hennekens CH, Manson JE, Colditz GA, Rosner B, Willett WC. Vitamin E consumption and the risk of coronary disease in women. N Engl J Med 1993;328:1444-49.

28. Rimm EB, Stampfer MJ, Ascherio A, Giovannucci E, Colditz GA, Willett WC. Vitamin E consumption and the risk of coronary heart disease in men. N Engl J Med 1993;328:1450-56.

29. Jha P, Flather M, Lonn E, Farkouh M, Yusuf S. The antioxidant vitamins and cardiovascular disease. A critical review of epidemiologic and clinical trial data [see comments]. Ann Intern Med 1995;123:860-72.

30. Hennekens CH, Buring JE, Manson JE, et al. Lack of effect of long-term supplementation with beta carotene on the incidence of malignant neoplasms and cardiovascular disease. N Eng J Med 1996;334:1145-49.

31. Omenn GS, Goodman GE, Thornquist MD, et al. Effects of a combination of beta carotene and vitamin A on lung cancer and cardiovascular disease. N Eng J Med 1996;334:1150-55.

32. Alpha-Tocopherol, Beta-Carotene Cancer Prevention Study Group. The effect of vitamin E and beta-carotene on the incidence of lung cancer and other cancers in male smokers. N Engl J Med 1994;330:1029-35.

33. Reaven P, Khouw A, Beltz W, Parthasarathy S, Witztum JL. Effect of dietary antioxidant combinations in humans: Protection of LDL by vitamin E, but not by B-carotene. Arterioscler Thromb 1993;13:590-600.

34. Dieber-Rotheneder M, Puhl H, Waeg G, Striegl G, Esterbauer H. Effect of oral supplementation with D-alpha-tocopherol on the vitamin E content of human low density lipoproteins and resistance to oxidation. J Lipid Res 1991;32:1325-32.

35. Reaven P, Ferguson E, Navab M, Powell F. Susceptibility of human low density lipoprotein to oxidative modification: Effects of variations in B-carotene concentration and oxygen tension. Arterioscler Thromb 1994;14:1162-12169.

36. Esterbauer H, Striegl G, Puhl H, Rotheneder M. Continuous monitoring of in vitro oxidation of human low density lipoprotein. Free Rad Res Comms 1989;6:67-75.

37. Shaish A, Daugherty A, O'Sullivan F, Schonfeld G, Heinecke JW. Beta-carotene inhibits atherosclerosis in hypercholesterolemic rabbits. J Clin Invest 1995;96:2075-82.

38. Stephens NG, Parsons A, Schofield PM, et al. Randomised controlled trial of vitamin E in patients with coronary disease: Cambridge Heart Antioxidant Study (CHAOS). The Lancet 1996;347:781-85.

DIETARY ANTIOXIDANTS AND CARDIOVASCULAR DISEASE

Aaron R. Folsom

Introduction

There is considerable evidence that oxidation of low density lipoproteins (LDL) plays a crucial step in atherogenesis [1]. There is also evidence that antioxidants help protect LDL from oxidation and can prevent atherosclerosis in animal models [1-3]. A number of observational studies and a few randomized trials have attempted to verify whether antioxidant intake from food and/or supplements may prevent the occurrence of cardiovascular events. Jha et al. recently published an excellent comprehensive overview of the relation of β-carotene, vitamin E, and vitamin C with cardiovascular disease occurrence [4]. In this report, I update the review through a Medline search over the past three years, and add recent studies on flavonoids, another family of antioxidants.

Discussion

Figure 1 shows the main outcome of prospective epidemiologic studies of β-carotene measured by questionnaires assessing food and/or supplement intake, or by analysis of baseline blood [5-14]. The relative risk for a "higher" versus "lower" level of β-carotene is depicted by the small rectangle and the 95% confidence interval, by the horizontal line. The majority of prospective studies show higher β-carotene levels associated with reduced risk of cardiovascular disease, with a number of individual relative risk estimates statistically significantly less than 1.0. Two [15-16] of four [15-18] prospective nested case-control studies of vitamin A metabolites in stored blood also observed significant negative associations with cardiovascular disease (not shown in Figure 1). In contrast, four randomized clinical trials of 20-50 mg/d of β-carotene in smokers [13,19], patients with skin cancer [12], smokers or asbestos workers [20], and physicians [21] found no evidence of benefit (Figure 2).

For vitamin E, prospective epidemiologic observations [5,6,10,13,14, 22,23] have often, but not uniformly, suggested benefit in preventing cardiovascular disease (Figure 3). However, only one [15] of six [15-18,24,25] prospective nested case-control studies has suggested stored blood levels of vitamin E are associated inversely with cardiovascular disease occurrence (not shown). As Figure 4 shows, randomized trials of 50 mg/d vitamin E in smokers [13,19] and 30 mg/d in a Chinese population [26] showed no benefit in

149

A. M. Gotto, Jr. et al. (eds.), Multiple Risk Factors in Cardiovascular Disease, 149–156.
© 1998 Kluwer Academic Publishers and Fondazione Giovanni Lorenzini. Printed in the Netherlands.

preventing cardiovascular disease. In contrast, the CHAOS project gave 400-800 IU/d to patients with angiographically demonstrated coronary artery disease and remarkably showed a nearly halving of subsequent cardiovascular disease events in an average follow-up of only 1.4 years [27].

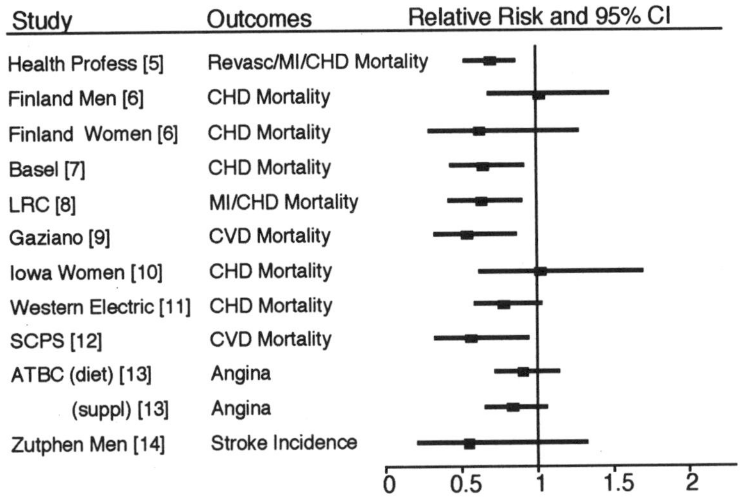

Figure 1. Prospective observational studies of β-carotene and CVD. Portions adapted from Jha et al. [4].

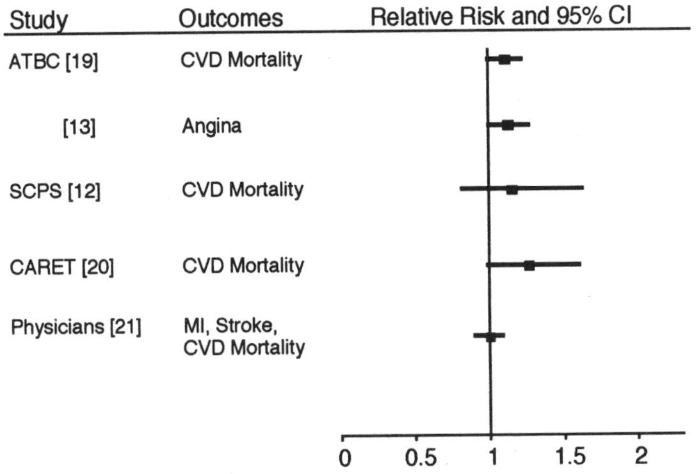

Figure 2. Randomized trials of β-carotene and CVD. Portions adapted from Jha et al [4].

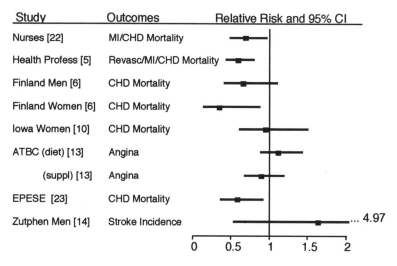

Figure 3. Prospective observational studies of vitamin E and CVD. Portions adapted from Jha et al. [4].

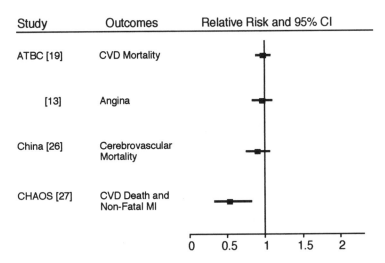

Figure 4. Randomized trials of vitamin E and CVD. Portions adapted from Jha et al. [4].

Prospective observational studies of vitamin C intake from diet and/or supplements [5-7,10,11,14,23,28-32] or via blood assessment have sometimes, though far from uniformly, shown potential benefit in preventing cardiovascular disease (Figure 5). The extremely sparse randomized trial data (Figure 6) show no benefit from 120-200 mg/d [26,33].

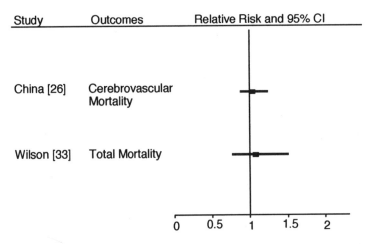

Study	Outcomes	Relative Risk and 95% CI
Health Profess [5]	Revasc/MI/CHD Mortality	
NHANES [28]	CVD Mortality	
Finland Men [6]	CHD Mortality	
Finland Women [6]	CHD Mortality	
Alameda [29]	CVD Mortality	
Basel [7]	CHD Mortality	
Gale [30]	Stroke Mortality	
Gale [30]	CHD Mortality	
Iowa Women [10]	CHD Mortality	
Western Electric [11]	CHD Mortality	
EPESE [23]	CHD Mortality	
Zutphen Men [14]	Stroke Incidence	... 2.66
Norway Postal [31]	Stroke Mortality	
Finland Men [32]	Acute MI	

Figure 5. Prospective observational studies of vitamin C and CVD. Portions adapted from Jha et al. [4].

Study	Outcomes	Relative Risk and 95% CI
China [26]	Cerebrovascular Mortality	
Wilson [33]	Total Mortality	

Figure 6. Randomized trials of vitamin C and CVD. Portions adapted from Jha et al. [4].

Recently, dietary intake of flavonoids, another family of antioxidant compounds [34], has been examined in three prospective studies. Foods high in flavonoids include tea, apples, onions, beans, soy, and red wine. Two [14,34,35] of the three [14,34-36] studies have suggested an inverse association of flavonoid intake with cardiovascular disease occurrence (Figure 7).

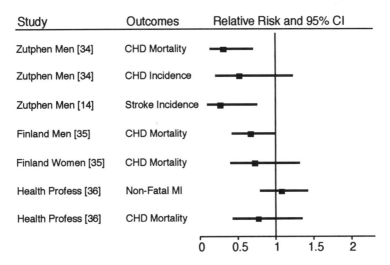

Figure 7. Prospective observational studies of flavonoids and CVD.

The epidemiologic observational data suggest stronger potential benefit of dietary antioxidants than do the extant randomized chemopreventive trials. Though statistical adjustments were generally performed, the observational studies may have overestimated benefit of antioxidants, due to 1) biases, for example by healthier participants selecting to take in higher levels of antioxidants, or 2) substitution of foods high in antioxidants for foods high in saturated fat. Trials may have suffered from 1) choosing the wrong dose (especially some of the vitamin E trials), 2) being too short, 3) or intervening too late in the course of cardiovascular disease development. It may also be that the multiple nutrients interacting together in foods are much more efficacious than vitamin supplements.

Additional trials, especially of vitamin E are needed, and several are underway [4]. In the meantime, evidence remains too weak to promote antioxidant supplementation widely. Rather, recommendations to limit animal products and saturated fat and to increase vegetables, fruit, nuts, and whole grains continue to be important public health messages.

Acknowledgement

Supported in part by Contract N01-HC-55019 from the U.S. National Heart, Lung, and Blood Institute and Grant R01 CA39742 from the National Cancer Institute.

References

1. Steinberg D, Parthasarathy S, Carew TE, Khoo JC, Witztum J. Beyond cholesterol. Modifications of low-density lipoprotein that increase its atherogenicity. N Engl J Med 1989; 320:915-24.

2. Steinberg D. Antioxidants in the prevention of human atherosclerosis. Summary of the proceedings of a National Heart, Lung, and Blood Institute Workshop; 1991 September 5-6; Bethesda, Maryland. Circulation 1992;85:2337-44.

3. Chisolm GM 3d. Antioxidants and atherosclerosis: A current assessment. Clin Cardiol 1991; 14:125-30.

4. Jha P, Flather M, Lonn E, Farkouh M, Yusuf S. The antioxidant vitamins and cardiovascular disease. A critical review of epidemiologic and clinical trial data. Ann Intern Med 1995;123: 860-72.

5. Rimm EB, Stampfer MJ, Ascherio A, Giovannucci E, Colditz GA, Willett WC. Vitamin E consumption and the risk of coronary heart disease in men. N Engl J Med 1993;328:1450-56.

6. Knekt P, Reunanen A, Jarvinen R, Seppanen R, Heliovaara M, Aromaa A. Antioxidant vitamin intake and coronary mortality in a longitudinal population study. Am J Epidemiol 1994;139:1180-90.

7. Gey KF, Moser UK, Jordan P, Stahelin HB, Eichholzer M, Ludin E. Increased risk of cardiovascular disease at suboptimal plasma concentrations of essential antioxidants: An epidemiological update with special attention to carotene and vitamin C. Am J Clin Nutr 1993; 57(5 Suppl.):787S-97S.

8. Morris DL, Kritchevsky SB, Davis CE. Serum carotenoids and coronary heart disease. The Lipid Research Clinics Coronary Primary Prevention Trial and Follow-up Study. JAMA 1994; 272:1439-41.

9. Gaziano JM, Manson JE, Branch LG, et al. Dietary beta-carotene and decreased cardio-vascular mortality in an elderly cohort [Abstract]. J Am Coll Cardiol 1992;19(Suppl.A):377A.

10. Kushi LH, Folsom AR, Prineas RJ, Mink PJ, Wu Y, Bostick RM. Dietary antioxidant vitamins and death from coronary heart disease in postmenopausal women. N Engl J Med 1996;334:1156-62.

11. Pandey DK, Shekelle R, Selwyn BJ, Tangney C, Stamler J. Dietary vitamin C and β-carotene and risk of death in middle-aged men. The Western Electric Study. Am J Epidemiol 1995;142: 1269-78.

12. Greenberg ER, Baron JA, Karagas MR, et al. Mortality associated with low plasma concentration of beta carotene and the effect of oral supplementation. JAMA 1996; 275:699-703.

13. Rapola JM, Virtamo J, Haukka JK, et al. Effect of vitamin E and beta carotene on the incidence of angina pectoris. A randomized, double-blind controlled trial. JAMA 1996;275: 693-98.

14. Keli SO, Hertog MG, Feskens EJ, Kromhout D. Dietary flavonoids, antioxidant vitamins, and incidence of stroke: The Zutphen study. Arch Intern Med 1996;156: 637-42.

15. Salonen JT, Nyyssonen K, Parviainen MT, et al. Low plasma beta carotene, vitamin E and selenium levels associated with accelerated carotid atherogenesis in hypercholesterolemic eastern Finnish men. Circulation 1993;87:1.

16. Street DA, Comstock GW, Salkeld RM, Schüep W, Klag MJ. Serum antioxidants and

myocardial infarction. Are low levels of carotenoids and a-tocopherol risk factors for myocardial infarction? Circulation 1994;90:1154-61.

17. Salonen JT, Salonen R, Penttilä I, et al. Serum fatty acids, apolipoproteins, selenium and vitamin antioxidants and the risk of death from coronary artery disease. Am J Cardiol 1985; 56:226-231.

18. Kok FJ, de Bruijn AM, Vermeeren R, et al. Serum selenium, vitamin antioxidants, and cardiovascular mortality: A 9-year follow-up study in the Netherlands. Am J Clin Nutr 1987; 45:462-468.

19. Anonymous. The effect of vitamin E and beta carotene on the incidence of lung cancer and other cancers in male smokers. The Alpha-Tocopherol, Beta Carotene Cancer Prevention Study Group. N Engl J Med 1994;330:1029-35.

20. Omenn GS, Goodman GE, Thornquist MD, et al. Effects of a combination of beta carotene and vitamin A on lung cancer and cardiovascular disease. N Engl J Med 1996;334:1150-55.

21. Hennekens CH, Burning JE, Manson JE, et al. Lack of effect of long-term supplementation with beta carotene on the incidence of malignant neoplasms and cardiovascular disease. N Engl J Med 1996;334:1145-49.

22. Stampfer MJ, Hennekens CH, Manson JE, Colditz GA, Rosner B, Willett WC. Vitamin E consumption and the risk of coronary disease in women. N Engl J Med 1993;328:1444-49.

23. Losonczy KG, Harris TB, Havlik RJ. Vitamin E and vitamin C supplement use and risk of all-cause and coronary heart disease mortality in older persons: The Established Populations for Epidemiologic Studies of the elderly. Am J Clin Nutr 1996;64:190-96.

24. Hense HW, Stender M, Bors W, Keil U. Lack of an association between serum vitamin E and myocardial infarction in a population with high vitamin E levels. Atherosclerosis 1993;103: 21-28.

25. Öhrvall M, Berglund L, Salminen I, Lithell H, Aro A, Vessby B. The serum cholesterol ester fatty acid composition but not the serum concentration of alpha tocopherol predicts the development of myocardial infarction in 50-year old men: 19 years follow-up. Atherosclerosis 1996;127:65-71.

26. Blot WJ, Li JY, Taylor PR, et al. Nutrition intervention trials in Linxian, China: Supplementation with specific vitamin/mineral combinations, cancer incidence, and disease-specific mortality in the general population. J Natl Cancer Inst 1993;85: 1483-92.

27. Stephens NG, Parsons A, Schofield PM, et al. Randomized controlled trial of vitamin E in patients with coronary disease: Cambridge Heart Antioxidant Study (CHAOS). Lancet 1996; 347:781-86.

28. Enstrom JE, Kanim LE, Klein MA. Vitamin C intake and mortality among a sample of the United States population. Epidemiology 1992;3:194-202.

29. Enstrom JE, Kanim LE, Breslow L. The relationship between vitamin C intake, general health practices, and mortality in Alameda County, California. Am J Public Health 1986;76:1124-30.

30. Gale CR, Martyn CN, Winter PD, Cooper C. Vitamin C and risk of death from stroke and coronary heart disease in cohort of elderly people. BMJ 1995;310:1563-66.

31. Vollset SE, Bjelke E. Does consumption of fruit and vegetables protect against stroke? [Letter] Lancet 1983;2:742.

32. Nyyssönen K, Parviainen MT, Salonen R, Tuomilehto J, Salonen JT. Vitamin C deficiency and risk of myocardial infarction: Prospective population study of men from eastern Finland. BMJ 1997;314:634-38.

33. Wilson TS, Datta SB, Murrell JS, Andrews CT. Relation of vitamin C levels to mortality in a geriatric hospital: A study of the effect of vitamin C administration. Age Aging 1973;2:163-

        71.

34.   Hertog MG, Fesken EJM, Hollman PCH, Katan MB, Kromhout D. Dietary antioxidant
        flavonoids and risk of coronary heart disease: The Zutphen Elderly Study. Lancet 1993;342:
        1007-11.

35.   Knekt P, Jarvinen R, Reunanen A, Maatela J. Flavonoid intake and coronary mortality in
        Finland: A cohort study. BMJ 1996;312:478-81.

36.   Rimm EB, Katan MB, Ascherio A, Stampfer MJ, Willett WC. Relation between intake of
        flavonoids and risk for coronary heart disease in male health professionals. Ann Intern Med
        1996;125:384-89.

Is "Antioxidant Status" a Risk Factor?

Daniel Steinberg

The question we are addressing is: "Should the susceptibility of low density lipoproteins (LDL) to oxidation *ex vivo* be added to the list of risk factors?" My answer will be "No....at least not yet." First of all, it has yet to be conclusively proved that the oxidative modification hypothesis of atherosclerosis applies to the human disease. Clinical trials have begun and an answer should be available within a few years but at the moment we are not sure. Second, it is not all clear that the efficacy of an antioxidant in protecting LDL against *ex vivo* oxidation predicts its efficacy in slowing the progression of atherosclerosis, even in animal models of the disease.

The Oxidative Modification Hypothesis

The basic idea of the oxidative modification hypothesis is summarized in Figure 1. It is universally accepted that the rate of progression of arterial lesions is proportional in some fashion to plasma LDL levels. The oxidative modification hypothesis adds a second term suggesting that the rate of progression is also proportional to the rate at which LDL undergoes oxidation [1,2]. Note that it is not specified where that oxidation takes place (because it is not yet known) nor exactly how it takes place (because it is not yet known). It is not likely that oxidation takes place within the plasma compartment, because even a very small concentration of plasma is enough to inhibit oxidation of LDL in any *ex vivo* system. Plasma is very rich in antioxidants, both water-soluble and lipid-soluble. It is known that oxidized LDL is present in human lesions and the oxidation may be occurring right there in the artery. However, it seems likely that it occurs also at other tissue sites, possibly at all sites of inflammation. If there were some magical way to measure the concentration of oxidized LDL in the artery wall or the rate at which it is generated there, then a measurement might exist that would qualify for addition to the list of risk factors. Unfortunately, it does not. The inclusion of a term relating to the number of "scavenger receptors," receptors that take up oxidized LDL is justified by the recent report of Suzuki et al. [3] showing that deletions of scavenger receptor A by targeted mutations decreases severity of atherosclerosis in apoE-deficient mice.

A. M. Gotto, Jr. et al. (eds.), Multiple Risk Factors in Cardiovascular Disease, 157–164.

RATE OF LESION PROGRESSION =

a [LDL level] + b [rate of LDL oxidation]

+ c [number of scavenger receptors]

+ d [?] + e [?] + ...

Figure 1. A hypothetical equation suggesting that the rate of progression of atherosclerotic lesions is in some fashion proportional not only to the level of LDL but also to the rate at which LDL undergoes oxidative modification, the level of expression of scavenger receptors that recognize oxidized LDL and probably a number of other factors that modulate the impact of LDL on the artery wall.

Measurements of the Susceptibility of LDL to Oxidation *Ex vivo*

In the absence of any such direct way of assessing LDL oxidation, investigators have instead measured the susceptibility of circulating LDL to oxidative modification *ex vivo*. LDL is purified from the plasma, subjected to standardized prooxidant conditions for a given time and at a given temperature (generally incubation with copper ion) and the rate and extent of LDL oxidation is assessed. The most widely used method, as introduced by Esterbauer and co-workers [4], is to follow the rate of diene conjugation (see Figure 2). Free radical attack on a polyunsaturated fatty acid causes an immediate shift of the double bonds to a conjugated configuration, which results in an increase in the absorption of light at 234 µm. Initially the rate of increase is very slow (although it is not zero), indicating that very little diene conjugation is occurring. Then there follows a very rapid increase in diene conjugation called the propagation phase. The time interval between the start of the incubation and the beginning of the propagation phase is called the lag time. During the lag phase the antioxidant compounds found in the LDL (e.g. vitamin E, retinol, lycopene) are trapping free radicals and thus protecting the polyunsaturated fatty acids from oxidation. After the limited amounts of endogenous antioxidant compounds have been consumed, then the chain reaction leading to rapid oxidation of the polyunsaturated fatty acids takes off. Finally, a plateau is reached and no further increase in diene conjugation occurs. The value at the plateau is in a sense just a measure of the total amount of polyunsaturated fatty acids in the sample that are available for oxidation. This value is analogous to the value of an enzymatic reaction that has gone all the way to completion; it is not an indication of the susceptibility of the substrate to oxidation, i.e. it is not a rate measurement.

　　　Other methods can be used, such as measurement of the initial rates of peroxide generation, measurement of the increase in electrophoretic mobility of the LDL particle over time, measurement of thiobarbituric acid-reactive substances as a function of time. All these measure "susceptibility of LDL to oxidation" in some sense and may be indicative. And these approaches are reasonable. If circulating LDL is more susceptible to oxidative modification, then, all else being equal, one would expect more oxidized LDL to be generated *in vivo* and the patient to be at higher risk. But is that really the case? What exactly is the evidence to support the jump from "susceptibility of LDL to oxidation" under arbitrarily chosen *ex vivo* conditions, on the one hand, and the risk of clinical coronary heart disease on the other?

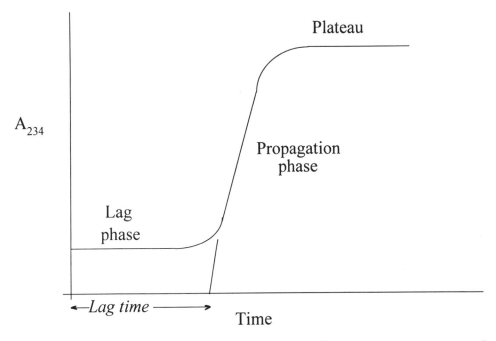

Figure 2. A theoretical curve demonstrating the change in diene conjugation (a measure of fatty acid oxidation) as a function of time during the oxidative modification of LDL. See text for discussion.

Correlation of "Oxidizability" of LDL with Susceptibility to Atherosclerosis in Animal Models

There are many studies showing that in a number of different animal models of atherosclerosis the administration of an antioxidant compound slows the progression of the disease [2]. This has been shown in the LDL receptor-deficient rabbit, in the cholesterol-fed rabbit, in the cholesterol-fed hamster, in the cholesterol-fed monkey, and in the apoE-deficient mouse. In those studies how good is the correlation between the level of protection afforded the plasma LDL against *ex vivo* oxidation and the extent of inhibition of atherosclerosis? Sasahara et al. studied the effects of probucol on atherosclerosis in cholesterol-fed monkeys [5]. There was a good deal of variability from animal to animal, affording an opportunity to look at the correlation between the level of protection of LDL against oxidation *ex vivo* and the level of protection against the development of lesions. As shown in Figure 3, there was a reasonably good negative correlation between the prolongation of the lag time and the extent of lesions. But still there was a great deal of scatter. When the data were examined without regard to the change in lag time, the difference between the probucol-treated group as a whole and the control group with respect to lesion formation was statistically significant only in the thoracic aorta. However, when the animals were arbitrarily divided into those with lag times above 400 minutes and those with lag times below 400 minutes there was a systematic, consistent difference with respect to lesion formation. As shown in Figure 4, with the animals divided in this fashion there was statistically significant protection against atherosclerosis at all levels of the aorta in those that showed a lag time of greater than 400 minutes. This study, then, suggested there may be a threshold level of protection necessary before an antioxidant can exert a significant antiatherosclerotic effect and that the "magic number" for protection might be at about a lag time of about 400 minutes.

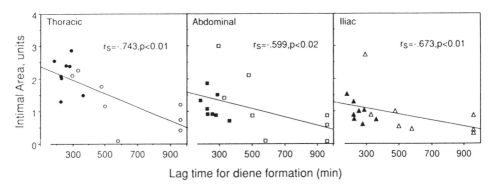

Figure 3. Negative correlation between diene conjugation lag time (abscissa) and extent of atherosclerotic lesions (ordinate) in cholesterol-fed monkeys: untreated, closed symbols; treated with probucol 1% in diet, open symbols. Reproduced with permission from Sasahara et el., 1994 [5].

It is important to stress at this point that probucol is known to have a number of biological effects in addition to its ability to act as an antioxidant in LDL. For example, it can induce the expression of the cholesterol ester-transfer protein [6] and it can stimulate the release of interleukin-1 [7]. The possibility that some of the antiatherosclerotic effects of probucol relate to these additional biological properties has not been ruled out. It should be noted also that these additional biological properties may actually be due to the antioxidant activity of the compound but the result of an action at the cellular level, rather than (or in addition to) a direct protection of LDL oxidation.

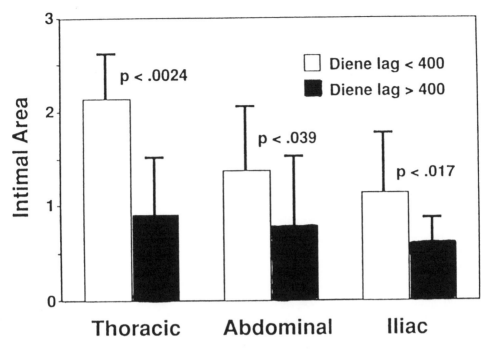

Figure 4. Comparison of the severity of lesions in cholesterol-fed monkeys arbitrarily divided into those with diene conjugation lag times greater than or less than 400 minutes (i.e. independent of treatment group) in the study by Sasahara et al. [5].

In view of this Fruebis et al. [8] undertook a study of a probucol analog that has antioxidant potency comparable to that of probucol but does not share the lipid-lowering effects of probucol (and presumably not the additional biological effects). A dose of the analog was chosen that would protect circulating LDL of the LDL-receptor deficient rabbit to the same extent as did probucol at 1% in the diet. As in the early studies with probucol [9], lesion formation was inhibited by about 50%. The analog, in contrast, had no effect on lesion formation despite a very similar, albeit somewhat lower, level of protection of LDL against *ex vivo* oxidation. The superiority of probucol may be attributable to its greater prolongation of lag time but it may also be due to the fact that the probucol has additional biological effects not shared by the analog.

Sparrow et al. [10] used an antioxidant of a very different molecular structure (N,N-diphenylphenylenediamine; DPPD) and found it effective in inhibiting atherogenesis in cholesterol-fed New Zealand white rabbits. This compound did not have any effect on plasma cholesterol levels. Its efficacy as an antioxidant was tested *ex vivo* by measuring the generation of thiobarburituric acid-reactive substances during incubation with copper ion.

The LDL from control animals had already reached a maximum TBARS value at the earliest time point measured (18 hours). In contrast, LDL from the DPPD-treated rabbits showed only a minimal increase in TBARS at 18 hours and even at 44 hours showed less than half the TBARS value of the LDL from DPPD-treated animals. While not exactly equivalent to a direct measurement of lag time in the diene conjugation assay, the observations suggest that the lag time was prolonged to at least 20 hours, i.e. more than 1,000 minutes. There was a highly significant 71% decrease in the area of atherosclerotic lesions and a 51% decrease in the total cholesterol content of the aorta. These results are consonant with the hypothesis that there is a threshold of protection and that the threshold is rather high.

Fruebis et al. studied the effects of vitamin E in LDL receptor-deficient rabbits [11]. The dosage was sufficient to increase plasma vitamin E 6-fold and to prolong the lag time from 123 minutes to 404 minutes. Despite this rather impressive protection against *ex vivo* oxidation of LDL, there was no effect on lesion formation.

O'Leary et al. examined the effects of probucol in inhibiting lesion formation in LDL receptor-deficient rabbits [12]. In their studies there was a rather good correlation between protection against lesion progression, on the one hand, and protection of the circulating LDL against *ex vivo* oxidation, on the other.

It is important to note that a good correlation between protection of LDL against *ex vivo* oxidation and protection against atherogenesis does not necessarily mean that the protection is the immediate result of preventing LDL oxidation. Obviously the level of the antioxidant compound will reflect the efficacy of its absorption and that will be reflected in part by the degree of antioxidant protection afforded to the plasma LDL. The antiatherosclerotic effects, on the other hand, may have little or nothing to do with that but rather simply depend upon the greater uptake of the antioxidant compound into tissues and one or more biological effects attributable to that.

REASONS WHY PROLONGATION OF *EX VIVO* LAG TIME MAY NOT PREDICT ANTIATHEROSCLEROTIC EFFICACY

The arbitrary conditions chosen to test resistance of LDL to oxidative challenge may not mirror the in vivo conditions. Most of the methods currently in use call for the isolation of LDL from the plasma. *In vivo* LDL in the plasma or in the interstitial fluid can interact with a number of potent antioxidants in the aqueous phase, notably including vitamin C. Vitamin C added to LDL during the measurement of diene conjugation markedly prolongs its lag time [13] because it can restore the vitamin E radical by reducing it and allowing it to trap another radical. There may be important analogous interactions with other plasma antioxidants and effects of this kind would obviously not be measured in the currently utilized protocols. Furthermore, the conditions chosen for oxidatively stressing the LDL may have little to do with the oxidative stresses the particle encounters *in vivo*. At this point the relative importance of various cell types and various oxidizing systems *in vivo* is not known but it is quite possible that metal-catalyzed oxidation plays a relatively minor part. For example, myloperoxidase-catalyzed oxidation and lipoxygenase-catalyzed oxidation do not necessarily depend upon free metal ions.

The effectiveness of antioxidants in preventing atherosclerosis may depend to a greater extent on their effects at the intracellular level. As discussed above, probucol has additional biological effects beyond its ability to protect LDL directly. The same may be true of other antioxidant compounds. Until we know more about the mechanisms of action involved we cannot presume that the important variable is the level of protection of LDL against oxidative modification when it has been isolated from the plasma.

The animal models in use may not be appropriate. For example, the lipoprotein levels in these models, such as the LDL receptor-deficient rabbit and the cholesterol-fed rabbit, may be so high that the effectiveness of antioxidants is masked and underestimated.

Prasad et al. [14] studied rabbits fed cholesterol at 0.5% and at 1.0% in the diet. At the lower cholesterol intake, with cholesterol levels in the plasma correspondingly lower, probucol inhibited lesion formation by 41%. In contrast, with cholesterol intake of 1.0% (and the same intake of probucol) the inhibition of lesion formation was only about 17%. The extent of lesions was of course much greater in the group fed 1% cholesterol.

Summary

There remain many unanswered questions about the quantitative relationship between antioxidant protection of LDL and protection of the arterial wall against lesion formation. Much more needs to be done at the level of animal models. Certainly it is too early to extrapolate to the human disease until clinical trial evidence supports the validity of the antioxidant hypothesis in the human disease. Unfortunately, because it is relatively easy to measure the resistance of LDL to oxidative modification, many papers are appearing that report rather modest differences in lag time yet interpret those differences to relate to resistance to atherogenesis. Often the differences in lag time are as small as 20 to 40%. Yet the experience with animal models is that the lag time has to be increased several-fold at a minimum before there is much effect on lesion formation. Of course, it is quite possible that even small differences over the much longer life history of the human lesion become relevant. Only time will tell. Meanwhile, it is to be hoped that systematic studies will be undertaken of: a) the quantitative relationship between plasma lipoprotein levels and the rate of progression of arterial lesions; and b) the quantitative relationship between prolongation of lag time (or other measures of resistance to LDL oxidation) and the degree of protection against progression of atherosclerotic lesions.

References

1.   Steinberg D, Parthasarathy S, Carew TE, Khoo JC, Witztum JL. Beyond cholesterol. Modifications of low-density lipoprotein that increase its atherogenicity [see comments]. N Engl J Med 1989;320:915-24.
2.   Steinberg D. Oxidative modification of LDL and atherogenesis. The 1995 Lewis A. Conner Memorial Lecture. Circulation 1997;95:1062-71.
3.   Suzuki H, Kurihara Y, Takeya M, et al. Resistance to atherosclerosis and susceptibility to

infection in scavenger receptor knockout mice. Nature 1997;386:292-96.

4.   Esterbauer H, Puhl H, Dieber-Rotheneder M, Waeg G, Rabl H. Effect of antioxidants on oxidative modification of LDL. Ann Med 1991;23:573-81.

5.   Sasahara M, Raines EW, Chait A, Carew TE, Steinberg D, Wahl PW, Ross R. Inhibition of hypercholesterolemia-induced atherosclerosis in the nonhuman primate by probucol. I. Is the extent of atherosclerosis related to resistance of LDL to oxidation? J Clin Invest 1994;94:155-64.

6.   McPherson R, Hogue M, Milne RW, Tall AR, Marcel YL. Increase in plasma cholesteryl ester transfer protein during probucol treatment. Relation to changes in high density lipoprotein composition. Aterioscler Thromb 1991;11:476-81.

7.   Ku G, Thomas CE, Akeson AL, Jackson RL. Induction of interleukin-1- beta expression from human blood monocyte-derived macrophages by 9-hydroxyoctadecadienoic acid. J Biol Chem 1992;267:14183-88.

8.   Fruebis J, Steinberg D, Dresel HA, Carew TE. A comparison of the antiatherogenic effects of probucol and of a structural analogue of probucol in low density lipoprotein receptor-deficient rabbits. J Clin Invest 1994;94:392-98.

9.   Carew TE, Schwenke DC, Steinberg D. Antiatherogenic effect of probucol unrelated to its hypocholesterolemic effect: evidence that antioxidants in vivo can selectively inhibit low density lipoprotein degradation in macrophage-rich fatty streaks and slow the progression of atherosclerosis in the Watanabe heritable hyperlipidemic rabbit. Proc Natl Acad Sci USA 1987;84:7725-29.

10.   Sparrow CP, Doebber TW, Olszewski J, Wu MS, Ventre J, Stevens KA, Chao YS. Low density lipoprotein is protected from oxidation and the progression of atherosclerosis is slowed in cholesterol-fed rabbits by the antioxidant N,N'-diphenyl-phenylenediamine. J Clin Invest 1992;89:1885-91.

11.   Fruebis J, Carew TE, Palinski W. Effect of vitamin E on atherogenesis in LDL receptor-deficient rabbits. Atherosclerosis 1995;117:217-24.

12.   O'Leary V, Tilling L, Fleetwood G, Stone D, Darley-Usmar V. The resistance of low density lipoprotein to oxidation promoted by copper and its use as an index of antioxidant therapy. Atherosclerosis 1995;119:169-79.

13.   Esterbauer H, Dieber-Rotheneder M, Waeg G, Puhl H, Tatzber F. Endogenous antioxidants and lipoprotein oxidation. Biochem Soc Trans 1990;18:1059-61.

14.   Prasad K, Kalra J, Lee P. Oxygen free radicals as a mechanism of hypercholesterolemic atherosclerosis: effects of probucol. International J Angio 1994;3:100-12.

George Steiner

Magnitude of the Problem of Atherosclerosis in Diabetes

Most studies have found that the incidence of coronary artery disease mortality in those with diabetes is between 2 and 4 times greater than that in the general population [1]. A similar increase is found in fatal and nonfatal cerebrovascular disease events [1]. Additionally the increase in the incidence of intermittent claudication, a reflection of peripheral arterial disease, in those with diabetes is even greater [2]. The increase in atherosclerosis seen in diabetes has been found in almost all populations, whether their basal incidence of atherosclerotic vascular disease is high or low [3-5]. While there is some controversy, it is generally felt that women lose some or all of their premenopausal protection from atherosclerosis if they have diabetes [1]. The increase in the incidence of coronary disease is found both in those with type 1 and those with type 2 diabetes [6-8]. However, the magnitude of the problem of atherosclerosis is by far greater in type 2 diabetes than it is in type 1 diabetes. At least a part, if not all, of the reasons for this is that the majority of diabetes is type 2 diabetes and that type 2 diabetes occurs in the older, and therefore more atherosclerosis-prone, population. In the United States, based on 1993 estimates of the total population, the prevalence of diabetes, the number of death certificates listing diabetes as a diagnosis and the recognition that 65% of deaths in diabetes are related to atherosclerosis, one can estimate that approximately 100,000 people die per annum with diabetes and atherosclerotic cardiovascular disease.

Dyslipoproteinemias and Hyperinsulinemia as Risk Factors for Atherosclerosis in Diabetes

Many factors have been suggested to play a role in increasing atherogenesis in diabetes. The basis for the suggestions comes from epidemiologic evidence, pathophysiologic studies, or reasonable postulates. No single factor should be looked upon as "the cause" for the problem. Rather, this is a multifactorial process. Many aspects of these risk factors have been reviewed by others [1,9,10] and this review will be confined to those aspects relating to insulin and lipoproteins.

Studies in general populations have indicated that hyperinsulinemia marks people who have an increased risk for coronary artery disease [11-15]. Interestingly, this

A. M. Gotto, Jr. et al. (eds.), Multiple Risk Factors in Cardiovascular Disease, 165–170.

association r ıay be either exclusive to, or stronger in men than in women. There is a well-recognized association between the insulin resistance syndrome and early coronary artery disease [16,17]. Many factors that may, themselves, increase the coronary risk are found in people with the insulin resistance syndrome. Some of these are hypertriglyceridemia, the presence of small dense low density lipoprotein (LDL), hypertension, alterations in blood coagulation factors, and abdominal obesity. One may ask whether it is the hyperinsulinemia or the insulin resistance that underlies these associations. In addition, many of the insulin assays have also detected proinsulin and its split products and it is not clear which one or ones of these may be "the risk factor" [18,19]. Many suggest that the contributions of proinsulin and of the split products may be very small in those without diabetes and, therefore, may not alter the conclusions in that population. However, in those with diabetes the contributions of proinsulin and split products to the insulin assay may be greater and, therefore, definite answers in that population may require assays that are specific for insulin. At the moment, there are some suggestions that hyperinsulinemia may also be accompanied by an increase in atherosclerosis in diabetes [20]. Clearly these observations raise two important questions in the treatment of diabetes. Should one treat the person by injecting exogenous insulin or by stimulating the pancreas to secrete more insulin? Should the treatment avoid hyperinsulinemia? There are no clear answers to either of these. The Diabetes Control and Complications Trial, which showed a clear reduction of *micro*vascular disease in those treated intensively (and therefore with higher doses) insulin than in those treated routinely (and therefore with lower doses). It also found that *macro*vascular disease was reduced, but this was not significant [21]. On the other hand, there are two smaller studies that failed to find any reduction, and even suggested an increase, in coronary disease, in those treated receiving higher doses of insulin [22,23].

The most frequent form of hyperlipoproteinemia in diabetes is hypertriglyceridemia [24]. This primarily reflects an increase in the numbers of the smaller (Sf 12-60) triglyceride-rich lipoproteins, a fraction that has been called intermediate density lipoprotein [25,26]. It is this fraction of the triglyceride-rich lipoproteins that has been associated with coronary artery disease in the general population [25].

Since hypercholesterolemia is no more frequent in those with diabetes than it is in those without [25,27], it should not be interpreted as implying that cholesterol is not important in increasing the risk of atherosclerosis in diabetes. In fact, the Multiple Risk Factor Intervention Trial demonstrated that the incidence of coronary artery disease in diabetes is curvilinearly related to the plasma cholesterol level in the same way as it is in those without diabetes [28]. It is noteworthy that although the shape of the curve relating these two variables is similar in both populations, the risk of coronary artery disease at any given cholesterol level in diabetes is four times greater than it is in those without diabetes. The reason for this increased risk at any given level of cholesterol is not yet clear. It may relate to changes that make the artery more susceptible to the atherogenic effects of LDL, or to changes that make any given amount of LDL more atherogenic. The latter could include the LDL in diabetes being glycated and oxidized [29-31]. It could also include the observation that in diabetes LDL is more frequently small and dense [32].

In those with diabetes, hypertriglyceridemia has been linked to an increased risk of coronary artery disease [33,34]. However, in only one study has high density lipoprotein (HDL) been measured simultaneously [34]. That study found that an increase in very low density lipoprotein (VLDL)-cholesterol and a decrease in HDL-cholesterol predicted an increase in the incidence of coronary artery disease in diabetes. Recently, we have observed that the severity of angiographically measured coronary artery disease in diabetes is related to the number of smaller (Sf 12-60) and larger (Sf 60-400) triglyceride-rich lipoprotein particles [35]. This relationship is independent of HDL.

We have suggested that hypertriglyceridemia and hyperinsulinemia are linked in a vicious cycle with atherogenic potential [36]. The basis for this comes from the observations that fasting triglyceride levels are positively correlated to insulin levels [36], that in the chronic hyperinsulinemic state the production of triglyceride-rich lipoproteins is increased [37,38], and that hypertriglyceridemia and insulin resistance are associated [39-41].

Intervention Studies

One would predict that, if dyslipoproteinemias play an important role in atherogenesis in diabetes, and if they have not already produced irreversible damage, correcting them would reduce the risk of atherosclerotic cardiovascular disease in that population. There is evidence that this is so in those without diabetes [42-45]. However, to date no studies have been completed that are designed specifically to address this prediction in diabetes [46].

A post hoc analysis of the few people with diabetes in the Helsinki Heart Study did suggest that, also in that population, treatment with gemfibrozil might reduce coronary artery disease [47]. However, this was not significant. Two recently published cholesterol lowering studies, the Scandinavian Simvastatin Survival Study (4S) and the CARE study, also conducted post hoc analyses of their diabetic participants [44,48]. Both report that cholesterol lowering led to a significant reduction in coronary artery disease. The characteristics of the CARE study have not yet been as fully described as those of the 4S study. The interpretation of the latter is limited by the post hoc nature of the analysis and by the characteristics of the participants. Only approximately 4% of the 4S population had diabetes. This is about one-quarter of the prevalence of diabetes in a Scandinavian population comparable age and suggests that there was some selection bias in the diabetics in the 4S study. This might have occurred because of the exclusion of anyone with plasma triglyceride levels exceeding 2.5 mmol/L from the study. It also points out one severe limitation on the implications of this study for diabetes. The 4S study does not address the most frequently observed form of dyslipoproteinemia in diabetes.

One study that is specifically designed to determine whether correcting the dyslipoproteinemia of diabetes will reduce coronary artery disease is currently well under way. It is the multinational Diabetes Atherosclerosis Intervention Study (DAIS) that is being conducted in collaboration with the World Health Organization. The details of its protocol have been published [49]. In summary, it is an angiographic study being conducted in both men and women with type 2 diabetes, who have the mild to moderate increases in plasma triglyceride and/or LDL that is typical of this form of diabetes. The participants may or may not have had previous clinical coronary disease. They undergo pretreatment quantitative angiography and are then treated with either placebo or micronized fenofibrate for a minimum of three years. At the end of this time, all will undergo repeat angiography. The two angiograms will be evaluated by a computer assisted system and compared to each other. In the near future we should know, from studies aimed specifically at those with diabetes, whether correcting the dyslipoproteinemias of diabetes will reduce the major health problem, atherosclerosis, facing that group of people.

References

1.   Haffner SM, Stern MP, Rewers M. Diabetes and atherosclerosis: Epidemiological considerations. In: Draznin B, Eckel RH, editors. Diabetes and atherosclerosis. Amsterdam: Elsevier Science, 1993:229-54.

2.   Widmer LK, Greensher A, Kannel WB. Occlusion of peripheral arteries: A study of 6400 working subjects. Circulation 1964;30:836-52.

3.   Fukuda H, Katsurada A, Iritani N. Nutritional and hormonal regulation of mRNA levels of lipogenic enzymes in primary cultures of rat hepatocytes. J Biochem (Tokyo) 1992;111:25-30.

4.   Howard BV, Lisse JR, Knowler WC, Davis MP, Pettitt DJ, Bennett PH. Diabetes and atherosclerosis in the Pima Indians. Mt Sinai J Med 1982;49:169-75.

5.   Diabetes Drafting Group. Prevalence of small vessel and large vessel disease in diabetic patients from 14 centres: The World Health Organization multinational study of vascular disease in diabetics. Diabetologia 1985;28:615-40.

6.   Krolewski AS, Kosinski EJ, Warram JH, et al. Magnitude and determinants of coronary artery disease in juvenile-onset, insulin-dependent diabetes mellitus. Am J Cardiol 1987;59:750-55.

7.   Krolewski AS, Warram JH, Valsania P, Martin BC, Laffel LM, Christlieb AR. Evolving natural history of coronary artery disease in diabetes mellitus. Am J Med 1991;90:56S-61S.

8.   Steiner G. Atherosclerosis, the major complication of diabetes. In: Vranic M, Hollenberg CH, Steiner G, editors. Comparison of type I and type II diabetes. New York: Plenum, 1985:277-97.

9.   Kannel WB, D'Agostino RB, Wilson PW, Belanger AJ, Gagnon DR. Diabetes, fibrinogen, and risk of cardiovascular disease: The Framingham experience. Am Heart J 1990;120:672-76.

10.   Pyorala K, Laakso M, Uusitupa M. Diabetes and atherosclerosis: An epidemiologic view. Diabetes Metab Rev 1987;3:463-524.

11.   Pyorala K. Hyperinsulinaemia as predictor of atherosclerotic vascular disease: Epidemiological evidence. Diabete Metab 1991;17:87-92.

12.   Pyorala K, Savolainen E, Kaukola S, Haapakoski J. Plasma insulin as coronary heart disease risk factor: Relationship to other risk factors and predictive value during 9 1/2-year follow-up of the Helsinki Policemen Study population. Acta Med Scand Suppl 1985;701:38-52.

13.   Fontbonne AM, Eschwege EM. Insulin and cardiovascular disease. Paris Prospective Study. Diabetes Care 1991;14:461-69.

14.   Fontbonne A, Eschwege E. Insulin-resistance, hypertriglyceridaemia and cardiovascular risk: The Paris Prospective Study. Diabete Metab 1991;17:93-95.

15.   Pyorala K. Hyperinsulinaemia as predictor of atherosclerotic vascular disease: Epidemiological evidence. Diabete et Metabolisme 1991;17:87-92.

16.   Reaven GM. Insulin resistance and compensatory hyperinsulinemia: Role in hypertension, dyslipidemia, and coronary heart disease. Am Heart J 1991;121:1283-88.

17.   Modan M, Or J, Karasik A, et al. Hyperinsulinemia, sex, and risk of atherosclerotic

cardiovascular disease. Circulation 1991;84:1165-75.

18. Wareham NJ, Byrne CD, Hales CN. Role of insulin and proinsulin in diabetic vascular disease. Metabolism 1995;44:76-82.

19. Bavenholm P, Karpe F, Proudler A, Tornvall P, Crook D, Hamsten A. Association of insulin and insulin propeptides with an atherogenic lipoprotein phenotype. Metabolism 1995;44:1481-88.

20. Ronnemaa T, Laakso M, Puukka P, Kallio V, Pyorala K. Atherosclerotic vascular disease in middle-aged, insulin-treated, diabetic patients. Association with endogenous insulin secretion capacity. Arteriosclerosis 1988;8:237-44.

21. The Diabetes Control and Complications Trial Research Group. The effect of intensive treatment of diabetes on the development and progression of long-term complications in insulin dependent diabetes mellitus. N Engl J Med 1993;329:977-86.

22. Janka HU, Ziegler AG, Standl E, Mehnert H. Daily insulin dose as a predictor of macrovascular disease in insulin treated non-insulin-dependent diabetics. Diabete Metab 1987;13:359-64.

23. Abraira C, Colwell J, Nuttall F, et al. Cardiovascular events and correlates in the Veterans Affairs Diabetes Feasibility Trial. Veterans Affairs Cooperative Study on Glycemic Control and Complications in Type II Diabetes. Arch Intern Med 1997;157:181-88.

24. Steiner G. The dyslipoproteinemias of diabetes. [Review] [40 refs]. Atherosclerosis 1994;110 Suppl:S27-33.

25. Steiner G, Schwartz L, Shumak S, Poapst M. The association of increased levels of intermediate-density lipoproteins with smoking and with coronary artery disease. Circulation 1987;75:124-30.

26. Reardon MF, Poapst ME, Steiner G. The independent synthesis of intermediate density lipoproteins in type III hyperlipoproteinemia. Metabolism 1982;31:421-27.

27. Harris MI. Hypercholesterolemia in diabetes and glucose intolerance in the U.S. population. Diabetes Care 1991;14:366-74.

28. Stamler J, Vaccaro O, Neaton JD, Wentworth D. Diabetes, other risk factors, and 12-yr cardiovascular mortality for men screened in the Multiple Risk Factor Intervention Trial. Diabetes Care 1993;16:434-44.

29. Picard S. Lipoprotein glyco-oxidation. Diabete Metab 1995;21:89-94.

30. Kawamura M, Heinecke JW, Chait A. Pathophysiological concentrations of glucose promote oxidative modification of low density lipoprotein by a superoxide-dependent pathway. Journal of Clinical Investigation 1994;94:771-78.

31. Lyons TJ, Lopes-Virella MF. Glycation related mechanisms. In: Draznin B, Eckel RH, editors. Diabetes and atherosclerosis. Amsterdam: Elsevier, 1993:169-90.

32. Feingold KR, Grunfeld C, Pang M, et al. LDL subclass phenotypes and triglyceride metabolism in non-insulin-dependent diabetes. Arterioscler Thromb 1992;12:1492-1502.

33. Fontbonne A, Eschwege E, Cambien F, et al. Hypertriglyceridaemia as a risk factor of coronary heart disease mortality in subjects with impaired glucose tolerance or diabetes. Results from the 11-year follow-up of the Paris Prospective Study. Diabetologia 1989;32:300-304.

34. Laakso M, Lehto S, Penttila I, Pyorala K. Lipids and lipoproteins predicting coronary heart disease mortality and morbidity in patients with non-insulin-dependent diabetes [see comments]. Circulation 1993;88:1421-30.

35. Tkac I, Kimball B, Lewis GF, Uffelman KD, Steiner G. The severity of coronary atherosclerosis in type 2 diabetes mellitus is related to the number of circulating

triglyceride-rich lipoprotein particles. Arterioscler Thromb Vasc Biol 1997; in press.

36. Steiner G, Vranic M. Hyperinsulinemia and hypertriglyceridemia, a vicious cycle with atherogenic potential. Int J Obes 1982;6(Suppl.1):117-24.

37. Streja DA, Marliss EB, Steiner G. The effects of prolonged fasting on plasma triglyceride kinetics in man. Metabolism 1977;26:505-16.

38. Steiner G, Haynes FJ, Yoshino G, Vranic M. Hyperinsulinemia and in vivo very-low-density lipoprotein-triglyceride kinetics. Am J Physiol 1984;246:E187-E192.

39. Steiner G, Morita S, Vranic M. Resistance to insulin but not to glucagon in lean human hypertriglyceridemics. Diabetes 1980;29:899-905.

40. Steiner G. Altering triglyceride concentrations changes insulin-glucose relationships in hypertriglyceridemic patients. Double-blind study with gemfibrozil with implications for atherosclerosis. Diabetes Care 1991;14:1077-81.

41. Zuniga-Guarjardo S, Steiner G, Shumak S, Zinman B. Insulin resistance and action in hypertriglyceridemia. Diabetes Res Clin Pract 1991;14:55-61.

42. Kjekshus J, Pedersen TR, Tobert JA. Lipid-lowering therapy for patients with or at risk of coronary artery disease. Current Opinion in Cardiology 1996;11:418-27.

43. Shepherd J, Cobbe SM, Ford I, et al. Prevention of coronary heart disease with pravastatin in men with hypercholesterolemia. N Engl J Med 1995;333:1301-07.

44. Sacks FM, Pfeffer MA, Moye LA, et al. The effect of pravastatin on coronary events after myocardial infarction in patients with average cholesterol levels. N Engl J Med 1996;335:1001-1009.

45. Anonymous. Randomised trial of cholesterol lowering in 4444 patients with coronary heart disease: The Scandinavian Simvastatin Survival Study (4S) [see comments]. Lancet 1994;344:1383-89.

46. Pyorala K, Steiner G. Will correction of dyslipoproteinaemia reduce coronary heart disease risk in patients with non-insulin-dependent diabetes? Need for trial evidence. [Review] [35 refs]. Annals of Medicine 1996;28:357-62.

47. Frick MH, Elo O, Haapa K, et al. Helsinki Heart Study: primary-prevention trial with gemfibrozil in middle-aged men with dyslipidemia. Safety of treatment, changes in risk factors, and incidence of coronary heart disease. N Engl J Med 1987;317:1237-45.

48. Pyorala K, Pedersen TR, Kjekshus J, Faergeman O, Olsson AG, Thorgeirsson G, The Scandinavian Simvastatin Survival Study (4S) Group. Cholesterol lowering with simvastatin improves prognosis of diabetic patients with coronary heart disease. Diabetes Care 1997;20:614-21.

49. Steiner G. The Diabetes Atherosclerosis Intervention Study (DAIS): A study conducted in cooperation with the World Health Organization. The DAIS Project Group. Diabetologia 1996;39:1655-61.

INSULIN RESISTANCE: WHAT, WHY, AND HOW

Gerald M. Reaven

Introduction

Over the past 20 years it has become increasingly clear that the ability of insulin to mediate glucose disposal varies widely from person to person, and that this difference plays a major role in development of what are often designated as diseases of Western civilization—Type 2 diabetes, hypertension, and coronary heart disease [1,2]. The general nature of this problem has been extensively reviewed [1,2], and in this presentation an effort will be made to look at it from a somewhat different perspective. In particular, attention will be directed to some background issues that, although rarely addressed, are intrinsic to our understanding of the syndromes associated with insulin resistance, and, in particular, Syndrome X [1,2]. More specifically, attention will be directed to answering three rhetorical questions.

What Do We Mean by Insulin Resistance?

Quantitative assessments of insulin action are almost uniformly made by techniques that primarily estimate the ability of insulin to mediate glucose uptake by muscle. As a consequence, the statement that "insulin resistance" exists usually means that a defined amount of insulin stimulates glucose uptake by muscle to a lesser degree than it does in an "insulin sensitive" person. However, there is no accepted definition of who is insulin resistant and who is insulin sensitive. Indeed, the data in Figure 1 emphasize the fact that there is an enormous variability in degree of insulin resistance in a healthy, nonobese population, and that this function is distributed continuously throughout the population. The most insulin resistant individuals in this study (the highest steady-state plasma glucose [SSPG] values in Figure 1) were able to maintain normal glucose tolerance, and prevent the development of Type 2 diabetes, by secreting large amounts of insulin. If it is possible to maintain this state of compensatory hyperinsulinemia, total muscle glucose disposal can be kept at a normal level. On the other hand, there are a series of questions related to insulin resistance that arise once this rather simplistic definition has been made.

A. M. Gotto, Jr. et al. (eds.), Multiple Risk Factors in Cardiovascular Disease, 171–179.

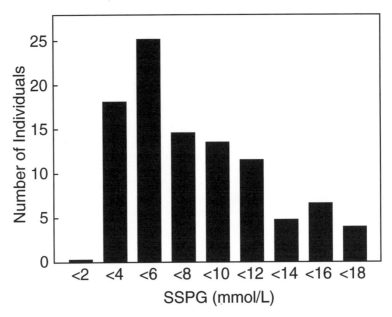

Figure 1. Frequency distribution of SSPG concentration in 94 healthy nonobese individuals. Volunteers were infused for 180 minutes with somatostatin (5µg/min), insulin (40mU/m^2/min), and glucose (280 mg/m^2/min). Since the steady-state plasma insulin concentrations were the same in all individuals, the SSPG concentration provides a direct estimate of the ability of insulin to mediate disposal of the infused glucose load; the higher the SSPG, the more insulin resistant the subject.

DIFFERENCES IN TISSUE SENSITIVITY TO INSULIN

Insulin, or insulin-like hormones, are present in most forms of life, and in the process of evolution has come their role in regulation of energy metabolism that we now recognize. As a corollary, although insulin receptors are present on multiple cell types, insulin action is dependent upon differentiation in signal transduction mechanisms that are cell-specific. Perhaps the most relevant example of this as concerns the pathophysiology of insulin resistance involves the difference between insulin action on the kidney and muscle. There is evidence that both endogenous and exogenous hyperinsulinemia increase sodium retention by the kidney and decrease urinary uric acid clearance [3-6]. The former effect may help explain the link between insulin resistance, hyperinsulinemia, and hypertension [2,7]. Indeed, evidence has been published showing that salt-sensitivity is associated with insulin resistance and/or compensatory hyperinsulinemia [8,9]. In the case of the decrease in urinary uric acid clearance, the fact that insulin has this capacity helps explain the recently described relationship between insulin resistance, compensatory hyperinsulinemia, and height of serum uric acid concentration [4]. In both of these examples the premise is that day-long increases in insulin response, as seen in nondiabetic individuals with muscle insulin resistance, leads to enhanced renal sodium retention and decreased urinary uric acid clearance. Obviously, this formulation is based on the premise that the sensitivity of the kidney to the effects of insulin on renal sodium and uric acid handling can be maintained in the face of muscle insulin resistance. This notion of differences in tissue sensitivity to insulin has been documented by results showing that the ability of insulin to increase renal sodium retention and decrease uric acid clearance is normal in individuals who have evidence of resistance to insulin action on glucose disposal by muscle [5,10].

A somewhat more complicated issue, related to differences in tissue insulin sensitivity, involves the liver. Perhaps the most common abnormality associated with muscle insulin resistance and compensatory hyperinsulinemia is an increase in hepatic very low density lipoprotein (VLDL)-triglyceride (TG) secretion and elevated plasma TG concentrations [11]. In order for these two events to exist simultaneously, i.e. a defect in insulin-stimulated glucose uptake by muscle and an increase in hepatic VLDL-TG secretion, the liver must remain normally sensitive to the interaction between ambient insulin and free fatty acid (FFA) concentrations in regulation of hepatic VLDL-TG synthesis [12] in the face of muscle insulin resistance. Fortunately, there is also published information showing that this is most likely the case [13].

DIFFERENCES IN TISSUE DOSE-RESPONSE CURVES

As indicated previously, the phrase "insulin resistance" is almost always used to refer to muscle. However, although only recently appreciated, adipose tissue appears to be as resistant to regulation by insulin as muscle [14,15]. The explanation for this belated recognition of adipose tissue insulin resistance is readily understood if one takes into account both the techniques usually used to assess resistance to insulin-mediated glucose disposal and the differences in the dose responses characteristics of insulin action on adipose tissue versus muscle. For example, we have shown [15] that a plasma insulin concentration of ~20 μU/mL will suppress by approximately 50% the release of free fatty acids (FFA) by adipose tissue; a circulating insulin concentration that has essentially no effect on stimulating glucose disposal by muscle. The infusion techniques conventionally used to quantify insulin resistance, i.e. the ability of insulin to stimulate glucose disposal by muscle, have almost uniformly been performed by maintaining steady-state insulin concentrations at least fourfold greater than the level needed to half-maximally suppress adipose tissue lipolysis. As a result, plasma FFA levels were maximally suppressed in all subjects, and differences in adipose tissue resistance to insulin could not be discerned. It is now clear that the degree of insulin resistance in muscle and adipose tissue is highly correlated [16], and that both defects contribute to the manifestations of Syndrome X. For example, the results shown in Figure 2 are from a study comparing day-long plasma, glucose, insulin, FFA, and glycerol concentrations in hypertriglyceridemic and normotriglyceridemic individuals [17]. Muscle insulin resistance in the hypertriglyceridemic subjects leads to a significant degree of compensatory hyperinsulinemia. However, the increase in plasma insulin concentration could not totally overcome the insulin resistance in adipose tissue, and there was also a modest increase in FFA and glycerol concentrations. When subjected to multiregression analysis, both circulating insulin and FFA concentrations were found to be independent predictors of the degree of hypertriglyceridemia.

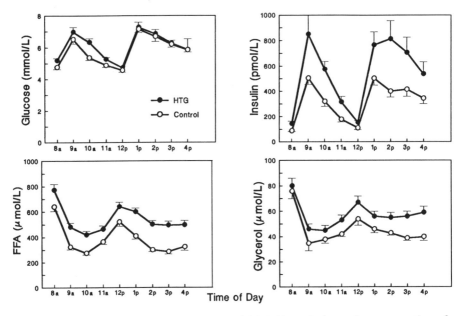

Figure 2. Plasma glucose, insulin, free fatty acid (FFA), and glycerol concentrations from 8:00 a.m. to 4:00 p.m. insulin resistant, in hypertriglyceridemic (●--●) and control (o--o) subjects. Blood was drawn at hourly intervals before and after breakfast (8 a.m.) and lunch (12 p.m.). Reprinted from reference 17 with permission of the authors and the journal.

Why Is Insulin Resistance Important?

The vast majority of patients with Type 2 diabetes are insulin resistant [1], and results of both cross-sectional and prospective studies have emphasized the importance of resistance to insulin-mediated glucose disposal as a defect leading to the development of Type 2 diabetes [18-21]. These observations, by themselves, testify to the importance of variations in insulin-mediated glucose disposal in the genesis of a common and serious disease; the prevalence of which is rapidly developing into an epidemic. However, as important as insulin resistance is in the pathophysiology of Type 2 diabetes, it assumes an even more powerful role if one focuses on its relationship to coronary heart disease (CHD). Up until quite recently, consideration of the metabolic risk factors contributing to CHD have almost entirely been confined to abnormalities of cholesterol metabolism. In that context, there is now general agreement that increases in low density lipoprotein (LDL)-cholesterol concentration increase risk of CHD. However, it is becoming increasingly evident that the cluster of abnormalities associated with insulin resistance (Syndrome X) may be as important, if not more important, as is hypercholesterolemia in increasing risk for CHD

[2,22].

How Does Insulin Resistance Increase Risk for CHD?

There are multiple factors associated with insulin resistance that increase risk for CHD [2,22]. For both intellectual and practical reasons it would be helpful to know the relative importance of these individual risk factors. Is insulin resistance or compensatory hyperinsulinemia the culprit? Both? Neither? A high TG and/or a low high-density lipoprotein (HDL)-cholesterol? The purpose of this section is to suggest that attempts to solve this issue may be misleading, and lead to more confusion than clarity. For this purpose, two examples will be cited.

INSULIN RESISTANCE VERSUS COMPENSATORY HYPERINSULINEMIA

Of relevance to the issue of what components of Syndrome X cause CHD is the recent report from the Insulin Resistance Atherosclerosis Study (IRAS) group [23]. The IRAS investigators quantified a variety of variables in a cross-sectional study of ~1500 individuals, and concluded that insulin resistance, but not hyperinsulinemia, correlated with intimal-medial thickness of the carotid artery as determined by B-mode ultrasonography. More specifically, they concluded that "insulin resistance may have an independent effect on atherogenesis," irrespective of any other associated variables. Although this may be true, caution should be exercised in drawing conclusions of pathophysiologic causality from epidemiologic observations. To begin with, consideration should be given to possible shortcomings of the statistical methods used. For example, the IRAS investigators conclude "that the relation of insulin sensitivity with atherosclerosis is stronger than that between insulin measures and atherosclerosis." However, this does no rule out the possibility that the compensatory hyperinsulinemia directly related to degree of insulin resistance in nondiabetic subjects [24,25] plays a role, direct or indirect, in the pathogenesis of atherosclerosis. The reproducibility of the method used to quantify insulin sensitivity in the IRAS study has been estimated to have a coefficient of variation of ~15% when the study is performed twice in the same person [26]. In contrast, the plasma insulin concentration two hours after an oral glucose tolerance test varied by more than 30% in half of a group of normal subjects studied 48 hours apart in a clinical research setting [27]. It is obvious that the more precisely two variables are measured, the greater the chances that a relationship between them might be discerned. In addition, the complexity involved in the regulation of the variable in question cannot be ignored. Thus, although methods used to quantify insulin sensitivity are complicated, the phenomenon measured is straightforward. Conversely, although measurement of plasma insulin concentration is quite simple, the variable in question is a complex result of degree of insulin resistance, plasma glucose concentration, and pancreatic insulin secretory response [25], not to mention differences in insulin catabolic rate. This issue is further confounded by the variable relationship that had to exist between insulin resistance and hyperinsulinemia in the IRAS study. Both diabetic and nondiabetic subjects were included, and the relationship between insulin resistance and the plasma insulin response to oral glucose varies dramatically as a function of degree of glucose tolerance. Specifically, there is an approximate 10-fold variability between degrees of insulin resistance in normal subjects, with a strong, direct relationship between degree of insulin resistance and extent of the plasma insulin response [24,25]. In contrast, there is much less variability in the degree of insulin resistance in patients with noninsulin-dependent diabetes mellitus (NIDDM) [1,28,29]. Indeed, the IRAS investigators could find no measurable insulin action in ~15% of the population, or ~210 subjects, primarily those with Type 2 diabetes. Thus, ~50% of the patients with Type 2 diabetes studied were absolutely insulin resistant by the technique used. Furthermore, the relationship between insulin resistance and plasma insulin response to glucose can range from a positive to a negative one in this heterogeneous population [29,30]. Consequently, it is necessary to question the conclusion that insulin resistance, rather than compensatory hyperinsulinemia, is responsible for Syndrome X.

On the other hand, this is not meant to imply that hyperinsulinemia, *per se*, rather than insulin resistance, is the "cause" of Syndrome X. Perhaps the simplest way to emphasize this point is to imagine the metabolic effects of infusing an insulin sensitive person with glucose. Such an intervention would lead to an increase in plasma insulin concentration, an increased rate of glucose disposal, a fall in plasma FFA and glycerol concentrations, and, in the absence of the essential substrate, a decline in hepatic VLDL-TG secretion and plasma TG concentration. Obviously, a situation which does not in the remotest mimic Syndrome X.

HYPERTRIGLYCERIDEMIA, SYNDROME X, AND CHD

An increase in plasma TG concentration is perhaps the most common metabolic characteristic of Syndrome X [31]. Despite the fact that the existence of an association between CHD and hypertriglyceridemia has been appreciated for more than 30 years [32], not everyone believes that there is a causal relationship between abnormal TG metabolism and CHD [33,34]. This is not due to lack of experimental data, but from an emphasis on the results of statistical analyses applied to large bodies of epidemiologic observations. The majority of studies aimed at defining the risk factors involved in the development of CHD have demonstrated a highly statistically significant relation between plasma TG concentration and risk of CHD [35]. When more sophisticated statistical methods are used to evaluate the relative impact of a number of individual factors that might be related to CHD, however, the relation between plasma TG concentration and CHD frequently loses statistical significance. For example, when attempts are made to differentiate between the risk factor status of changes in concentration of total or LDL-cholesterol, HDL-cholesterol, or TG, it is often concluded that an increase in plasma TG concentration is not an independent risk factor for CHD. More specifically, when both HDL-cholesterol and TG concentrations have been measured and multivariate analysis used, a low HDL-cholesterol concentration almost always emerges as an independent risk factor for CHD, whereas a high TG concentration rarely does. The conclusion that hypertriglyceridemia is not an independent risk factor for CHD appears to be widely accepted, and supports the frequently cited view that increases in plasma TG concentration are only of clinical relevance when the magnitude of the change increases risk of pancreatitis. The appropriateness of the multivariate statistical analyses that have been used to evaluate the relation between plasma TG concentration and CHD has been comprehensively reviewed by Austin [35]. As she emphasized, several conditions must be satisfied before conclusions based on multivariate analyses can be considered valid. In particular, great care must be exercised when two variables in question are themselves closely related. This is certainly true of this particular situation, because a high plasma TG and a low HDL-cholesterol concentration frequently occur in the same individual. When this happens, considerable caution must be exercised before deciding that one of a pair of closely related variable is statistically significant by multivariate analysis and the other is not. When two variables, in this case plasma TG and HDL-cholesterol concentrations, are highly correlated, it is essential that our ability to measure the true value of each variable precisely is equally good in order to obtain meaningful information from multivariate analysis. This requirement is not met in the case of TG and HDL-cholesterol; that is, the individual variability in TG measurements is substantially greater. When both the inverse correlation between TG and HDL-cholesterol concentrations, and the difference in the precision with which these two measurements can be made are considered, the predicted result from using multivariate analysis would be to underestimate the relation between hypertriglyceridemia and CHD. In other words, the fact that a low HDL-cholesterol concentration, but not a high plasma TG concentration, emerges from multivariate analysis as an independent CHD risk factor is almost a self-fulfilling prophecy. Furthermore, when an attempt is made to factor in the differences between the inter- and intraindividual variability in the measurements of TG and HDL-cholesterol concentrations, it appears that they are equally correlated with risk of CHD [35]. Thus, the conclusion that hypertriglyceridemia is not an independent risk factor for CHD is likely an artifact of the statistical approach that led to it.

However, even if a high plasma TG concentration, *per se,* does not lead to atherosclerosis, it is well established that hypertriglyceridemia is closely associated with a low HDL-cholesterol concentration, smaller and denser LDL-particles, enhanced postprandial lipemia, and higher levels of PAI-1 [2,22]. Although not addressed in this communication, the ample evidence that establishes the link between CHD and the changes known to be associated with hypertriglyceridemia has recently been reviewed [22,31,36]. Based on the above considerations it seems reasonable to suggest that the focus should not be on whether or not hypertriglyceridemia is an independent risk factor for CHD, but rather on the notion that this central feature of Syndrome X, and/or its associated abnormalities, play an extremely important role in the genesis of CHD.

Conclusion

Insulin resistance and its associated abnormalities are involved in the pathogenesis and clinical course of Type 2 diabetes, hypertension, and CHD. Although the overall prevalence of these diseases is slowly growing or stable in most Western countries, they are increasing at an alarming rate in underdeveloped countries, as well as in individuals of non-European descent living in developed countries. It does not seem excessive to conclude that it is time to focus more on understanding these events and attempting to intervene in an effort to halt this epidemic related to insulin resistance. In this review an effort has been made to contribute to this process by addressing issues which, although not often considered in discussion of insulin resistance and its consequence, are important in expanding our understanding of these phenomena.

References

1.   Reaven GM. Insulin resistance in noninsulin-dependent diabetes mellitus: Does it exist and can it be measured? Am J Med 1983; 74:3-17.
2.   Reaven GM. Role of insulin resistance in human disease. Diabetes 1988;37:1495-1607.
3.   DeFronzo RA, Cooke C, Andres R, Faloona GR, David PJ. The effect of insulin in renal handling of sodium, potassium, calcium and phosphate in man. J Clin Invest 1995;55:845-55.
4.   Facchini F, Chen Y-DI, Hollenbeck CB, Reaven GM. Relationship between resistance to insulin-mediated glucose uptake, urinary uric acid clearance, and plasma uric acid concentration. J Am Med Assoc 1991;266:3008-11.
5.   Quinones GA, Natali A, Baldi S, Frascerra S, Sanna G, Ciociaro D, Ferrannini E. Effect of insulin on uric acid excretion in humans. Am J Physiology 1995; 268:E1-5.
6.   Muscelli E, Natali A, Bianchi S, et al. Effect of insulin on renal sodium and uric acid handling in essential hypertension. Am J Hyperten 1996;9:746-52.
7.   Reaven GM. Insulin resistance, hyperinsulinemia, hypertriglyceridemia, and hypertension: Parallels between human disease and rodent models. Diabetes Care/Review 1991;14:195-202.
8.   Sharma AM, Schorr U, Distler A. Insulin resistance in young salt-sensitive normotensive subjects. Hypertension 1993;21:273-79.
9.   Zavaroni I, Coruzzi P, Bonini L, et al. Association between salt sensitivity and insulin concentrations in patients with hypertension. Am J Hyperten 1995;8:855-58.
10.   Skott P, Vaag A, Bruun NE, et al. Effect of insulin on renal sodium handling in hyperinsulinemia Type 2 (non-insulin-dependent) diabetic patients with peripheral insulin resistance. Diabetologia 1991;34:275-81.
11.   Olefsky JM, Farquhar JW, Reaven GM. Reappraisal of the role of insulin in hypertriglyceridemia. Am J Med 1974;57:551-60.
12.   Reaven GM, Mondon CE. Effect of in vivo plasma insulin levels on the relationship between perfusate free fatty acid concentration and triglyceride secretion by perfused rat livers. Horm Metab Res 1984;16:230-32.
13.   Bernstein RJ, Davis BM, Olefsky JM, Reaven GM. Hepatic insulin responsiveness in patients with endogenous hypertriglyceridemia. Diabetologia 1978;14:249-53.
14.   Fraze E, Donner CC, Swislocki ALM, Chiou Y-AM, Chen Y-DI, Reaven GM. Ambient plasma free fatty acid concentrations in noninsulin-dependent diabetes mellitus: Evidence for insulin resistance. J Clin Endocrinol Metab 1985;61:807-11.
15.   Swislicki ALM, Chen Y-DI, Golay A, Chang M-O, Reaven GM. Insulin suppression of plasma-free fatty acid concentration in normal individuals and patients with Type 2 (non-insulin-dependent) diabetes. Diabetologia 1987;30:622-26.
16.   Pei D, Chen Y-DI, Hollenbeck CB, Bhargave R, Reaven GM. Relationship between insulin-mediated glucose disposal by muscle and adipose tissue lipolysis in healthy volunteers. J Clin Endocrinol Metab 1995;80:3368-72.
17.   Jeng C-Y, Fuh MM-T, Sheu WH-H, Chen Y-DI, Reaven GM. Hormone and substrate

modulation of plasma triglyceride concentration in primary hypertriglyceridemia. Endocrinol Metab 1994;1:15-21.

18. Sicree RA, Zimmet PZ, King HOM, Coventry JS. Plasma insulin response among Nauruans: Prediction of deterioration in glucose tolerance over 6 yr. Diabetes 1987; 36:179-86.

19. Haffner SM, Stern MP, Mitchell BD, Hazuda HP, Patterson JK. Incidence of type II diabetes in Mexican Americans predicted by fasting insulin and glucose levels, obesity, and body-fat distribution. Diabetes 1990;39:283-88.

20. Warram JH, Martin BC, Krolewski AS, Soeldner JS, Kahn CR. Slow glucose removal rate and hyperinsulinemia precede the development of type II diabetes in the offspring of diabetic parents. Ann Intern Med 1990;113:909-15.

21. Lillioja S, Mott DM, Spraul M, et al. Insulin resistance and insulin secretory dysfunction as precursors of non-insulin-dependent diabetes mellitus. N Engl J Med 1993;329:1988-92.

22. Reaven GM. Pathophysiology of insulin resistance in human disease. Physiol Rev 1995;75: 473-86.

23. Howard G, O'Leary DH, Zaccaro D, et al. for the IRAS Investigators. Insulin sensitivity and atherosclerosis. Circulation 1996;93:1809-17.

24. Hollenbeck CB, Reaven GM. Variation in insulin-stimulated glucose uptake in healthy individuals with normal glucose tolerance. J Clin Endocrinol Metab 1987; 64:1169-73.

25. Reaven GM, Brand RJ, Chen Y-DI, Mathur AK, Goldfine I. Insulin resistance and insulin secretion are determinants of oral glucose tolerance in normal individuals. Diabetes 1993;42: 1324-1332.

26. Abbat SL, Fujimoto WY, Brunzell JD, Kahn SE. Effect of heparin on insulin-glucose interactions measured by the minimal model technique: Implications for reproducibility using this method. Metabolism 1993;42:353-57.

27. Olefsky JM, Reaven GM. Insulin and glucose responses to identical oral glucose tolerance tests performed forty-eight hours apart. Diabetes 1974;23:449-53.

28. Reaven GM, Chen Y-DI, Donner CC, Fraze E, Hollenbeck CB. How insulin resistant are patients with non-insulin-dependent diabetes mellitus? J Clin Endocrinol Metab 1985;61:32-36.

29. Reaven GM, Hollenbeck CB, Chen Y-DI. Relationship between glucose tolerance, insulin secretion, and insulin action in non-obese individuals with varying degrees of glucose tolerance. Diabetolgia 1989;32:53-55.

30. Reaven GM, and Miller R. Study of the relationship between glucose and insulin responses to an oral glucose load in man. Diabetes 1968;17:560-69.

31. Reaven GM. Hypertriglyceridemia: The central feature of Syndrome X. Cardiovascular Risk Factors 1996;6:29-35.

32. Albrink MJ, Meigs W, Man EB. Serum lipids, hypertension and coronary artery disease. Am J Med 1961:31:4-23.

33. Hulley SB, Rosenman RH, Bawol RD, Brand RJ. Epidemiology as a guide to clinical decisions. The association between triglyceride and coronary heart disease. N Engl J Med 1993;302:1383-89.

34. Criqui MH, Heiss G, Cohn R. Plasma triglyceride level and mortality from coronary heart disease. N Engl J Med 1993;328:1220-25.

35. Austin MA. Plasma triglyceride and coronary heart disease. Arterioscler Thromb 1991;11:2-14.

36. Reaven GM. Are triglycerides important as a risk factor for coronary heart disease? Heart Dis Stroke 1993;2:44-48.

D. Tschoepe

Epidemiological Considerations

The vascular morbidity rather than the mortality of patients with diabetes mellitus increases with increasing population's age in most industrialized countries which not only precipitates the incidence of type 2 diabetes, but predominantly the incidence figures of clinical apparent degenerative vasculopathies such as coronary artery disease [1-3]. Mainly this fatal situation drives the socioeconomic burden of diabetes mellitus [4,5].

The results of different population-based trials such as Framingham, PROCAM, DIS, or the Multiple Risk Factor Intervention Trial (MRFIT) show that patients with diabetes are also responsive to classical risk factors, but the imposition of hypertension, smoking, or lipid abnormalities on diabetes significantly exaggerates the incidence of cardiovascular disease and mortality. Diabetes is a risk factor by itself, but beyond the epidemiological risk associations it remains unclear from a pathogenetic point of view how these risk factors translate into clinical endpoints and by which mechanism diabetes might increase the incidence, kind, and prognosis of vascular complications [6-10].

One pathogenetic mechanism is attributed to the general finding that diabetes is associated with a hypercoagulable state. Hyperactive platelets at injured endothelial interfaces act together with an increased availability of thrombotic precursors, reduced coagulation inhibitors and diminished fibrinolysis [11-15]. This could help to explain that more than 75% of the diabetes population dies from thrombotic complications superimposed to preexisting atherosclerosis [3].

Diabetes mellitus must therefore be included into the group of arterial atherothrombotic diseases, the clinical prognosis of which becomes determined by hemostaseological control mechanisms of thrombogenesis. In the UKPDS study nearly 20% of the type 2 diabetes patients presented with electrocardiografical signs of ischemia at study entry and this figure increased up to 30% after six years study duration. Along with this a 12.1% prevalence of severe macroangiopathic ischemic events was observed in this cohort of initially included 4,209 patients. Macrovascular events accounted for more than 50% of total mortality and this underscores that the clinically relevant endpoint in the type 2 diabetic population is determined by the vascular component [16]. Atherosclerosis develops more aggressively, faster and interacts with a more sticky blood. Recent data point to the possibility that these alterations start to occur prior to the clinical manifestation of the

A. M. Gotto, Jr. et al. (eds.), Multiple Risk Factors in Cardiovascular Disease, 181–190.
© 1998 Kluwer Academic Publishers and Fondazione Giovanni Lorenzini. Printed in the Netherlands.

metabolic disease being implemented in a much wider network of classical risk factors such as hypertension, dyslipoproteinemia, or obesity in front of a genetically programmed susceptibility addressed to as metabolic syndrome [17].

In patients with diabetes mellitus the natural course of arterial ischemic events at atherosclerotic lesion sites such as myocardial infarction is significantly aggravated and results in a much higher death rate reflecting a combination from advanced microangiopathic impairment of parenchymatous organ function and overshooting rheological and hemostaseological mechanisms of ischemia. This also results in a particularly worsened short- and long-term success (patency) and complication rate following specific angiological revascularization maneuvers such as thrombolysis, by-pass surgery, or angioplasty which clearly depends upon changes of the cellular hemostasis and the plasmatic coagulation and fibrinolysis system [15,18-26].

The Prethrombotic State

Blood from patients with diabetes tends to clot shorter than "normal" blood. Interestingly, this affects the high-flow arterial circulation branch rather than the low-flow veins leading to a lowered threshold for triggering the coagulation process in favor of thrombotic occlusion of a damaged nutritive artery of an parenchymatous organ such as the heart. The thrombotic tendency results from complex changes of the cellular and plasmatic coagulation system and the respective inhibitors [13,21,27-31]. Increased availability of precursor substrates such as factor VII, VIIIc, X, fibrinogen, or tissue factor parallels reduced concentrations of anticoagulant molecules such as antithrombin, protein C/S, or thrombomodulin [11,32-34]. Reduced repair fibrinolysis results from increases in inhibitors such as PAI-1 with potentially reduced profibrinolytic tPA [35-40]. In type 2 diabetes insulin or insulin like activity such as insulin growth factor 1 (IGF- 1) appear to enhance PAI-1 concentrations [41-46], but this also occurs in the healthy population as demonstrated by the MONICA project [47]. This mechanism could potentially link the insulin resistance/hyperinsulinemia of the metabolic syndrome with the precipitation of atherosclerotic vascular disease [48,49]. What factors are controlling the clinical outcome in what patients within what circulation area remains somewhat unclear, but increases in fibrinogen together with increases in PAI-1 seem to dominate the coagulation system in metabolic syndrome patients. These factors are known to strongly correlate to cardiovascular outcome [50-52]. Patency rates from interventional maneuvers such as thrombolysis or PTCA may also be affected [20,53]. A genetic basis for these findings may be represented by a genetic variant of the PAI-1 promoter gene which associates with increased triglyceride levels thus becoming a candidate gene which indicates an increased cardiovascular risk in metabolic syndrome patients presenting with the low HDL-high triglyceride dyslipoproteinemia [54,55]. In type 2 diabetics increased platelet PAI-1 is suggested to further accelerate the thrombogenesis by local delivery of high antifibrinolytic concentrations leading to a particular rigid lysis resistant thrombus [37]. This adds significantly to the role of platelets in initiating and promulgating the instable coronary syndrome, particularly in diabetes patients [56-58] and clearly indicates the regulating role of the cellular hemostasis system components which manage local coagulation demand and delivery. Vessel wall matrix proteins and endothelial cells as well as corpuscular blood elements such as thrombocytes rule pro- and anticoagulant activity of the proteolytic enzymatic activation cascade which is nested at cellular membranes.

Endothelial Dysfunction and Platelet Hyperreactivity

Endothelial cell-derived mediators contribute to the regulation of local vasomotion and vessel wall permeability. Under normal (resting) conditions it prevents adherence of flow marginated leukocytes and thrombocytes thus managing its own cell reactivity in a paracrine manner [14,59]. Reduced prostacyclin and NO synthesis or release may significantly contribute to disturbed blood vessel wall interaction in diabetes mellitus. In addition, NO resistance of target smooth muscle cells and increased quenching by increases in reactive oxygen radicals may further contribute to early endothelial dysfunction such as constrictive vasomotor responses or increased thrombogenicity long before morphological alterations appear [59-64]. Increases in soluble endothelial cell-derived adhesion molecules may reflect early disturbances, but do not directly relate to the quality of glucose control, at least in type 2 diabetes [65]. However, *in vitro* increased glucose concentration induces transcription of such proteins [66-68], but clinically endothelial cell procoagulant activity appears to be predominantly dependent upon an off-balance of pro- and antifibrinolytic molecules such as PAI-1 and tPA. Furthermore, advanced glycation endproducts (AGE) do interfere with the endothelial production of antithrombotic thrombomodulin, but significantly induce the most powerful coagulation inducer "tissue factor" [69-72].

Platelets act as "first responsive elements" to endothelial cell disturbances. Platelet activation results from the dominance of activating over inhibitory agonists which clearly governs the situation in diabetes patients. Following activation platelets undergo a complex downstream molecular activation cascade with the key features of adhesion molecule expression and activation such as the fibrinogen receptor molecule GpIIbIIIa and generation of procoagulant surfaces [73-75]. In summary, platelet-dependent reactions may initiate the final occlusive infarction thrombus (trigger), as their release products may amplify the local atherosclerotic vessel damage (accelerator), but can definitely impair the capillary microcirculation ("embolic sowering;" for review [76-78]). In diabetes, accumulating evidence has suggested a state of primary platelet hyperreactivity ("diabetic thrombocytopathy") resulting from a changed bone marrow synthesis (for review [79]). Increased constitutive functional capacity could lower the threshold for intravasal activation explaining the finding of increased fractions of circulating activated platelets exposing adhesion molecules such as P-selectin for the attachment of white blood cells or to activated endothelium. This phenomenon was found in recent onset type 1 diabetes patients [80], but also in type 2 diabetes patients with high triglycerides and low HDL-cholesterol suffering from the metabolic syndrome [81].

Clinical Consequences

Near normoglycemic glucose control does not necessarily correct all aspects of the specific thrombotic diathesis in diabetes mellitus [82]. This fits with the key question whether the concept of tight glucose control alone achieves improvement of clinically relevant outcome figures [3]. The DCCT trial has conclusively shown that microvascular morbidity such as retinopathy, nephropathy, or neuropathy will be significantly lowered and there exists no reasonable doubt that this will apply for patients of either diabetes type. However, macrovascular events or overall mortality were not significantly affected. The price to pay for these benefits of near normoglycemic control was a significantly increased rate of severe hypoglycemia which undoubtedly must be looked upon as a particular negative factor for the vascular prognosis [83]. In fact, it has been repeatedly hypothesized that adrenergic crisis following hypoglycemia could precipitate micro- and potentially macrovascular endpoints particularly in elderly patients with preexisting severe vascular disease [84]. In this population of elderly type 2 diabetics the impact of tight glucose control continues to be an issue of controversy. The initial findings of crosscorrelation of cardiovascular events with the concomitant HbA1 value in the Framingham cohort were supported by the Scandinavian observation studies showing a worse prognosis with increasing tertiles of HbA1 for mid- to long-term cardiovascular mortality [85]. It must be emphasized that this does not prove to be evidence in favor of the concept of near normoglycemia in type 2 patients, since these trials were observational rather than interventional. In contrast, a variety of recent population based observational studies failed to link vascular outcome to the degree of metabolic control, but clearly to the control of classical risk factors such as dyslipoproteinemia or hypertension [86,87]. Furthermore, the VA feasibility trial for glucose control in noninsulin-dependent diabetes mellitus showed a negative influence of controlling for glucose upon cardiovascular outcome [88]. All this heterogeneous database forms a rational for a completely individualized therapeutic approach which avoids maniac glucose control, but rather includes all components of the vascular risk factor network identified in the individual patient explicitly including life quality measures ("risk factor management"). Glucose control represents the mandatory baseline therapy, but should be supplemented by educational advice for a healthier life style (exercise, no smoking, etc.), dietary modification ("lower cholesterol, increase unsaturated fatty acids," "antioxidants"), and pharmacological risk factor intervention forming a concept of integrated rather than monofactorial care.

Among these, antihypertensive, antihyperlipidemic, and antiplatelet agents have proven value for the preventive treatment for patients with diabetes mellitus who respond better to either interventional strategy by a factor of 2 to 3 [89]. A particular benefit will be achieved in diabetes patients with the aggressive control of cholesterol levels both in primary and secondary prevention settings as shown with the CARE (data on file) and 4S-cohort data [56,90]. It can be assumed that these added benefits largely depend on protective effects upon endothelial function leading to a passivation of blood vessel wall interaction and improved local vasomotor responses [91].

The use of antiplatelet agents interferes with the hyercoagulable state which potentially translates risk factors pathogenetically into manifest atherothrombotic endpoints.

Consecutively, the use of these agents has proven value both for the prevention of microvascular and macrovascular endpoints in patients with diabetes mellitus [92-95]. Thus, unless existing contraindications, we advocate the use of this group of agents (e.g. acetylsalicylic acid, thienopyridins, picotamid, rrr-α-tocopherol) at the earliest possible point, at least in type 2 patients where subtle clinical investigation nearly always identifies vessel wall damage even in the absence of clinical symptoms. Whether other components of the prethrombotic state in diabetes mellitus can be effectively reversed and achieve clinical significance remains unclear at present and requires further investigation.

References

1. Barinas E for the BERI investigators. International analysis of insulin-dependent diabetes mellitus mortality: A preventable mortality perspective. Am J Epidemiol 1995;142:612-18.
2. Kuller LH. Magnitude of the problem. In: Proceedings of the National Heart, Lung, and Blood Institute. Symposium on Rapid Identification and Treatment of Acute Myocardial Infarction. Issues and Answers. NIH Publication No. 91-3035: 1991;3-24.
3. Savage JP. Cardiovascular complications of diabetes mellitus: What we know and what we need to know about their prevention. Ann Int Med 1996;124:123-26
4. Bransome ED. Financing the care of diabetes mellitus in the U.S. Diab Care 1992; 15(Suppl.1):1-5.
5. Jacobs J, Sena M, Fox N. The cost of hospitalization for the late complications of diabetes in the United States. Diab Med 1990;8:523-29.
6. Agewall S, Fagerberg B, Attvall S, et al. Microalbuminuria, insulin sensitivity and haemostatic factors in non-diabetic treated hypertensive men. Risk Factor Intervention Study Group. J Intern Med 1995;237:195-203.
7. Brand FN, Abbott RD, Kannel WB. Diabetes, intermittent claudication, and risk of cardiovascular events. The Framingham Study. Diabetes 1989;38:504-9.
8. Colwell JA for the ADA. Consensus statement. Role of cardiovascular risk factors in prevention and treatment of macrovascular disease in diabetes. Diab Care 1989;12:573-79.
9. Diabetes Epidemiology Research International Mortality Study Group. International evaluation of cause-specific mortality and IDDM. Diabetes Care 1991;14:55-60.
10. Songer TJ, DeBerry K, LaPorte RE, Tuomilehto J. International comparisons of IDDM mortality. Diab Care 1992;15(Suppl.1):15-21.
11. Ceriello A. Coagulation activation in diabetes mellitus: The role of hyperglycaemia and therapeutic prospects. Diabetologia 1993;36:1119-25.
12. Ceriello A, Taboga C, Tonutti L, et al. Post-meal coagulation activation in diabetes mellitus: The effect of acarbose. Diabetologia 1996;39:469-73.
13. Chan P, Pan WH. Coagulation activation in type 2 diabetes mellitus: The higher coronary risk of female diabetic patients. Diabetes Med 1995;12:504-7.
14. Cohen RA. Dysfunction of vascular endothelium in diabetes mellitus. Circulation 1993; 87(Suppl.5):67-76.
15. Gray RP, Hendra TJ, Patterson DLH, Yudkin JS. "Spontaneous" platelet aggregation in whole blood in diabetic and non diabetic survivors of acute myocardial infarction. Thromb Haemostas 1993;70:932-36.
16. Prospective Diabetes Study Group. Perspectives in diabetes. U.K. Prospective diabetes study 16. Overview of 6 years' therapy of type II diabetes: A progressive disease. Diabetes 1995;44:

1249-58.

17. Donahue RP, Abbott RD, Reed DM, Yano K. Postchallenge glucose concentration and coronary heart disease in men of Japanese ancestry. Honolulu Heart Program. Diabetes 1987; 36:689-92.

18. Alderman EL for the BARI investigators. Comparison of coronary artery bypass surgery with angioplasty in patients with multivessel disease. N Engl J Med 1996;335:217-25.

19. Fava S, Azzopardi J, Muscat HA, Fenech FF. Factors that influence outcome in diabetic subjects with myocardial infarction. Diabetes Care 1993;16:1615-18.

20. Gray RP, Yudkin JS, Patterson DL. Enzymatic evidence of impaired reperfusion in diabetic patients after thrombolytic therapy for acute myocardial infarction: A role for plasminogen activator inhibitor? Br Heart J 1993;70:530-36.

21. Gries FA, Petersen Braun M, Tschoepe D, van de Loo J. Hemostasis and diabetic angiopathy. Pathophysiology and therapeutic concepts. Georg Thieme Verlag: Stuttgart-New York, 1993.

22. Herlitz J, Wognsen GB, Emanuelsson H, et al. Mortality and morbidity in diabetic and nondiabetic patients during a 2-year period after coronary artery bypass grafting. Diabetes Care 1996;19:698-703.

23. Jacoby RM, Nesto RW. Acute myocardial infarction in the diabetic patient: Pathophysiology, clinical course and prognosis. J Am Coll Cardiol 1992;20:736-44.

24. Kip KE, Faxxon DP, Detre KM, Yeh W, Kelsey SF, Currier JW for the NHLBI PTCA Registry. Coronary angioplasty in diabetic patients. The National Heart, Lung and Blood Institute Percutaneous Transluminal Coronary Angioplasty Registry. Circulation 1996;94: 1818-25.

25. Sprafka JM, Burke GL, Folsom AR, McGovern PG, Hahn LP. Trends in prevalence of diabetes mellitus in patients with myocardial infarction and effect of diabetes on survival. The Minnesota Heart Survey. Diabetes Care 1991;14:537-43.

26. Stein B, Weintraub WS, Gebhart SSP, et al. Influence of diabetes mellitus on early and late outcome after percutaneous transluminal coronary angioplasty. Circulation 1995;91:979-89.

27. Banga JD, Sixma JJ. Diabetes mellitus, vascular disease and thrombosis. Clin Haematol 1986; 15:465-92.

28. Colwell JA. Vascular thrombosis in type II diabetes mellitus. Diabetes 1993;42:8-11.

29. Frade LJG, de la Calle H, Alava I, Navarro JL, Creighton LJ, Gaffney PJ. Diabetes mellitus as a hypercoagulable state: Its relationship with fibrin fragments and vascular damage. Thromb Res 1987;47:533-40.

30. Ostermann H, van de Loo J. Factors of the hemostatic system in diabetic patients. A survey of controlled studies. Hemostasis 1986;16:386-416.

31. Vague P, Raccah D, Juhan Vague I. Hemobiology, vascular disease, and diabetes with special reference to impaired fibrinolysis. Metabolism 1992;41(5Suppl.1):2-6.

32. Carter M, Stickland MH, Mansfield MW, Grant PJ. ß-fibrinogen gene-455 G/A polymorphism and fibrinogen levels. Risk factors for coronary artery disease in subjects with NIDDM. Dia Care 1996;19:1265-68.

33. Gruden G, Cavallo Perin P, Romagnoli R, Olivetti C, Frezet D, Pagano G. Prothrombin fragment 1 + 2 and antithrombin III-thrombin complex in microalbuminuric type 2 diabetic patients. Diabetic Med 1994;11(5):485-88.

34. Kannel WB, D'Agostino RB, Wilson PW, Belanger AJ, Gagnon DR. Diabetes, fibrinogen, and risk of cardiovascular disease: The Framingham experience. Am Heart J 1990;120:672-76.

35. Auwerx J, Bouillon R, Collen D, Geboers J. Tissue-type plasminogen activator antigen and plasminogen activator inhibitor in diabetes mellitus. Arteriosclerosis 1988;8(1):68-72.

36.   Gough SC, Grant PJ. The fibrinolytic system in diabetes mellitus. Diabet Med 1991;8:898-905.

37.   Jokl R, Laimins M, Klein RL, Lyons TJ, Lopes-Virella MF, Colwell JA. Platelet plasminogen activator inhibitor 1 in patients with type II diabetes. Diabetes Care 1994;17:818-23.

38.   Juhan Vague I, Alessi MC, Vague P. Increased plasma plasminogen activator inhibitor 1 levels. A possible link between insulin resistance and atherothrombosis. Diabetologia 1991; 34:457-62.

39.   Ostermann H, Tschoepe D, Greber W, Meyer Rusenberg HW, van de Loo J. Enhancement of spontaneous fibrinolytic activity in diabetic retinopathy. Thromb Haemost 1992;68:400-3.

40.   Ulvenstam G, Aberg A, Bergstrand R, et al. Long-term prognosis after myocardial infarction in men with diabetes. Diabetes 1985;34:787-92.

41.   McGill JB, Schneider DJ, Arfken CL, Lucore CL, Sobel BE. Factors responsible for impaired fibrinolysis in obese subject and NIDDM patients. Diabetes 1994;43:104-9.

42.   Nordt TK, Schneider DJ, Sobel BE. Augmentation of the synthesis of plasminogen activator inhibitor type-1 by precursors of insulin. A potential risk factor for vascular disease. Circulation 1994;89:321-30.

43.   Padayatty SJ, Orme S, Zenobi PD, Stikland MH, Belchetz PE, Grant PJ. The effects of insulin-like growth factor-1 on plasminogen activator inhibitor-1 synthesis and secretion: Results from in vitro and in vivo studies. Thromb Haemostas 1993;70: 1009-13.

44.   Schneider DJ, Nordt TK, Sobel BE. Attenuated fibrinolysis and accelerated atherogenesis in type II diabetic patients. Diabetes 1993;42:1-7.

45.   Schneider DJ, Nordt TK, Sobel BE. Stimulation by proinsulin of expression of plasminogen activator inhibitor type-I in endothelial cells. Diabetes 1992;41:890-95.

46.   Schneider DJ, Sobel BE. Augmentation of synthesis of plasminogen activator inhibitor type 1 by insulin and insulin-like growth factor type I: Implications for vascular disease in hyperinsulinemic. Proc Natl Acad Sci USA 1991;88:9959-63.

47.   Eliasson M, Asplund K, Evrin PE, Lindahl B, Lundblad D. Hyperinsulinemia predicts low tissue plasminogen activator activity in a healthy population: The Northern Sweden MONICA Study. Metabolism 1994;43:1579-86.

48.   Bressler P, Bailey SR, Matsuda M, DeFronzo RA. Insulin resistance and coronary artery disease. Diabetologia 39:1345-50.

49.   Suzuki M, Shinozaki K, Kanazawa A, et al. Insulin resistance as an independent risk factor for carotid wall thickening. Hypertension 1996;28:593-98.

50.   ECAT angina pectoris study. Baseline associations of haemostatic factors with extent of coronary arteriosclerosis and other coronary risk factors in 3000 patients with angina pectoris undergoing coronary angiography. Eur Heart J 1993;14:8-17.

51.   Hamsten A, Defaire U, Walldius G, et al. Plasminogen activator inhibitor in plasma: risk factor for recurrent myocardial infarction. Lancet 1987;2:3-9.

52.   Meade TW. Thrombosis and cardiovascular disease. Ann Epidemiol 1992;2:353-64.

53.   Gray RP, Patterson DL, Yudkin JS. Plasminogen activator inhibitor activity in diabetic and nondiabetic survivors of myocardial infarction. Arterioscler Thromb 1993;13:415-20.

54.   Mansfield MW, Stickland MH, Grant PJ. Plasminogen activator inhibitor-1 (PAI-1) promoter polymorphism and coronary artery disease in non-insulin-dependent diabetes. Thromb Haemost 1995;74:1032-34.

55.   Panahloo A, Mohamed-Ali V, Lane A, Green F, Humphries SE, Yudkin JS. Determinants of plasminogen activator inhibitor 1 activity in treated NIDDM and its relation to a polymorphism in the plasminogen activator inhibitor 1 gene. Diabetes 1995;44:37-42.

56.   Genest J Jr, Cohn JS. AIMTI: Clustering of cardiovascular risk factors: Targeting high-risk
        individuals. Am J Cardiol 1995;76:8A-20A.
57.   Mizuno K, Satomura K, Miyamoto A, et al. Angioscopic evaluation of coronary- artery
        thrombi in acute coronary syndromes. N Engl J Med 1992;326:287-91.
58.   Silva JA, Escobar A, Collins TJ, Ramee SR, White CJ. Unstable angina. A comparison of
        angioscopic findings between diabetic and nondiabetic patients. Circulation 1995;92:1731-36.
59.   McGorisk GM, Treasure CB. Endothelial dysfunction in coronary heart disease. Curr Op
        Cardiol 1996;11:341-50.
60.   McVeigh GE, Brennan GM, Johnston GD, et al. Impaired endothelium-dependent and
        independent vasodilation in patients with type 2 (non-insulin-dependent) diabetes mellitus.
        Diabetologia 1992;35:771-76.
61.   Nitenberg A, Valensi P, Sachs R, Dali M, Aptecar E, Attali JR. Impairment of coronary
        vascular reserve and ACH-induced coronary vasodilation in diabetic patients with
        angiografically normal coronary arteries and normal left ventricular systolic function. Diabetes
        1993;42:1017-25.
62.   Stehouwer CDA, Nauta JJP, Zeldenrust GC, Hackeng WHL, Donker AJM, Den Ottolander
        GJH. Urinary albumin excretion, cardiovascular disease, and endothelial dysfunction in non-
        insulin-dependent diabetes mellitus. Lancet 1992;340:319-23.
63.   Yudkin JS. Coronary heart disease in diabetes mellitus: Three new risk factors and a unifying
        hypothesis. J Intern Med 1995;238:21-30.
64.   Zeiher AM, Drexler H, Wollschläger H, Just H. Modulation of coronary vasomotor tone in
        humans: Progressive dysfunction with different early stages of coronary atherosclerosis.
        Circulation 1991;83:391-401.
65.   Steiner M, Reinhardt KM, Krammer B, Ernst B, Blann D. Increased levels of soluble adhesion
        molecules in type-2 diabetic patients. Thromb Haemostas 1994;72:979-84.
66.   Lorenzi M, Cagliero E. Pathobiology of endothelial and other vascular cells in diabetes
        mellitus. Call for Data. Diabetes 1991;40:653-59.
67.   Lorenzi M. Glucose toxicity in the vascular complications of diabetes: The cellular
        perspective. Diab Metab Rev 1992;8:85-103.
68.   Maiello M, Boeri D, Podesta F, et al. Increased expression of tissue plasminogen activator and
        its inhibitor and reduced fibrinolytic potential of human endothelial cells cultured in elevated
        glucose. Diabetes 1992;41:1009-15.
69.   Iwashima Y, Sato T, Watanabe K, et al. Elevation of plasma thrombomodulin level in diabetic
        patients with early diabetic nephropathy. Diabetes 1990;39:983-88.
70.   Kario K, Matsuo T, Kobayashi H, Matsuo M, Sakata T, Miyata T. Activation of tissue factor-
        induced coagulation and endothelial cell dysfunction in non-insulin-dependent diabetic patients
        with microalbuminuria. Arterioscler Thromb Vasc Biol 1995;15:1114-20.
71.   Stern DM, Esposito C, Gerlach H, et al. Endothelium and regulation of coagulation. Diabetes
        Care 1991;14:160-66.
72.   Takahashi H, Ito S, Hanano M, et al. Circulating thrombomodulin as a novel endothelial cell
        marker: comparison of its behavior with von Willebrand factor and tissue-type plasminogen
        activator. Am J Hematol 1992;41(1):32-39.
73.   Aoki I, Shimoyama K, Aoki N, et al. Platelet-dependent thrombin generation in patients with
        diabetes mellitus: Effects of glycemic control in coagulability in diabetes. J Am Coll Cardiol
        1996;27(3):560-66.
74.   Lupu C, Calb M, Ionescu M, Lupu F. Enhanced prothrombin and intrinsic factor X activation
        on blood platelets from diabetic patients. Thromb Haemost 1993;70:579-83.

75. Tschoepe D, Esser J, Schwippert B, et al. Large platelets circulate in an activated state in diabetes mellitus. Sem Thromb Haemostas 1991;17:433-39.

76. Fitzgerald DJ, Roy L, Catella F, Fitzgerald GA. Platelet activation in unstable coronary disease. N Engl J Med 1986;315:983-89.

77. Fuster V, Badimon L, Badimon JJ, Chesebro JH. The pathogenesis of coronary artery disease and the acute coronary syndromes. N Engl J Med 1992;326:242-50.

78. Tschöpe D, Rösen P, Schwippert B, Gries FA. Platelets in diabetes: The role in the hemostatic regulation in atherosclerosis, Sem Thromb Hemostas 1993;19:122-28.

79. Tschoepe D, Lampeter E, Schwippert B. Megakaryocytes and platelets in diabetes mellitus. Hämostaseologie 1996;16:144-50.

80. Tschoepe D, Driesch E, Schwippert B, Nieuwenhuis HK, Gries FA. Exposure of adhesion molecules on activated platelets in patients with newly diagnosed IDDM is not normalized by near-normoglycemia. Diabetes 1995;44:890-94.

81. Tschoepe D, Hesse S, Rauch U, Schwippert B. Monocyte-platelet-co-aggregation is associated with low HDL/high triglyceride dyslipoproteinemia in NIDDM patients. Diabetes 1996; 45(Suppl.2):270A.

82. Knobl P, Schernthaner G, Schnack C, et al. Haemostatic abnormalities persist despite glycaemic improvement by insulin therapy in lean type 2 diabetic patients. Thromb Haemost 1995;73:165-66.

83. The Diabetes Control and Complications Trial Research Group. The effect of intensive treatment of diabetes on the development and progression of long-term complications in insulin dependent diabetes mellitus. N Engl J Med 1993;329:977-86.

84. Moskalets E, Galstyan G, Starostina E, Antsiferov M, Chantelau E. Association of blindness to intensification of glycemic control in insulin dependent diabetes mellitus. J Diab Compl 1994;8:45-50.

85. Laakso M. Glycemic control and the risk for coronary heart disease in patients with non-insulin-dependent diabetes mellitus. The Finnish Studies. Ann Int Med 1996;124 1/2:127-30.

86. Meigs JB, Singer DE, Sullivan LM, Dukes KA, D'Agostino RB, Nathan DM. Metabolic control and prevalent cardiovascular disease in non-insulin-dependent diabetes mellitus (NIDDM): The NIDDM patient outcome research team. Am J Med 1997;102:38-47.

87. Smith DA. Comparative approaches to risk reduction of coronary heart disease in Tecumseh non-insulin dependent diabetic population. Diabetes Care 1986;9:601-8.

88. Abraira C, Colwell J, Nuttwall F, et al. Cardiovascular events and correlates in the veterans Affairs Diabetes feasibility trial. Veterans Affairs Cooperative Study on Glycemic Control and Complications in Type II Diabetes. Arch Intern Med 1997;157:181-88.

89. Yudkin J. How can we best prolong life? Benefits of coronary risk factor reduction in non-diabetic and diabetic subjects. BMJ 1993;306:1313-18.

90. Pyörälä K, Pedersen TR, Kjekshus J, Olsson AG, Thorgeirsson G for the Scandinavian Simvastatin Survival Study (4S) Group. Cholesterol lowering with simvastatin improves prognosis of diabetic patients with coronary heart disease: A subgroup analysis of the Scandinavian Simvastatin Survival Study (4S). Diabetes Care 1997;20:614-20.

91. Anderson TJ, Meredith IT, Yeung AC, Frei B, Selwyn AP, Ganz P. The effect of cholesterol-lowering and antioxidant therapy on endothelium-dependent coronary vasomotion. New Engl J Med 1995;332:488-93.

92. Antiplatelet Trialist Collaboration. Collaborative overview of randomised trials of antiplatelet therapy-I: Prevention of death, myocardial infarction, and stroke by prolonged antiplatelet therapy in various categories of patients. Br Med J 1994;308: 81-106.

93.   Colwell JA. Antiplatelet drug and prevention of macrovascular disease in diabetes mellitus.
       Metabolism 1992;41:7-10.
94.   Patrono C, Davi G. Antiplatelet agents in the prevention of diabetic vascular complications.
       Diab Metab Rev 1993;9:177-88.
95.   Steering Committee of the Physicians Health Study Research Group: Final report on the
       aspirin component of the ongoing physicians health study. N Engl J Med 1989;321:129-35.

DYSLIPIDEMIA, DIABETES, AND CELL ADHESION MOLECULES

Yasunori Abe, Bassem El-Masri, Kay T. Kimball, Henry Pownall, Karin Osmundsen, C. Wayne Smith, and Christie M. Ballantyne

Introduction

One of the key initial events in the development of atherosclerosis is the adhesion of monocytes to endothelial cells with subsequent transmigration into the vascular intima. Leukocyte and vascular cell adhesion molecules such as selectins, integrins, vascular cell adhesion molecule 1 (VCAM-1), and intercellular adhesion molecule 1 (ICAM-1) play critical roles in the adhesion of monocytes to endothelial cells. Immunohistochemical studies of human tissues showed that these cell adhesion molecules (CAMs) are expressed at increased levels in atherosclerotic plaques [1-4]. In this review we examine evidence that CAMs may play an important role in the accelerated atherosclerosis seen in patients with diabetes mellitus and dyslipidemia.

Background

Several lines of evidence suggest that either dyslipidemia or diabetes mellitus may enhance expression of CAMs on vascular cells. Cybulsky and Gimbrone demonstrated that VCAM-1 was upregulated in endothelial cells adjacent to atherosclerotic plaques of hereditary hypercholesterolemic and high cholesterol-fed rabbits [5]. Richardson et al. reported enhanced expression of E-selectin and VCAM-1 on aortic endothelial cells of alloxan-induced diabetic rabbits [4]. These results are supported by several *in vitro* studies. Lysophosphatidylcholine, a component of oxidized low-density lipoprotein (LDL), induced expression of CAMs [6], and low high-density lipoprotein (HDL) [7] and oxidized fatty acids [8] augmented expression of CAMs in response to cytokines in cultured endothelial cells. Advanced glycation endproducts, a potential pathogenic substance for vascular complications of diabetes mellitus, induced expression of CAMs in a similar *in vitro* system [9].

Patients with diabetes mellitus frequently have abnormalities in lipid metabolism. These patients have high triglycerides, low HDL cholesterol, and abnormalities in levels and components of fatty acids. The combination of abnormalities in lipid and carbohydrate metabolism may contribute to premature and extensive atherosclerosis, which is often found in diabetic patients, by further potentiating expression of CAMs in vascular walls.

A. M. Gotto, Jr. et al. (eds.), Multiple Risk Factors in Cardiovascular Disease, 191–198.

Thus, CAMs are potential molecular markers for early and ongoing atherosclerosis. However, assessment of expression of CAMs in man has been hampered by the difficulty of quantitative assessment of CAM expression *in vivo*.

CAMs are also present in the circulation as soluble forms, which lack membrane-spanning and cytoplasmic domains that are present in the membrane-bound forms. Although the origins, metabolism, and functional significance of soluble CAMs (sCAMs) are not fully understood, quantitative assessment of the levels of sCAMs is straightforward. These levels have been noted to be elevated in certain pathological conditions such as sepsis, autoimmune diseases, and allograft rejection, when tissue expression of the membrane-bound forms of CAMs is also known to be upregulated. Thus, the levels of sCAMs may serve as surrogate markers that reflect the cellular expression of CAMs.

We have previously shown that patients with severe elevations of either LDL cholesterol or triglyceride levels have increased levels of sCAMs and that aggressive reductions in LDL cholesterol with 3-hydroxy-3-methylglutaryl coenzyme A (HMG-CoA) reductase inhibitor therapy over 6 months in patients with high LDL cholesterol significantly reduce the levels of soluble E-selectin (sE-selectin) without changing the levels of soluble ICAM-1 (sICAM-1) or soluble VCAM-1 (sVCAM-1) [10]. Previous reports by others have shown that sCAMs are elevated in patients with diabetes mellitus [11-13]. Although we noted that hypertriglyceridemic patients had an increased frequency of other risk factors, such as diabetes mellitus, the sample size of our previous studies was not large enough to examine the associations between sCAMs and the risk factors that are frequently concurrently seen with hypertriglyceridemia.

Methods and Results

A subsequent study was performed to explore further the following questions in regard to the relationship between hypertriglyceridemic dyslipidemia (high triglyceride/low HDL), diabetes mellitus, and levels of sCAMs:

1)   Is hypertriglyceridemic dyslipidemia independently associated with increased levels of sCAMs when other risk factors such as diabetes mellitus, gender, and hypertension are considered?

2)   Does treatment of hypertriglyceridemic dyslipidemia with a highly purified formulation of the ethyl esters of n-3 fatty acids, Omacor, influence levels of sCAMs in patients with or without diabetes mellitus?

Two groups of subjects (n=59) were recruited and gave informed consent to participate in a protocol approved by the Institutional Review Board for Human Subjects Research, Baylor College of Medicine; the procedures followed in the study were in accordance with institutional guidelines. Hypertriglyceridemic subjects (n=41) aged 18–70 years were enrolled after a 6-week initial dietary phase (American Heart Association Step I Diet). Patients were randomized to receive placebo (n=21) or Omacor (n=20) for 6 weeks while continuing the Step I Diet. One Omacor patient was lost to follow-up, and one placebo patient did not have specimens available for measurement of sCAMs; the remaining 39 patients are included in the following analyses. After 6 weeks of treatment with Omacor or placebo, 31 patients, including those randomized to placebo, received Omacor 4 g/day for > 6 months. Of these patients, 27 had serum available after > 6 months of treatment (7 months [n=18] or 12 months [n=9]) for measurement of sCAMs.

sICAM-1, sVCAM-1, and sE-selectin concentrations were measured by using monoclonal antibody–based ELISA (R & D Systems, Minneapolis, MN) on frozen serum collected at baseline from all subjects and after treatment from the patients who received medications (placebo and Omacor). Assays of all samples and controls were performed in duplicate. Concentrations of samples were determined by analyzing standards with known concentrations of recombinant adhesion molecules coincident with samples and plotting of signal versus concentration.

We found that sICAM-1, sE-selectin, and sVCAM-1 were significantly increased in the serum of patients with severe hypertriglyceridemia (n=39) in comparison with normal controls (n=20) even after adjusting for consideration of noninsulin-dependent diabetes mellitus (NIDDM), clinical atherosclerosis, hypertension, and smoking. Among the 39 patients with hypertriglyceridemia that we studied, 11 patients had NIDDM, and these patients had higher levels of sE-selectin and sICAM-1 than patients without diabetes. In multivariable analyses, NIDDM remained a strong predictor for higher sICAM-1 and sE-selectin, and male gender was also a predictor for higher levels of sICAM-1, sE-selectin, and sVCAM-1. However, levels of sVCAM-1 were not significantly different between the two subsets of patients. Prolonged treatment (4 g daily for > 7 months) with Omacor led to a significant reduction in triglycerides and total cholesterol and an increase in HDL cholesterol. Accordingly, the levels of sICAM-1 and sE-selectin were decreased by 9% and 16%, respectively, with more impressive reductions of 27% and 32% noted in the patients with NIDDM. A significant decrease in the level of sVCAM-1 was seen only in patients with NIDDM.

Discussion

HIGH TRIGLYCERIDE/LOW HIGH-DENSITY LIPOPROTEIN CHOLESTEROL

Although considerable controversies surround the issue of hypertriglyceridemia as a risk factor for atherosclerosis, recent studies have shown that premature atherosclerosis can occur in patients with familial chylomicronemia caused by mutations in the lipoprotein lipase gene [14]. Defective lipolysis, which results in marked increases in triglycerides and decreases in HDL, may increase susceptibility to atherosclerosis in humans. The results of our study, which show that patients with increased levels of triglycerides and low HDL cholesterol have increased levels of sCAMs, are consistent with previous *in vitro* studies that have shown that oxidized fatty acids increase endothelial expression of CAMs in response to cytokines whereas high levels of HDL inhibit the endothelial expression of CAMs in response to cytokines [7]. Omacor contains 3.3 IU/g of vitamin E, which may have prevented the enhanced oxidation of fatty acids seen in some studies with fish oils [15]. These data suggest that increased expression of CAMs may be a mechanism whereby high triglyceride/low HDL promotes atherogenesis.

Increased levels of triglycerides and low HDL are frequently seen in diabetes mellitus, and several epidemiological studies have suggested that elevated triglyceride and low HDL may be particularly adverse for the development of coronary artery disease in patients with diabetes mellitus. Our results suggest that the combination of high triglyceride/low HDL and abnormalities of glucose metabolism may both act to increase the level of CAM expression. The improvement of hypertriglyceridemic lipidemia seems to be particularly beneficial in patients with NIDDM, since the reduction in the levels of sICAM-1 and sE-selectin were greatest in patients with NIDDM and the reduction of sVCAM-1 was seen only in diabetic patients. However, since docosahexaenoic acid and eicosapentaenoic acid are known to inhibit the expression of E-selectin and VCAM-1 induced by cytokines or lipopolysaccharide on cultured endothelial cells [16], it is unclear whether the reduction in the levels of sE-selectin and sICAM-1 was due to the improvement in dyslipidemia or to direct effects of n-3 fatty acids.

DIABETES MELLITUS

Fasching et al. looked at the levels of circulating adhesion molecules in NIDDM as potential mediators of diabetic macroangiopathy [17]. They found that serum concentrations of sICAM-1, sVCAM-1, and sE-selectin were elevated by 36%, 14%, and 70% respectively in NIDDM patients compared with controls. Circulating adhesion molecule concentrations were not different between NIDDM patients requiring insulin and those not requiring insulin, or between NIDDM patients with and NIDDM patients without clinical symptoms of macroangiopathy. In this report, sVCAM-1 was found to increase significantly with age in NIDDM patients and in healthy controls, but sICAM-1 and sE-selectin were not; similar findings have been reported in nondiabetic patients with coronary and peripheral vascular disease [18]. The similarity between CAM concentrations in NIDDM patients with and without symptomatic macroangiopathy may be due to the high incidence of subclinical atherosclerosis in patients with NIDDM [19].

In a study by Cominacini et al., patients with insulin-dependent diabetes mellitus (IDDM), NIDDM, or hyperlipidemia had increased sE-selectin concentrations compared with healthy control subjects ($p < 0.01$), whereas ICAM-1 concentrations were elevated only in the patients with NIDDM ($p < 0.01$); VCAM-1 concentrations were not significantly different among groups [12]. This study also showed a positive correlation between plasma E-selectin concentration and glycated hemoglobin in IDDM and NIDDM patients, which is of particular interest because sE-selectin and sVCAM-1 have recently been shown to mediate angiogenesis [20].

In a study by Steiner et al. involving 60 NIDDM patients, sE-selectin and sVCAM-1 concentrations were increased compared with those in controls, and no correlation was found between sCAM levels and glycemic control [11]. However, E-selectin was significantly correlated with LDL cholesterol, which was not the case in the study by Cominacini et al [12].

In a study of 25 men and women with NIDDM, Ceriello et al. examined the contribution of metabolic control and oxidative stress to increased levels of circulating

ICAM-1 [13]. Compared with controls, patients with NIDDM had significantly increased levels of hemoglobin A_{1c} (HbA$_{1c}$), malondialdehyde (MDA), and sICAM-1 at baseline and after 3 months of improved metabolic control. Concentrations of sICAM-1 and HbA$_{1c}$ were significantly correlated in the patients at both time points. Significant correlations were also found between concentrations of sICAM-1 and MDA and between concentrations of MDA and Hb$_{A1c}$. As demonstrated in multiple regression analysis, both glucose and oxidative stress appear to contribute to the increase in sICAM-1.

Our study found a gender difference in the levels of sCAMs among the patients. The baseline levels of all three sCAMs that we studied were significantly higher in male patients than in female patients. In multivariable analyses, male gender remained a strong predictor of higher sCAMs. Blann et al. reported that levels of sE-selectin in normal subjects were significantly higher in males than in females, although they did not find any significant differences in levels of sICAM-1 or sVCAM-1 [21]. 17-estradiol has been shown by two groups to reduce interleukin-1 (IL-1)–induced adhesion of CAMs at the mRNA level by inhibiting transcription *in vitro* [22,23], with conflicting results reported by a third group using different methods [24]. Our results support the hypothesis that estrogen may suppress CAM expression *in vivo,* and this may partially explain why the incidence of atherosclerosis in premenopausal women is reduced compared with men.

We have previously postulated that increased levels of sCAMS may be related to the extent of atherosclerosis, the activity of atherosclerosis, or endothelial dysfunction [10]. We have recently observed from a large epidemiological study, the Atherosclerosis Risk in Communities (ARIC) trial, that patients who developed coronary artery disease events or who had carotid artery disease had increased levels of sCAMs as compared with cohort controls after adjustment for all measured risk factors [25].

Although one may postulate that the increased levels of sCAMs in patients with hypertriglyceridemia at baseline are due to an extensive burden of asymptomatic atherosclerosis, it is highly improbable that treatment of dyslipidemia with fish oils could lead to a significant reduction in the extent of atherosclerosis within 12 months. Lipid lowering with statins has not reduced the extent of atherosclerosis as assessed by carotid ultrasound by 12 months [26]. Therefore, it is unlikely that the reduction in the levels of sE-selectin and sICAM-1 by fish oil therapy in the hypertriglyceridemic patients was secondary to regression of atherosclerotic lesions. In our previous study, levels of sE-selectin but not sICAM-1 were significantly decreased after treatment of hypercholesterolemia with a statin for 6 months [10]. Since E-selectin is expressed exclusively by endothelial cells following activation, the levels of sE-selectin should reflect the activation state of endothelial cells. Thus, our previous and current studies suggest that levels of sE-selectin in the serum of dyslipidemic patients may be a marker of endothelial cell activation or dysfunction. On the other hand, since ICAM-1 is expressed by a wide variety of cell types, including intimal smooth muscle cells as well as endothelial cells, the interpretation of changes in levels of sICAM-1 are more complicated and may be related to the "activity" of multiple cell types in atherosclerotic lesions.

In contrast to sICAM-1 and sE-selectin, sVCAM-1 levels were not reduced by therapy with fish oils. This was somewhat surprising, because previous *in vitro* studies had suggested that fish oil would inhibit cytokine-induced expression of VCAM-1 [16]. Although triglyceride levels were improved substantially by therapy, they remained elevated, and perhaps normalization of triglyceride would be required to reduce levels of sVCAM-1. As previously mentioned, it is unlikely that fish oil therapy for < 1 year significantly changed the extent of atherosclerosis, which has been shown to correlate to the levels of VCAM-1 in one study [27].

In conclusion, the levels of sE-selectin, sICAM-1, and sVCAM-1 in the serum of patients with hypertriglyceridemia were increased, and multivariable analyses showed that this increase was independent of other risk factors. The association of NIDDM with hypertriglyceridemia further enhanced the levels of sE-selectin and sICAM-1 but not sVCAM-1. Marked reduction of triglyceride and increase of HDL cholesterol by concentrated fish oil therapy led to a reduction in the levels of sE-selectin and sICAM-1, which was most prominent in patients with NIDDM. The levels of sVCAM-1 were reduced only in patients with NIDDM. These results support previous *in vitro* data suggesting that disorders of triglyceride and HDL metabolism may promote atherogenesis through effects on CAMs, which are most pronounced in patients with NIDDM, and that treatment of dyslipidemia with fish oils may alter vascular cell activation.

Acknowledgments

This work was supported in part by National Institutes of Health grant HL-42550 (CWS, CMB), American Heart Association Established Investigator Award (CMB), Pronova Biocare, and the Zeneca–Baylor College of Medicine Strategic Research Alliance. The authors would like to acknowledge Rima Farhat Maghes and Kerrie Jara for editorial assistance in the preparation of this manuscript.

References

1.   Poston RN, Haskard DO, Coucher JR, Gall NP, Johnson-Tidey RR. Expression of intercellular adhesion molecule-1 in atherosclerotic plaques. Am J Pathol 1992;140:665-73.
2.   Davies MJ, Gordon JL, Gearing AJH, Pigott R, Woolf N, Katz D, Kyriakopoulos A. The expression of the adhesion molecules ICAM-1, VCAM-1, PECAM, and E-selectin in human atherosclerosis. J Pathol 1993;171:223-29.
3.   O'Brien KD, Allen MD, McDonald TO, et al. Vascular cell adhesion molecule-1 is expressed in human coronary atherosclerotic plaques: Implications for the mode of progression of advanced coronary atherosclerosis. J Clin Invest 1993;92:945-51.
4.   Richardson M, Hadcock SJ, DeReske M, Cybulsky MI. Increased expression in vivo of VCAM-1 and E-selectin by the aortic endothelium of normolipemic and hyperlipemic diabetic rabbits. Arterioscler Thromb 1994;14:760-69.
5.   Cybulsky MI, Gimbrone MA Jr. Endothelial expression of a mononuclear leukocyte adhesion molecule during atherogenesis. Science 1991;251:788-91.
6.   Kume N, Cybulsky MI, Gimbrone MA Jr. Lysophosphatidylcholine, a component of atherogenic lipoproteins, induces mononuclear leukocyte adhesion molecules in cultured human and rabbit arterial endothelial cells. J Clin Invest 1992;90:1138-44.

7. Cockerill GW, Rye K-A, Gamble JR, Vadas MA, Barter PJ. High-density lipoproteins inhibit cytokine-induced expression of endothelial cell adhesion molecules. Arterioscler Thromb Vasc Biol 1995;15:1987-94.

8. Khan BV, Parthasarathy SS, Alexander RW, Medford RM. Modified low density lipoprotein and its constituents augment cytokine-activated vascular cell adhesion molecule-1 gene expression in human vascular endothelial cells. J Clin Invest 1995;95:1262-70.

9. Schmidt AM, Hori O, Chen JX, et al. Advanced glycation endproducts interacting with their endothelial receptor induce expression of vascular cell adhesion molecule-1 (VCAM-1) in cultured human endothelial cells and in mice: A potential mechanism for the accelerated vasculopathy of diabetes. J Clin Invest 1995;96:1395-403.

10. Hackman A, Abe Y, Insull W Jr, et al. Levels of soluble cell adhesion molecules in patients with dyslipidemia. Circulation 1996;93:1334-38.

11. Steiner M, Reinhardt KM, Krammer B, Ernst B, Blann AD. Increased levels of soluble adhesion molecules in type 2 (non-insulin dependent) diabetes mellitus are independent of glycaemic control. Thromb Haemost 1994;72:979-84.

12. Cominacini L, Fratta Pasini A, Garbin U, et al. Elevated levels of soluble E-selectin in patients with IDDM and NIDDM: Relation to metabolic control. Diabetologia 1995;38:1122-24.

13. Ceriello A, Falleti E, Bortolotti N, et al. Increased circulating intercellular adhesion molecule-1 levels in type II diabetic patients: The possible role of metabolic control and oxidative stress. Metabolism 1996;45:498-501.

14. Benlian P, De Gennes JL, Foubert L, Zhang H, Gagné SE, Hayden M. Premature atherosclerosis in patients with familial chylomicronemia caused by mutations in the lipoprotein lipase gene. N Engl J Med 1996;335:848-54.

15. Hau M-F, Smelt AHM, Bindels AJGH, et al. Effects of fish oil on oxidation resistance of VLDL in hypertriglyceridemic patients. Arterioscler Thromb Vasc Biol 1996;16:1197-202.

16. De Caterina R, Cybulsky MI, Clinton SK, Gimbrone MA Jr, Libby P. The omega-3 fatty acid docosahexaenoate reduces cytokine-induced expression of proatherogenic and proinflammatory proteins in human endothelial cells. Arterioscler Thromb 1994;14:1829-36.

17. Fasching P, Waldhäusl W, Wagner OF. Elevated circulating adhesion molecules in NIDDM—potential mediators in diabetic macroangiopathy [letter]. Diabetologia 1996:39: 1242-44.

18. Blann AD, McCollum CN. Circulating endothelial cell/leukocyte adhesion molecules in atherosclerosis. Thromb Haemost 1994;72:151-54.

19. Pujia A, Gnasso A, Irace C, Colonna A, Mattiolo PL. Common carotid arterial wall thickness in NIDDM subjects. Diabetes Care 1994;17:1330-36.

20. Koch AE, Halloran MM, Haskell CJ, Shah MR, Polverini PJ. Angiogenesis mediated by soluble forms of E-selectin and vascular cell adhesion molecule-1. Nature 1995;376:517-19.

21. Blann AD, Daly RJ, Amiral J. The influence of age, gender and ABO blood group on soluble endothelial cell markers and adhesion molecules. Br J Haematol 1996;92:498-500.

22. Caulin-Glaser T, Watson CA, Pardi R, Bender JR. Effects of 17β-estradiol on cytokine-induced endothelial cell adhesion molecule expression. J Clin Invest 1996;98:36-42.

23. Nakai K, Itoh C, Hotta K, Itoh T, Yoshizumi M, Hiramori K. Estradiol-17β regulates the induction of VCAM-1 mRNA expression by interleukin-1β in human umbilical vein endothelial cells. Life Sci 1994;54:PL221-27.

24. Cid MC, Kleinman HK, Grant DS, Schnaper HW, Fauci AS, Hoffman GS. Estradiol enhances leukocyte binding to tumor necrosis factor (TNF)-stimulated endothelial cells via an increase in TNF-induced adhesion molecules E-selectin, intercellular adhesion molecule type 1, and

vascular cell adhesion molecule type 1. J Clin Invest 1994;93:17-25.

25.   Hwang S, Ballantyne CM, Sharrett AR, et al. Circulating adhesion molecules VCAM-1, ICAM-1, and E-selectin in carotid atherosclerosis and incident coronary heart disease cases: The Atherosclerosis Risk in Communities (ARIC) study. Circulation. In press.

26.   Furberg CD, Adams HP Jr, Applegate WB, et al. for the Asymptomatic Carotid Artery Progression Study (ACAPS) Research Group. Effect of lovastatin on early carotid atherosclerosis and cardiovascular events. Circulation 1994;90:1679-87.

27.   Peter K, Nawroth P, Conradt C, et al. Circulating vascular cell adhesion molecule-1 correlates with the extent of human atherosclerosis in contrast to circulating intercellular adhesion molecule-1, E-selectin, P-selectin, and thrombomodulin. Arterioscler Thromb Vasc Biol 1997; 17:505-12.

NOVEL THERAPEUTIC APPROACHES TO INSULIN RESISTANCE/DIABETIC DYSLIPIDEMIA

Cesare R. Sirtori and Franco Pazzucconi

Introduction

Diagnosis of diabetes is based today not only on clear cut hyperglycemia (dependent or nondependent from insulin) but also on clinical syndromes, where hyperglycemia is only part of the picture. In the "insulin resistance syndrome" (IRS) also known as "syndrome X" or "metabolic syndrome" [1], hyperglycemia is mild to moderate, but elevated fasting or postprandial insulinemia leads to a variety of metabolic and clinical consequences, frequently to early coronary heart disease (CHD) [2]. In the IRS, the well-known diabetes associated lipid/lipoprotein abnormalities become predominant, in addition to the frequent concomitant occurrence of abdominal obesity and increased blood pressure [3]. Lipoprotein changes are characterized by triglyceride (TG) enrichment in the different lipoproteins, generally associated with reduction of high density lipoprotein (HDL) cholesterol [4].

A number of studies have recently indicated that hypertriglyceridemia may antedate the occurrence of clinical type II diabetes [5] and that long-term mortality in patients with noninsulin dependent diabetes (NIDDM) is only weakly related to hypercholesterolemia and fasting glycemia, whereas postprandial glycemia, fasting triglyceridemia, and elevated blood pressure seem to have a significant impact on mortality, as recently shown in the NIDDM Policy Group Study [6] (Table 1).

The role of insulin in the atherogenic process is still incompletely understood. Excess insulin may affect the arterial wall by enhancing arterial smooth muscle cell proliferation and cholesterol ester accumulation. By increasing low density lipoprotein (LDL) receptor activity it may stimulate delivery of cholesterol to cells [4] and, in addition, potentially raise cholesterol retention by decreasing HDL-mediated efflux [7]. An elevated activity of hepatic lipase may lead to high very low density lipoprotein (VLDL)/reduced HDL, thus suggesting this enzyme as a potential target for pharmacological management [8]. IRS and diabetic dyslipidemia are characterized by a procoagulant state, associated with increased concentrations of thrombogenic factors, such as factor VII, factor X, and the inhibitor of tissue plasminogen activator (PAI-1) [9]. It may thus be that the best correlation between the IRS and increased CHD risk may not be found in altered glucose/insulin levels, but rather in the accompanying lipid/lipoprotein alterations (Table 2).

A. M. Gotto, Jr. et al. (eds.), Multiple Risk Factors in Cardiovascular Disease, 199–208.
© 1998 Kluwer Academic Publishers and Fondazione Giovanni Lorenzini. Printed in the Netherlands.

Table 1. NIDDM Policy Group Study: 11 Years Mortality According to Category of Glucose Control [10]. 1,139 participating patients 30-55 years. In the 11 years of follow up 15% had MI; 19.82% died.

Control of Glycemia and Prevalence of MI or Mortality				
	Good	Border	Poor	P for Trend
FBG mM	4.4-6.1	≤ 7.8	> 7.8	-
MI	123	147	183	
Mortality	164	222	203	-
PP-BG mM	4.4-8.0	≤ 10	≥ 10	
MI	120	165	200	**
Mortality	167	199	202	*
TG mM	< 1.7	≤ 2.2	> 2.2	
MI	138	157	180	
Mortality	161	238	240	*
BP mmHg	≤ 149/90	≤ 160/95	> 160/95	
MI	109	147	216	**
Mortality	178	175	244	-
No Significant Effect of Cholesterolemia				

FBG: fasting blood glucose; MI: myocardial infarction; PP-BG: postprandial blood glucose; TG: triglycerides; BP: blood pressure.

The frequent long-term failure of sulfonylureas in NIDDM, particularly in obese individuals [10] also supports the search of new types of antidiabetic medications. Lipid changes, mainly hypertriglyceridemia may, in fact, not only antedate NIDDM (by 10 years or longer) [5], but may also be linked to poor suppressibility of raised free fatty acid (FFA) levels by insulin, that in itself may predispose to insulin resistance [11]; insulin resistance may finally predict the risk of hypertriglyceridemia (risk ratio, RR 3.5), low HDL-C (RR 1.6) and hypertension (RR 2.0) [12].

Table 2. Dyslipidemia/Insulin Resistance. Targets of Therapy

Dyslipidemia in NIDDM characterized by

    TG enrichment in all lipoproteins; reduced HDL-C levels [4]

    Increased postprandial lipemia

    Small LDL

    Excess E4 with hypercholesterolemia/CHD [13]

    Reduced suppressibility of FFA by insulin [12]

Correlation between CHD risk and:

    Insulin resistance?

    Insulin levels?

    The reverse (excess TG)?

New Therapeutic Approaches to the Modulation of Insulin-Dependent Pathways of Glucose/Lipid Metabolism

A number of new drugs have entered clinical evaluation for a potential use in NIDDM, IRS, and the possible associated dyslipidemia. These may be divided into:
- inhibitors of lipolysis and of fatty acid oxidation
- α-glucosidase inhibitors
- stimulators of energy expenditure
- insulin sensitizing agents

The first three classes of drugs, acting either via an indirect effect on energy consumption, ranging from inhibition of lipolysis or fatty acid oxidation, to reduction of polysaccharide breakdown in the intestine (α-glucosidase inhibitors) or via a direct metabolic stimulation (β_3-adrenergic agonists), have received limited development.

INHIBITORS OF LIPOLYSIS

Inhibitors of lipolysis, particularly acipimox, with a long lasting action, may provide a potentially useful therapeutic tool in IRS. At least one report shows complete correction by acipimox in a case of the polycystic ovary syndrome, with severe hypertriglyceridemia, hyperglycemia, and IRS [14]. However, in carefully conducted studies in NIDDM, very frequent administrations (up to 2-hour intervals) of acipimox, failed to achieve a sustained 24-hour suppression of FFA levels [15].

INHIBITORS OF FATTY ACID OXIDATION

Inhibitors of fatty acid oxidation, such as etomoxir and clomoxir, may be effective in enhancing glucose uptake [16], and in reducing hepatic production [17], thus as a result improving insulin sensitivity. Administration of these drugs, on the other hand, leads to higher levels of circulating fatty acids, potentially leading to arrhythmias [18].

α-GLYCOSIDASE INHIBITORS

α-glycosidase inhibitors finally prevent abnormally high increments of postprandial blood glucose, reduce hyperinsulinemia and, in specific conditions, can improve insulin resistance [19]. The lipid lowering activity of acarbose is generally of a modest degree [20]. An improved hypotriglyceridemic response was recently described for voglibose, a new low-dose disaccharidase inhibitor [21].

$β_3$-ADRENERGIC AGONISTS

Finally, $β_3$-adrenergic agonists, as stimulators of energy expenditure, may have a role in obesity management, but as yet their metabolic activities have not received sufficient support from available animal and clinical studies [22].

SULFONYLUREAS

The list of potentially useful drugs should not, finally, leave out the sulfonylureas for which recently, evidence of peripheral effects has been given.

Insulin Sensitizing Agents: Metformin and Thiazolidinediones

Drugs affecting glucose metabolism, without stimulating insulin release, are best exemplified by metformin, an antidiabetic agent in use for over 30 years and now approved for therapy in the United States. Metformin has no effect on insulin release from the pancreas; in fact it reduces post-load insulin secretion, both in NIDDM and in normoglycemic individuals, and it can significantly improve fasting and post-load hyperglycemia [23]. A variety of studies have investigated the mechanism of metformin and it is now well established that metformin can act at the intestinal level by promoting local glycolysis (partly resulting in a mild rise of plasma lactic acid levels) [24], and in the periphery by stimulating glucose transporter (GLUT) activity, mainly GLUT-1 versus GLUT-4 [25]. By this combination of mechanisms, metformin will *per se* improve diabetic hyperglycemia, also resulting in reduced triglyceridemia and increased HDL cholesterol, these last effects being most likely independent of the diabetic condition [26]. A recent U.S. study indicated that the mechanism of metformin may be linked to a reduced hepatic glucose output; this study is probably flawed by the presence of variable glycemic levels without establishing a clamp condition [27]. In this same study it was, however, also clearly established that a 60% increase of glucose clearance in muscle is achieved in drug-treated obese NIDDM patients (Figure 1).

Additional properties of metformin are: a reduction of elevated PAI-1 levels, thus providing the only pharmaceutical agent, aside from anabolic steroids, affecting this parameter, and a stimulated peripheral arterial flow [23], possibly NO mediated [28], and potentially of help in peripheral vascular disease [29].

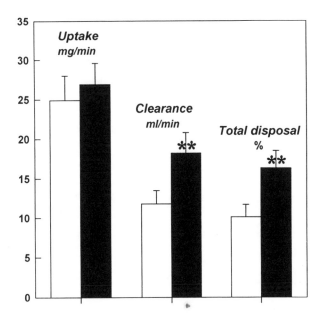

Figure 1. Metformin treatment in obese NIDDM patients significantly increases glucose clearance and total disposal (+60%) in skeletal muscle [27].

THIAZOLIDINEDIONES OR GLITAZONES

Thiazolidinediones or glitazones, have a clear hypoglycemic effect in various animal models of NIDDM and insulin resistance [30]. At therapeutic doses, three effects are apparent:

- an enhanced expression of GLUT-4 in the adipose tissue and muscle [31]
- increased levels of liver fructose-2,6-bisphosphate, a physiological activator of 6-phosphofructo-1-kinase, rate limiting in glycolysis [32]
- stimulated activity of PPAR (peroxisome proliferator associated receptor)-γ in the adipose tissue [33]

This last mechanism, unique among hypoglycemic agents, may possibly result in a lipid modulating activity, different from other antidiabetic medications (Table 3). Thiazolidinediones are, in fact, chemically distant derivatives of clofibrate and while exerting no activity on PPAR-α in the liver (the major target of fibrates), they do indeed activate PPAR-γ in the adipose tissue, thus leading not only to increased adipocyte differentiation [34], but also to an increased adipose tissue lipoprotein lipase activity [35]. This last mechanism should result in a reduction of triglyceridemia, that has not, however, been corroborated by clear cut clinical findings (Figure 2). Troglitazone does not, in fact, appear to exert a dose-related TG lowering/HDL raising effect in adult onset NIDDM [36]. Glitazones, on the other hand, display an interesting regulatory activity on leptin secretion, i.e. by improving the coordinate regulation of plasma leptin levels and glucose disposal rates in obese patients, where these two parameters are frequently dissociated [37].

Table 3. Pharmacology of Thiazolidinedione Derivatives (Glitazones)

- Lower glucose by improving insulin action, not by stimulating secretion

- Increase liver and muscle glycogen synthase [30]

- Improve Glut-1 and Glut-4 expression in adipose tissue and muscle [31,33]

- Increase liver fructose; 2,6-bisphosphate, activator of 6-phosphofructo-1-kinase, rate limiting in glycolysis [32]

- Increase adipocyte differentiation (PPAR γ activation) [33,34]

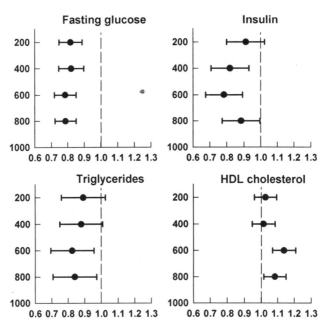

Figure 2. Troglitazone at doses between 200 and 800 mg/day significantly decreases fasting glucose and insulin at all doses tested, whereas triglyceride reduction is statistically significant only beyond 400 mg/day and so is the rise of HDL cholesterolemia. These last two effects do not appear to be clearly dose-related [36].

Sulfonylureas: New Vistas on the Mechanism

Sulfonylureas are ambiguous characters in the fight against diabetes and the associated enhanced risk of heart disease. Their major mechanism is, in fact, that of blocking ATP regulated K^+ channels, thus leading to cell depolarization, increased Ca^{++} uptake and insulin exocytosis [38]. Recent evidence also suggests that sulfonylureas may activate a novel Cl^- ion channel, by inhibit Na/K/ATPase or acting by PKC-dependent mechanisms [39]. Studies on sulfonylureas have been associated with tremendous steps forward in the understanding of the molecular mechanisms. Sulfonylureas have in fact high affinity receptors on pancreatic β-cells, explaining most of their local mechanisms [40]; alterations of these receptors lead to a familial hypoglycemic syndrome [41], up to now the only clinical syndrome only explained by an altered receptor to a class of synthetic drugs.

While the blocking of K^+ channels may in itself seem an atherogenic mechanism, in view of the well recognized vasodilatory role of K^+ channels, sulfonylureas exhibit other contrasting properties. They do antagonize, as expected, the vascular relaxation induced by cromakalim, minoxidil and diazoxide, but also the vascular contractions induced by $PGF_{2\alpha}$, at similar concentrations as papaverine [42].

Closure of ATP regulated K^+ channels may also be useful in specific clinical conditions. Myocardial hypoxia can lead to unregulated K^+ channel opening and this can be effectively antagonized by glibenclamide. In a controlled clinical investigation glibenclamide antagonized, in fact, the occurrence of brief episodes of arrhythmias and ventricular tachycardia in NIDDM patients with coronary heart disease, an effect not exerted by, e.g. metformin [43]. Glibenclamide, in addition, does not abolish preconditioning during demand ischemia [44].

Finally, recent evidence suggests that sulfonylureas, may also act peripherally. Glimepiride, a novel sulfonylurea, exerts a powerful stimulating activity *in vitro* and in addition, on myocardial glucose transport [45] gliclazide can improve peripheral glucose disposal by unclear mechanisms, apparently unrelated to changes in skeletal muscle GLUT-4 levels [46].

Conclusions

This review has attempted to focus on new developments and future openings in the field of drugs for NIDDM and IRS, with their associated lipid disorders. Different from a previous review [47], the outlook seems more optimistic. While drugs such as the β_3-receptor agonists, the inhibitors of fatty acid oxidation and the inhibitors of lipolysis do not seem to have added much in terms of therapeutic novelty, both metformin and glitazones display novel mechanisms, potentially of help in the treatment of NIDDM associated vascular disorders.

Metformin can effectively improve peripheral insulin resistance, reduce glycemia and triglyceridemia, and also correct other parameters, such as the elevated PAI-1 levels. Insulin sensitizers such as the glitazones activate the PPAR-γ system, thus making them somewhat close to fibrates and potentially beneficial in the diabetes associated lipid disorders. In addition, more recent evaluation of sulfonylureas indicates that even these drugs may be to some extent improve peripheral glucose handling. These and other observations support more detailed clinical studies, investigating the effectiveness of different treatments in the clinical management of NIDDM. It should be finally underlined that drug intervention studies, in particularly the ongoing UK Prospective Diabetes Study (UKPDS), carried out on NIDDM patients with fasting glucose 108-270 mg/dl, on a strict diet plus insulin with or without sulfonylureas/metformin (intensive treatment), has not shown any apparent ill effects, or an increased cardiovascular mortality [48].

References

1.   De Fronzo RA, Ferrannini E. Insulin resistance: A multifaceted syndrome responsible for NIDDM, obesity, hypertension, dyslipidemia, and atherosclerotic cardiovascular disease. Diabetes Care 1991;14:173-94.

2.   Modan M, Or J, Karasik A, et al. Hyperinsulinemia, sex, and risk of atherosclerotic cardiovascular disease. Circulation, 1991;84:1165-75.

3.   Goldschmid MG, Barrett-Connor E, Edelstein SL, Wingard DL, Cohn, BA, Herman WH. Dyslipidemia and ischemic heart disease mortality among men and women with diabetes. Circulation 1994;89:991-97.

4.   Bierman EL. Atherogenesis in diabetes. Arterioscl Thromb 1992;12:647-56.

5.   Sane T, Taskinen M-R. Does familial hypertriglyceridemia predispose to NIDDM? Diabetes Care 1993;16:1494-1501.

6.   Hanefeld M, Fischer S, Julius U, et al. Risk factors for myocardial infarction and death in newly detected NIDDM: The Diabetes Intervention Study, 11-year follow-up. Diabetologia 1996;39:1577-83.

7.   Oppenheimer MJ, Sundquist K, Bierman EL. Downregulation of high-density lipoprotein receptor in human fibroblasts by insulin and IGF-1. Diabetes 1989;38:117-22.

8.   Kasim SE, Kingston K, Jen K.-LC, Khilnani S. Significance of hepatic triglyceride lipase activity in the regulation of serum high density lipoproteins in type II diabetes mellitus. J Clin Endocrinol Metab 1987;65:183-87.

9.   Juhan-Vague I, Alessi MC. Plasminogen activator inhibitor-1 and atherothrombosis. Thromb Haemost 1993;70:138-43.

10.   Rodger W. Non-insulin-dependent (type II) diabetes mellitus. Can Med Assoc J 1991;145: 1571-81.

11.   Yki-Jarvinen H, Taskinen MR. Interrelationships among insulin's antilipolytic and glucoregulatory effects and plasma triglycerides in nondiabetic and diabetic patients with endogenous hypertriglyceridemia. Diabetes 1988;37:1271-78.

12.   Haffner SM, Valdez RA, Hazuda HP, Mitchell BD, Morales PA, Stern MP. Prospective analyses of the insulin-resistance syndrome (syndrome X). Diabetes 1992;41:715-22.

13.   Laakso M, Kesäniemi A, Kervinen K, Jauhiainen, Pyörälä K. Relation of coronary heart disease and apolipoprotein E phenotype in patients with non-insulin dependent diabetes. Br Med J 1991;303:1159-62.

14.   Kumar S, Durrington PN, Bhatnagar D, Laing I. Suppression of non-esterified fatty acids to treat type A insulin resistance syndrome. Lancet 1994;343:1073.

15.   Saloranta C, Taskinen MR, Widén E, Härkönen M, Melander A, Groop L. Metabolic consequences of sustained suppression of free fatty acids by acipimox in patients with

NIDDM. Diabetes 1993;42:1559-66.

16.   Hubinger A, Weikert G, Wolf HP, Gries FA. The effect of etomoxir on insulin sensitivity in type 2 diabetic patients. Horm Metab Res 1992;115-18.

17.   Ratheiser K, Schneeweiss B, Waldhäusl W, et al. Inhibition by etomoxir of carnitine palmitoyl transferase reduces hepatic glucose production and plasma lipids in non-insulin-dependent diabetes mellitus. Metabolism 1991;40:1185-90.

18.   Wolf HPO, Eistetter K, Ludwig G. Phenylalkyloxirane carboxilic acids, a new class of hypoglycaemic substances: Hypoglycaemic and hypoketonaemic effects of sodium 2-[5-4-chlorophenyl)-pentyl]-oxirane-2-carboxylate (B807-27) in fasted animals. Diabetologia 1982; 22:456-63.

19.   Balfour JA, McTavish D. Acarbose. An update on its pharmacology and therapeutic use in diabetes mellitus. Drugs 1993;46:1025-54.

20.   Leonhardt W, Hanefeld M, Fischer S, Schulze J, Spengler M. Beneficial effects on serum lipids in noninsulin dependent diabetics by acarbose treatment. Arzneim-Forsch Drug Res 1991;41:735-38.

21.   Shinozaki K, Suzuki M, Ikebuchi M, Hirose J, Hara Y, Harano Y. Improvement of insulin sensitivity an dyslipidemia with a new α-glucosidase inhibitor, voglibose, in nondiabetic hyperinsulinemic subjects. Metabolism 1996;45:731-37.

22.   Arch JRS, Wilson S. Prospects for β_3-adrenoceptor agonists in the treatment of obesity and diabetes. Int J Obesity 1996;20:191-99.

23.   Sirtori CR, Pasik C. Re-evaluation of a biguanide, metformin - mechanism of action and tolerability. Pharmacol Res 1994;30:187-228.

24.   Bailey CJ, Mynett KJ, Page T. Importance of the intestine as a site of metformin-stimulated glucose utilization. Br J Pharmacol 1994;112:671-75.

25.   Hundahl HS, Ramlal T, Reyes R, Leiter LA, Klip A. Cellular mechanism of metformin action involves glucose transporter translocation from an intracellular pool to the plasma membrane in L6 muscle cells. Endocrinology 1992;131:1165-73.

26.   Sirtori CR, Tremoli E, Sirtori M, Conti F, Paoletti R. Treatment of hypertriglyceridemia with metformin: Effectiveness and analysis of results. Atherosclerosis 1977;26:583-92.

27.   Stumvoll M, Nurjahan N, Perriello G, Dailey G, Gerich JE. Metabolic effects of metformin in non-insulin-dependent diabetes mellitus. N Engl J Med 1995;333:550-54.

28.   Butterfield J. The circulation in diabetes, from HL523 to the NO era. Lancet 1993;342:533-36.

29.   Sirtori CR, Franceschini G, Gianfranceschi G, et al. Metformin improves peripheral vascular flow in non hyperlipidemic patients with arterial disease. J Cardiovasc Pharmacol 1984;6:914-23.

30.   Hofmann C, Lorenz K, Colca JR. Glucose transport deficiency in diabetic animals is corrected by treatment with the oral antihyperglycaemic agent pioglitazone. Endocrinology 1991;129: 1915-25.

31.   El-Kebbi IM, Roser S, Pollet RJ. Regulation of glucose transport by pioglitazone in cultured muscle cells. Metabolism 1994;43:953-58.

32.   Murano K, Inoue Y, Emoto M, Kaku K, Kaneko T. CS-045, a new oral antidiabetic agent, stimulates fructose-2,6-bisphosphate production in rat hepatocytes. Eur J Pharmacol 1994; 254:257-62.

33.   Saltiel AR, Olefsky JM. Thiazolidinediones in the treatment of insulin resistance and type II diabetes. Diabetes 1996;45:1661-69.

34.   Tafuri SR. Troglitazone enhances differentiation, basal glucose uptake, and Glut1 protein

levels in 3T3-L1 adipocytes. Endocrinology 1996;137:4706-12.

35. Schoonjans K, Staels B, Auwerx J. Role of the peroxisome proliferator-activated receptor (PPAR) in mediating the effects of fibrates and fatty acids on gene expression. J Lipid Res 1996;37:907-25.

36. Kumar S., Boulton AJM, Beck-Nielsen H, et al. Troglitazone, an insulin action enhancer, improves metabolic control in NIDDM patients. Diabetologia 1996;39:701-9.

37. Nolan JJ, Olefsky JM, Nyce MR, Considine RV, Caro JF. Effect of troglitazone on leptin production. Diabetes 1996;45:1276-78

38. Rorsman P, Berggren P-O, Bokvist K, Efendic S. ATP-regulated K^+ channels and diabetes mellitus. NIPS 1990;5:143-47

39. Satin LS. New mechanisms for sulfonylurea control of insulin secretion. Endocrine 1996;4: 191-98.

40. Aguilar-Bryan L, Nichols CG, Wechsler SW, et al. Cloning of the β cell high-affinity sulfonylurea receptor: A regulator of insulin secretion. Science 1995;268:423-26.

41. Thomas PM, Cote GJ, Wohllk N, et al. Mutations in the sulfonylurea receptor gene in familial persistent hyperinsulinemic hypoglycemia of infancy. Science 1995;268:426-29.

42. Oyama Y, Kawasaki H, Hattori Y, Kanno M. Attenuation of endothelium-dependent relaxation in aorta from diabetic rats. Eur J Pharmacol 1986;131:75-78.

43. Cacciapuoti F, Spiezia R, Bianchi U, Lama D, D'Avino M, Varricchio M. Effectiveness of glibenclamide on myocardial ischemic ventricular arrhythmias in non-insulin-dependent diabetes mellitus. Am J Cardiol 1991;67:843-47.

44. Correa SD, Schaefer S. Blockade of K_{ATP} channels with glibenclamide does not abolish preconditioning during demand ischemia. Am J Cardiol 1997;79:75-78.

45. Bähr M, Von Holtey M, Müller G, Eckel J. Direct stimulation of myocardial glucose transport and glucose transporter-1 (GLUT1) and GLUT4 protein expression by the sulfonylurea glimepiride. Endocrinology 1995;136:2547-53.

46. Vestergaard H, Weinreb JE, Rosen AS, Bjørbaek C, Hansen L, Pedersen O, Kahn BB. Sulfonylurea therapy improves glucose disposal without changing skeletal muscle GLUT4 levels in noninsulin-dependent diabetes mellitus subjects: A longitudinal study. J Clin Endocrinol Metab 1995;80:270-75.

47. Sirtori CR. Insulin resistance in diabetic dyslipidemia: Therapeutic approach. In Baba S, Kaneko T, editors. Diabetes. Excerpta Medica: Amsterdam, 1995:1162-65.

48. United Kingdom Prospective Diabetes Study (UKPDS). Br Med J 1995;310:1005-6.

HYPERTENSION AND THROMBOSIS, GENETIC DETERMINANTS OF CARDIOVASCULAR DISEASE

Roger R. Williams, Steven C. Hunt, Paul N. Hopkins, Lily Wu, and Jean-Marc Lalouel

Introduction and Summary Overview

Applying our growing understanding of genes that promote hypertension in humans should lead to more accurate diagnoses and more effective treatment. Furthermore in some cases it can already help us prevent avoidable early deaths. This discussion covers several dominant endocrine syndromes causing severe hypertension and preventable early deaths. We also discuss a very common genetic variant at the angiotensinogen locus that seems to be a gene for "salt sensitive hypertension."

Uncommon dominant genes for severe hypertension and early stroke (GRA and Liddle's Syndrome) and pheochromocytomas present a genetic paradigm for preventing early deaths through genetic diagnoses, effective therapy tailored to the underlying genetic mechanism, and family screening. MedPed ("Make Early Diagnoses to Prevent Early Deaths in Medical Pedigrees") is one practical approach to finding and helping persons with treatable, serious, uncommon, dominant disorders.

Common and ordinary essential hypertension is promoted by a genetic variant (A for G at DNA position -6 in the promoter region of the angiotensinogen locus (AGT) which is in strong linkage disequilibrium with a previously reported variant (amino acid residue T for M at 235). Homozygous (AA) carriers represent about 15% of Caucasians, 55% of Japanese, and 67% of Blacks, roughly in parallel to hypertension prevalence by racial background. This updated review of AGT studies includes genetic association and linkage to hypertension, pre-eclampsia, left ventricular hypertrophy, and hypertensive cardiomyopathy; expression of the A(-6) promoter variant in cultured cells; and results by AGT genotype of recent clinical trials of nonpharmacologic interventions for high blood pressure. AGT is a paradigm for common chronic disease genes.

Atherosclerosis seems to be promoted by thrombogenic factors such as fibrinogen, factor VIIc, and plasminogen activator inhibitor-1. Structural gene loci have been identified and studied without consensus to date regarding any dramatic contribution of these loci to atherosclerosis.

A. M. Gotto, Jr. et al. (eds.), Multiple Risk Factors in Cardiovascular Disease, 209–215.

Genes for Thrombogenic Factors

Fibrinogen, factor VII, and PAI(1) seem to predict the risk of developing coronary thrombosis [1,2]. Structural genes have been studied for all three [2-4]. Polymorphisms at the structural gene loci for these three factors have been reported to have modest but significant effect on factor levels or on risk of atherosclerosis. However obesity, dyslipidemia and smoking have been reported to have even stronger effects. Perhaps the most intriguing findings suggest that some of these environmental factors may interact with genes for these thrombogenic components of atherogenic risk [3].

Due to strict requirements for collection and handling of blood specimens, thrombotic factors are more difficult to study in large populations than the standard risk factors such as cholesterol or hypertension. However the future genetic determinants of atherosclerosis seem likely to include some accounting of factors in this discipline.

Dominant Genes Causing Severe Hypertension and Early Deaths

Figure 1 summarizes possible genetic mechanisms for hypertension that involve the renin-aldosterone system. While evidence is insufficient for kallakrein (KALL), angiotensin converting enzyme (ACE), and renin (REN), there is substantial evidence for a causal role for the three that are highlighted (AGT, GRA, and Liddle's Syndrome).

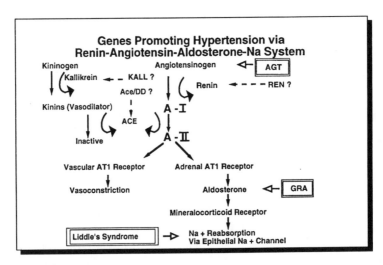

Figure 1. Genes Promoting Hypertension Via Renin-Angiotensin-Aldosterone-Sodium System

Two severe dominant forms of hypertension (GRA and Liddle's Syndrome) lead to early severe hypertension and strokes. Our understanding of these disorders has led to informative diagnostic tests and effective therapy tailored to the specific pathophysiology.

If these conditions are not properly diagnosed affected patients will die of early strokes in the 4th decade of life due to severe hypertension that is unresponsive to customary therapy.

Glucocorticoid remediable aldosteronism (GRA) results from a dominant "gain of function" mutation [5] on chromosome 8 inducing high levels of abnormal adrenal steroids 18-hydroxycortisol and 18-oxocortisol. This unusual chimeric mutation combines fragments of two genes, the aldosterone synthase gene and the steroid 11-beta-hydroxylase gene. The nucleotide sequences of these two genes are 95% identical. Because they have identical intron-exon boundaries and are located next to each other on chromosome 8, they can undergo unequal crossing over during recombination, producing the mutant gene with sequences and functions of both genes combined into the variant. Treatment with glucocorticoids (like dexamethasone or prednisone) can often suppress aldosterone, abnormal steroids, and the severe blood pressure elevations. Persons with the gene for GRA have been reported to have severe hypertension and relatives dying of cerebral hemorrhage in their forties. GRA has also been reported to fail to respond to ordinary antihypertensive medications but can respond to prednisone (suppress hormone production), spironolactone (competitively inhibit aldosterone receptor), or amiloride (inhibit distal renal epithelial sodium channel response to mineralocorticoid action).

Liddle's Syndrome is caused by dominant mutations [6] at the locus coding for the beta subunit of the epithelial sodium channel on chromosome 16p. A genetically activated channel is not maintained in a properly closed state. Plasma renin activity is low and sometimes hypokalemia may also be seen in this syndrome as in GRA. However Liddle's Syndrome causes suppression of aldosterone secretion in contrast to the hyperaldosteronism seen in GRA. Increased reabsorption of sodium with subsequent exchange of sodium for potassium in the distal nephron seem to explain the hypertension and hypokalemia. Both of these features of Liddle's Syndrome respond to triamterine or amiloride which specifically inhibit the epithelial sodium channel. Unlike GRA, this syndrome does not respond to spironolactone which inhibits the minaralocorticoid receptor. Kidney transplant has also been reported to eliminate the problem.

Several dominant genes [7,8] promote hormone secreting tumors called pheochromocytomas which can lead to serious medical problems or death. Periodic secretion of catecholamines causes episodic headaches, palpitations, pallor, perspiration, unusually labile blood pressure, and a hypertensive response to anesthesia or drugs. They can also secrete other substances such as serotonin, gastrin, cholecystokinin, somatostatin, and insulin-like growth factor. Three dominant syndromes causing pheochromocytoma include multiple endocrine neoplasia type II (MEN-II) linked to chromosome 10, neurofibromatosis (NF) on chromosomes 17 and 22, and von Hippel-Lindau disease (VHL) on chromosome 3. MEN-II tumors can include medullary thyroid carcinoma, parathyroid, and pheochromocytoma. While 90% of "pheos" arise in the adrenal medulla, 10% are extra-adrenal and have been reported most often from the abdomen, but also from the chest, neck, base of the brain, bladder, heart, and testicle. About 5% are malignant and are difficult to diagnose because benign "pheos" may be multicentric and malignant "pheos" lack the distinct histological certainty of other cancers. While the first "pheo" in a family may be difficult to diagnose, there is hope for finding other relatives who carry one of these serious dominant genes through genetic testing as demonstrated by at least one published family study of MEN-II and VHL. Once a gene carrier is found, advances in imaging techniques offer hope for finding and removing tumors even before serious clinical manifestations. These include computed tomography (CT), magnetic resonance imaging (MRI), and scintigraphy with iodine-131 labeled meta-iodobenzylguanidine (MIBG) which concentrates in adrenergic vesicles and light up tumors on scans.

The MedPed Approach: Screen Relatives to Prevent Early Deaths

For serious dominantly inherited syndromes for which methods are available for both diagnosis and treatment (like GRA, Liddle's, MEN-II, VHL, and NF), detailed family history charting and sequential relative screening should be performed for all first degree relatives and as many other relatives as possible on the affected side of the family including aunts and uncles, grandparents, nieces and nephews, cousins, and their offspring.

Because extensive relative screening is often not done for treatable dominant disorders, a pilot humanitarian effort has been organized to demonstrate how to help collect family history data and promote screening of relatives in high risk families. This nonprofit effort to save lives in high risk families is called Med Ped ("Make Early Diagnoses and Prevent Early Deaths in MEDical PEDigrees"). It has been applied to 15,000 families with heterozygous familial hypercholesterolemia (FH) in 25 countries and is now expanding to other treatable dominant disorders [9]. If you find or know of a proband with a treatable dominant disorder like FH, GRA, Liddle's Syndrome, MEN-II, or VHL, call MedPed Toll free (1-888-2Hi-Chol) to ask for free help to find affected relatives and to educate physicians who care for them.

Angiotensinogen: A Common Gene for "Salt Sensitive" Hypertension

Commonly occurring hypertension is also thought to result from the effects of milder effects of multiple genes in combination with environmental factors [10]. Large studies underway such as the National Heart Lung and Blood Institute (NHLBI) Family Blood Pressure Program are likely to produce a list of several common genes contributing to hypertension.

Variants of the gene for angiotensinogen (AGT) on chromosome 1 seem to promote hypertension, probably in a manner consistent with several theories of "salt sensitive hypertension." Several different types of studies support the importance of this gene:

1. Genetic linkage studies in selected hypertensive sibships have found statistically significant "excess sharing of alleles" (i.e. evidence of genetic linkage) in Utah, Paris, Japan, and England [11-13].

2. Genetic association studies have found significantly increased frequencies of the M235T variant of the AGT locus in essential hypertensives compared to controls in Utah, Paris, and Japan [11-12], but not in England [13] or in Black populations studied to date [14].

3. In pre-eclamptic women versus normotensive pregnant controls, the M235T

variant was significantly more frequent [14] (i.e. genetic linkage of AGT with pre-eclampsia).

4. Angiotensinogen levels in plasma were higher in TT than MM genotypes in women in Utah, Paris and in pre-eclamptic study participants [12,14].

5. The AGT M235T variant is much more common in Black and Asian populations than in Caucasian populations [11,14].

6. Persons who were homozygous (TT) for the AGT M235T variant show blunted renal vascular response to intravenous angiotensin II (Ang-II) infusion. Furthermore obesity, which also suppressed renovascular response to Ang-II infusion, was found to interact significantly with genotype such that, among the M235T homozygotes, obesity had a greater blunting effect on renal vascular response. [15].

7. Blood pressure tends to be higher in normotensive persons with higher angiotensinogen levels [16-17].

8. Pre-hypertensive persons in the NHLBI Trials of Hypertension Prevention with the AGT (235TT, -6AA) variant, developed hypertension significantly more often in the usual care group and less often in the sodium restriction and weight reduction groups [18].

9. In a Dutch clinical trial of "Saga Salt" (a salt substitute low in sodium and higher in potassium, calcium, and magnesium) unmedicated hypertensive persons with the AGT (235TT, -6AA) variant, showed better drop in blood pressure over time than those with the other genotypes [18].

10. Gene expression studies [19-20] report increased transcription rates for the hormone precursor angiotensinogen from the promoter variant AGT (-6AA) and not for AGT (235TT) which is in linkage disequilibrium with the apparently causal variant (-6AA).

In summary, the angiotensinogen gene (AGT) has been genetically linked to essential hypertension in several diverse populations, and genetically associated with both essential hypertension and pre-eclampsia in several populations. Higher levels by genotype and higher transcription rates for the AGT (-6AA) variant suggest a pathophysiologic mechanism involving increased production of the substrate angiotensinogen. Homozygous carriers of this AGT variant show blunting of renal response to infusion of angiotensin II (thought be some to be a sign of "salt sensitive hypertension"). Normotensive persons with the AGT variant tend to have higher blood pressure. Sodium restriction and weight reduction seem to be more beneficial as a measures to prevent hypertension in persons with the variant (-6AA, 235TT) AGT genotypes. A low sodium-high potassium salt substitute seems to be more beneficial as a measure to prevent or treat hypertension in persons with the AGT genotypes associated with hypertension.

Long-term compliance with medication and especially diet are often poor in persons with hypertension. Making a specific genetic diagnosis has proven in some studies to improve awareness of the need for intervention and compliance with long-term therapy. Early evidence suggests that the AGT gene may identify a subset of "sodium sensitive" pre-hypertensives in whom compliance with salt restriction may be especially beneficial. If your physician said you needed to follow a challenging low sodium diet to avoid or treat hypertension, would you like to know your genotype status for a locus that might predict how effective your dietary compliance would be? Practical questions like this will be the focus of future genetic studies of hypertension

References

1. Neinrich J, Balleisen L, Schulte H, Assman G, van de Loo J. Fibrinogen and factor VII in the prediction of coronary risk. Results from the PROCAM study in healthy men. Arterioscler Thromb 1994;14:54-59.
2. Humphries SE, Green FR, Temple A, et al. Genetic factors determining thrombosis and fibrinolysis. Ann Epidemiol 1992;2:371-85.
3. Wiman B. Plasminogen activator inhibitor 1 (PAI-1) in plasma: Its role in thrombotic disease. Thromb Haemost 1995;74:71-76.
4. Thomas AE, Green FR, Lamlum H, Humphries SE. The association of combined alpha and beta fibrinogen genotype on lasma fibrinogen levels in smokers and non-smokers. J Med Genet 1995;32:585-89.
5. Lifton RP, et al. A chimaeric 11β-hydroxylase/aldosterone synthase gene causes glucocorticoid-remediable aldosteronism and human hypertension.
    Nature 1992;355:262-65.
6. Shimkets RA, et al. Liddle's Syndrome: Heritable human hypertension caused by mutations in the β subunit of the epithelial sodium channel. Cell 1994;79:1-8.
7. Neumann HPH, et al. Consequences of direct genetic testing for germline mutations in the clinical management of families with multiple endocrine neoplasia, type II. JAMA 1995;274:1149-51.
8. Sheps SG. Pheochromocytoma: Evaluation. In: Izzo JL, Black HR, editors. Hypertension Primer. Am Heart Assoc 1993: 268-70.
9. Williams RR, Hamilton-Craig I, Kostner GM, et al. MED-PED: An integrated genetic strategy for preventing early deaths. In: Berg K, Boulyjenkov V, Christen Y, editors. Genetic approaches to noncommunicable diseases. Heidelberg: Springer-Verlag, 1996: 35-45.
10. Williams RR, et al. Multigenic hypertension: Evidence for subtypes and hope for haplotypes. J Hypertension 1990;8(Suppl.7):s39-46.
11. Jeunemaitre X, et al. Molecular basis of human hypertension: Role of angiotensinogen. Cell 1992;71:169-80.
12. Hata A, et al. Angiotensinogen as a risk factor for essential hypertension in Japan. JCI 1993; 93:1285-87.
13. Caulfield M, et al. Linkage of the angiotensinogen gene to essential hypertension. New Engl J Med 1994;330:1629-33.
14. Ward K, et al. A molecular variant of angiotensinogen associated with preeclampsia. Nature Genet 1993;4:59-61.
15. Hopkins PN, et al. Blunted renal vascular response to angiotensin II is associated with a common variant of angiotensinogen gene and obesity. J Hypertension 1996;14:199-207.
16. Walker WG, Whelton PK, Saito H, Russel RP, Hermann J. Relation between blood pressure and renin, renin substrate, angiotensin II, aldosterone and urinary sodium and potassium in 574 ambulatory subjects. Hypertension 1979;1:287-91.
17. Manatunga AK, Jones JJ, Pratt JH. Longitudinal assessment of blood pressures in black and

white children. Hypertension 1993;22:84-89.

18.   Williams RR, Genetics of hypertension, oral presentation at the National High Blood Pressure Education Program 25th Anniversary Symposium, National Institutes of Health, Bethesda, Maryland, 4 April 1997. Submitted for publication.

19.   Jeunemaitre X, Inoue I, Williams C, et al. Haplotypes of angiotensinogen in essential hypertension. Am J Hum Genet 1997;60:1448-60.

20.   Inoue I, Nakajima T, Williams CS, et al. A nucleotide substitution in the promoter of human angiotensinogen is associated with essential hypertension and affects basal transcription *in vitro*. J Clin Invest 1997;99:1786-97.

LIPOPROTEINS AND CARDIOVASCULAR RISK: FROM GENETICS TO PREVENTION OF CORONARY HEART DISEASE

Paul Cullen, Harald Funke, Helmut Schulte, and Gerd Assmann

Introduction

Dyslipidemia is said to be present when lipid or lipoprotein levels lie within a range which is known from epidemiological studies to be associated with secondary complications, in particular atherosclerosis of the coronary arteries, or when a lipid or lipoprotein grossly deviates from the norm as in abetalipoproteinemia, hypobetalipoproteinemia, or the high density lipoprotein (HDL) deficiency syndromes. In most cases, dyslipidemia is due not to a single genetic or environmental factor, but to a combination of the effects of several genes of small effect (polygenes) and environment. In other cases, however, dyslipidemia is caused by a mutation in a single gene of large effect. In such cases, the extent and nature of the phenotype depends primarily on the identity of the gene involved, but is also modulated to an important degree by the nature of the mutation and the genetic and environmental background against which this mutation occurs. In addition, many cases of hyperlipidemia are secondary to other disorders such as hypothyroidism or renal dysfunction. Such disorders may also unmask or exacerbate a genetic lipoprotein disorder. Examples of the latter are the unmasking of type III hyperlipidemia by diabetes mellitus or the exacerbation of familial hypercholesterolemia by hypothyroidism.

Genetic Epidemiology of Dyslipidemia

Only a minor part of the genetic component of the population variance in lipid parameters can be explained by disorders in single genes of large effect. The bulk of variation is due to a number of genes (polygenes), each of which accounts for only a small part of overall genetic variance. The challenge of current genetics is to unravel these complex genetic effects. A strategic approach to achieve this aim is outlined in Figure 1. In this approach, candidate genes are first identified based on biochemical knowledge of so-called "intermediate" phenotypes (e.g. raised low density lipoprotein (LDL) cholesterol, homocysteine, or fibrinogen levels). These genes are then screened for genetic variation and the phenotypic effects of the variant are assessed *in vivo* and *in vitro*. The technique of pool-screening is very useful in rapidly screening populations of interest for presence or enrichment of rare mutations in genes of interest [1]. Using this technique, a carrier can be

217

A. M. Gotto, Jr. et al. (eds.), Multiple Risk Factors in Cardiovascular Disease, 217–228.
© 1998 Kluwer Academic Publishers and Fondazione Giovanni Lorenzini. Printed in the Netherlands.

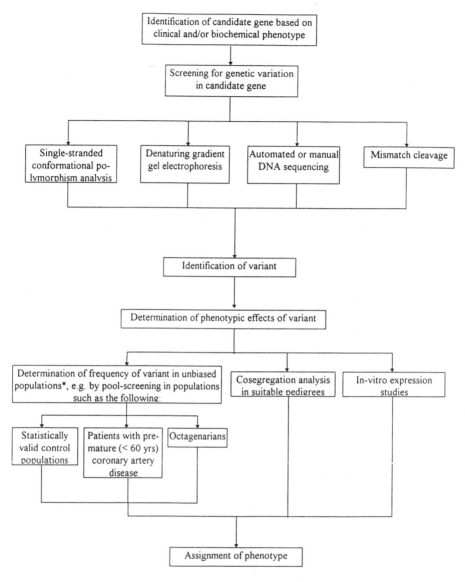

* By convention, variants with a population frequency of greater than 1% are referred to
as polymorphisms, those with a lesser frequency are termed mutations. Both polymorphisms and mutations may be either neutral (e.g. in the third base of a synonymous
codon) or associated with phenotypic effects

Figure 1. Genetic epidemiology: Strategy for the identification of genetic defects affecting
lipid phenotype, risk of atherosclerosis, or life expectancy. Identification of candidate gene
based on clinical or biochemical phenotype or both.

detected in a pool consisting of DNA samples from several thousand individuals. By selecting appropriate populations (e.g. patients with premature myocardial infarction or very elderly individuals), an association of a particular DNA variant with coronary artery disease or decreased (or increased) life expectancy can be detected. Using this strategy, differences in the frequencies of a number of genes affecting lipid metabolism between a control population from the Münster Heart Study (PROCAM) and patients with coronary artery disease before the age of 60 years. For example, in the coronary artery disease patients, the Arg3500Gln mutation in apolipoprotein B, which is responsible for familial defective apolipoprotein B, was found to be three times as common, while the Arg158Cys polymorphism in apolipoprotein E (E-2 allele) was found to be slightly less common (odds ratio 0.8) than in the Münster Heart Study controls.

Dyslipidemia and Risk of Coronary Heart Disease (CHD)

For many years, epidemiological evidence of a link between high LDL cholesterol, low HDL cholesterol, and coronary heart disease has been accumulating [2-7]. More recently, solid support for the causal nature of this link has been provided by large well-conducted trials showing that lowering LDL, both in patients with no history of angina pectoris (primary prevention) [8], and in patients with established CHD (secondary prevention) [9,10], reduces the incidence of fresh coronary events including coronary death. In the 4S study (secondary prevention) [10], total mortality was also reduced significantly. In addition, evidence from angiographic trials has convincingly shown that LDL cholesterol lowering may hinder progression, and perhaps even cause regression, of coronary atherosclerosis [11-27]. Evidence relating to the role of triglycerides in CHD has been more complex. In the Münster Heart Study, however, there was clear evidence of increased CHD risk in persons with a combination of high triglyceride and low HDL cholesterol [28]. In addition, it is not known whether the observed relationship between triglycerides and CHD is direct or indirect. Hypertriglyceridemia may contribute to CHD via a direct atherogenic effect of VLDL. Alternatively, hypertriglyceridemia may simply be part of a complex that includes other atherogenic lipoprotein profiles such as low HDL cholesterol, the presence of small, dense LDL, or the presence of large apoE-enriched VLDL particles.

Global Risk

An important step in recent years has been the development of the concept of global risk. Treatment decisions should almost never be based solely on lipid levels but must also take into account other risk factors. One of the most significant long-term achievements of the Münster Heart Study has been the development of an algorithm for calculation of global risk in middle-aged men, which takes into account the independent risk factors of age, systolic blood pressure, LDL cholesterol, HDL cholesterol, triglycerides, cigarette smoking, presence of diabetes mellitus, and family history of myocardial infarction (Table 1) [28].

Table 1. Coefficients of the Multiple Logistic Function Calculated in the Münster Heart Study

Variable	Coefficient
Age in years	+0.1001
Systolic blood pressure in mmHg	+0.0118
LDL cholesterol in mg/dl	+0.0152
HDL cholesterol in mg/dl	-0.0450
ln(triglycerides in mg/dl)	+0.3346
Cigarette smoking, 0 = no, 1 = yes	+0.9266
Diabetes mellitus, 0 = no, 1 = yes	+0.4015
Family history of myocardial infarction, 0 = no, 1 = yes	+0.4193
Angina pectoris, 0=no, 1=yes	+1.3190

Incidence of major coronary event in 8 years = $1/[1 + \exp(-y)]$ with $y = -12.3199 + \Sigma$ (variable coefficient)

Treatment Goals in Hyperlipidemia

In three major intervention trials (4S, WOSCOPS, CARE), cholesterol lowering has been achieved by statins, drugs which lower LDL cholesterol and triglyceride and increase HDL cholesterol and which have become the drugs of choice for treatment of hypercholesterolemia. The availability of these drugs has allowed persistent lowering of LDL cholesterol on the order of 30% with commonly used doses.

In the near future, statins of greater efficacy will be available which will allow even greater reductions in LDL cholesterol, effectively permitting titration to any desired level in most patients. This possibility has reopened the questions of treatment goals in LDL cholesterol lowering. Should absolute target LDL levels be defined, or is the important issue the extent by which LDL is lowered? Data from epidemiological studies including the Münster Heart Study indicates a log-linear relationship between the level of LDL cholesterol and CHD risk (Figure 2). Thus, when relative risk of CHD is plotted against cholesterol, a straight line relationship is obtained (Figure 3). However, the effect of lowering cholesterol on CHD risk depends on an individual's global risk of CHD. Thus, as shown in Figure 3, a person with a total cholesterol of 280 mg/dl but no other risk factors ("average risk") may have the same CHD risk as a person with a total cholesterol of 200 mg/dl but with other risk factors ("high risk"). In both cases, prolonged lowering of cholesterol by 40 mg/dl is associated with an approximate halving of CHD risk. Data from large scale intervention trials and indicate that this log-linear relationship between LDL cholesterol and CHD risk also applies to levels achieved by treatment (diet, drugs) and that 6 years of cholesterol reduction produces an approximate 30% reduction in CHD risk [8-10].

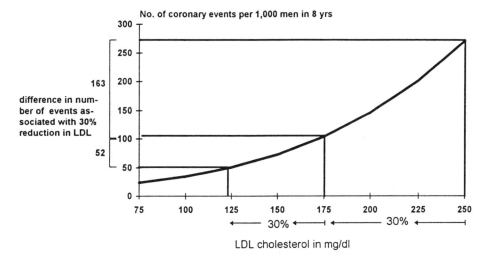

Figure 2. Münster Heart Study (PROCAM), 8-year risk of a coronary event according to LDL cholesterol in middle-aged men with angina pectoris (246 events, 4,501 men aged 40-65 years, results standardized to age 50 years). Statins produce a similar proportional lowering of LDL cholesterol (shown beneath X axis) irrespective of the baseline LDL cholesterol level (X axis). Thus the absolute reduction in LDL cholesterol is lower for a given baseline LDL cholesterol. In addition, because of the log-linear relationship between LDL cholesterol and CHD risk, the absolute difference in CHD risk associated with the same absolute difference in LDL cholesterol is greater at higher baseline levels of LDL cholesterol. For these reasons, all other things (pre-existing CHD, other risk factors) being equal, a prolonged 30% difference in baseline LDL cholesterol of 175 mg/dl versus 250 mg/dl is associated with almost 4 times as much benefit as a prolonged 30% difference of 125 mg/dl versus 175 mg/dl.

Since the relationship between statin dosage and cholesterol lowering is log-linear, a higher dose of statin (or a statin with higher efficacy) is necessary to reduce cholesterol in the high (non-LDL-associated) risk individual from, for example, 195 mg/dl to 155 mg/dl than to reduce cholesterol in the average (non-LDL-associated) risk individual from 310 mg/dl to 270 mg/dl (Figure 3). In both cases this would be expected to produce an approximate halving in the absolute coronary risk. Thus different doses of statin may be required to produce the same degree of risk reduction, depending on global risk (including LDL cholesterol) at baseline. Studies in China and Japan indicate that the log-linear relationship between cholesterol and CHD risk is maintained down to values as low as 120 mg/dl and, probably, even 80 mg/dl (Figure 4). Even at these extremely low levels, there is no evidence of a threshold below which the relationship no longer holds. The relevance of these findings to clinical practice, however, remains to be determined.

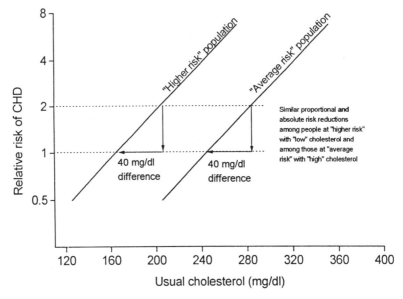

Figure 3. Diagram to indicate that similar proportional and absolute reductions in CHD risk are expected with the same absolute cholesterol reductions in individuals at the same absolute risk [29,30].

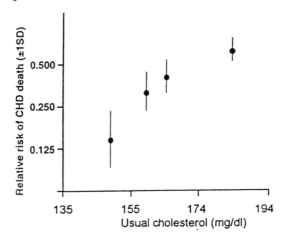

Figure 4. No "threshold" below Western cholesterol normal range. Shanghai prospective study in low cholesterol population of 9,000 urban Chinese followed for 8-13 years [31]. Risk is plotted on a doubling (i.e. log) scale. The "usual" cholesterol was derived from the baseline cholesterol by correction for "regression dilution" bias.

Several epidemiological studies have shown a U- or J-shaped relationship between total and LDL cholesterol and all-cause mortality with an excess of deaths primarily among men with total cholesterol levels below a cut-off of approximately 200 mg/dl or LDL cholesterol levels below a cut-off of approximately 130 mg/dl, in both community-based [5,32-45] and occupational [46-55] cohorts. This finding is not universal, however, and was not detected in a number of studies performed in younger [56-59], and in healthy [60] or nonsmoking [61] middle-aged cohorts. Data from the Münster Heart Study clearly shows that this increase in mortality at low cholesterol levels was seen in smokers only and was explained by an increase in death due to smoking-related cancers (Figure 5). In the CARE study, no benefit was seen in lowering LDL cholesterols below 125 mg/dl at baseline. However, this result may reflect the play of chance in a retrospective analysis of a small subgroup. From a theoretical point of view there is no reason to expect a cutoff for any level of LDL cholesterol within this range. Nevertheless, the benefits of treatment at low levels of cholesterol may become so small that they are outweighed by side effects of treatment and by the large number of persons who have to be treated in order to prevent one event. Despite this, in persons at high risk, treatment of LDL cholesterols of 125 mg/dl may be indicated.

The question arises with regard to treatment goals for LDL cholesterol in the secondary prevention of CHD: absolute levels or percentage lowering? Although an answer cannot be given which applies to every patient, a consensus view may be formulated:

(a)   In patients at high global risk of CHD (including patients with established CHD), LDL cholesterol should be lowered as far as possible. If initial levels are markedly elevated this is likely to require combination therapy with diet and drugs.

(b)   The benefits to be expected from lowering LDL cholesterol levels of below 125 mg/dl in patients with a history of MI may be small. However, patients with other risk factors in addition to a history of MI (e.g. diabetes, high blood pressure, overweight) may benefit to a worthwhile extent from LDL cholesterol lowering. More research is needed to conclusively answer this question and treatment decisions in such patients must currently be made on an individual basis.

Since the important factor in determining a person's chance of developing CHD is his or her global risk, and not just the LDL cholesterol level, every attempt should be made to modify other adverse variables by losing excess weight, giving up smoking, exercising, etc. Moreover, since these risk factors interact in an approximately multiplicative rather than an additive fashion, small changes in a number of risk variables may produce a disproportionately large overall beneficial effect.

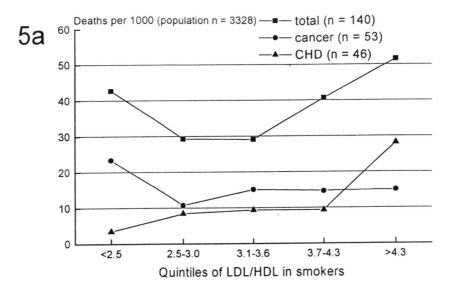

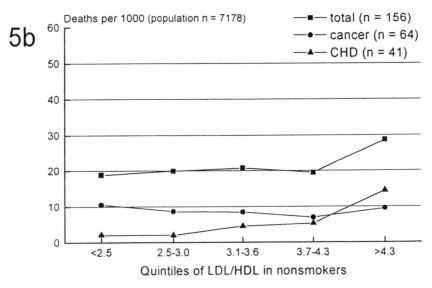

Figure 5. Age-standardized total, cancer-related, and CHD death according to quintiles of LDL cholesterol/HDL cholesterol ratio in male smokers (5a) and nonsmokers (5b) aged 35 to 65 years in the Münster Heart Study (PROCAM). Population = number of men on whom data were available as shown, total = total number of deaths, cancer = number of deaths due to cancer, CHD = number of deaths due to coronary heart disease.

References

1. Rust S, Funke H, Assmann G. Mutagenically separated PCR (MS-PCR): A highly specific one step procedure for easy mutation detection. Nucleic Acids Res 1993;21:3623-29.

2. Neaton JD, Blackburn H, Jacobs D, et al. Serum cholesterol level and mortality findings for men screened in the Multiple Risk Factor Intervention Trial. Multiple Risk Factor Intervention Trial Research Group [see comments]. Arch Intern Med 1992;152:1490-1500.

3. Law MR, Wald NJ, Wu T, Hackshaw A, Bailey A. Systematic underestimation of association between serum cholesterol concentration and ischemic heart disease in observational studies - data from the BUPA study. BMJ 1994;308:363-66.

4. Pekkanen J, Nissinen A, Punsar S, Karvonen MJ. Short and long term association of serum cholesterol with mortality. The 25 year follow-up of the Finnish cohorts of the Seven Countries Study. Am J Epidemiol 1992;135:1251-58.

5. Anderson KM, Castelli WP, Levy D. Cholesterol and mortality: 30 years of follow-up from the Framingham study. JAMA 1987;257:2176-80.

6. Assmann G, Schulte H. Role of triglycerides in coronary artery disease: Lessons from the Prospective Cardiovascular Munster Study. Am J Cardiol 1992;70:10H-13H.

7. Wilson PFW, Abbott RD, Castelli WP. High density lipoprotein cholesterol and mortality - the Framingham study. Arteriosclerosis 1988;8:737-41.

8. Shepherd J, Cobbe SM, Ford I, et al. Prevention of coronary heart disease with pravastatin in men with hypercholesterolemia. New Engl J Med 1995;333:1301-7.

9. Sacks FM, Pfeffer MA, Moye LA, et al. The effect of pravastatin on coronary events after myocardial infarction in patients with average cholesterol levels. New Engl J Med 1996;335:1001-9.

10. Scandinavian Simvastatin Survival Study Group. Randomised trial of cholesterol lowering in 4444 patients with coronary heart disease: The Scandinavian Simvastatin Survival Study (4S). Lancet 1994;344:1383-89.

11. Yamamoto A, Kojima SI, Haradashiba M, et al. Plasmapheresis for prevention and regression of coronary atherosclerosis. Ann N Y Acad Sci 1995;748:429-40.

12. Brown G, Albers JJ, Fisher LD, et al. Regression of coronary artery disease as a result of intensive lipid- lowering therapy in men with high levels of apolipoprotein B. New Engl J Med 1990;323:1289-98.

13. Kane JP, Malloy MJ, Ports TA, Phillips NR, Diehl JC, Havel RJ. Regression of coronary atherosclerosis during treatment of familial hypercholesterolemia with combined drug regimens. JAMA 1990;264:3007-12.

14. Watts GF, Lewis B, Brunt JNH, et al. Effects on coronary artery disease of lipid-lowering diet, or diet plus cholestyramine, in the St. Thomas' Atherosclerosis Regression Study (STARS). Lancet 1992;339:563-69.

15. Alaupovic P, Knightgibson C, Mack WJ, Kramsch DM, Hodis HN, Blankenhorn DH. Effect of lovastatin on apoA-containing and apoB-containing lipoprotein families - a report from the Mevacor Atherosclerosis Regression Study. Circulation 1992;86:743.

16. Blankenhorn DH, Azen SP, Kramsch DM, et al. Coronary angiographic changes with lovastatin therapy - the Monitored Atherosclerosis Regression Study (MARS). Ann Intern Med 1993;119:969-76.

17. Alaupovic P, Hodis HN, Knightgibson C, et al. Effects of lovastatin on apoa- and apob-containing lipoproteins - families in a subpopulation of patients participating in the monitored atherosclerosis regression study (MARS). Arterioscler Thromb 1994;14:1906-14.

18.   Waters D, Higginson L, Gladstone P, et al. Effects of monotherapy with an HMG-CoA reductase inhibitor on the progression of coronary atherosclerosis as assessed by serial quantitative arteriography - the Canadian Coronary Atherosclerosis Intervention Trial. Circulation 1994;89:959-68.

19.   Sacks FM, Pasternak RC, Gibson CM, Rosner B, Stone PH. Effect on coronary atherosclerosis of decrease in plasma-cholesterol concentrations in normocholesterolemic patients. Lancet 1994;344:1182-86.

20.   Ornish D, Brown SE, Scherwitz LW, et al. Can life style changes reverse coronary heart disease. Lancet 1990;336:129-33.

21.   Ornish D, Brown SE, Billings JH, et al. Can life-style changes reverse coronary atherosclerosis - 4-year results of the life-style heart trial. Circulation 1993;88:385.

22.   Haskell WL, Alderman EL, Fair JM, et al. Effects of intensive multiple risk factor reduction on coronary atherosclerosis and clinical cardiac events in men and women with coronary-artery disease - the Stanford Coronary Risk Intervention Project (SCRIP). Circulation 1994;89:975-90.

23.   Oliver MF, Defeyter PJ, Lubsen J, et al. Effect of simvastatin on coronary atheroma: The Multicentre Anti-Atheroma Study (MAAS). Lancet 1994;344:633-38.

24.   Thompson GR, Maher VMG, Matthews S, et al. Familial Hypercholesterolemia Regression Study - a randomized trial of low density lipoprotein apheresis. Lancet 1995;345:811-16.

25.   Pitt B, Mancini GBJ, Ellis SG, Rosman HS, Park JS, McGovern ME. Pravastatin limitation of atherosclerosis in the coronary-arteries (PLAC-I) - Reduction in atherosclerosis progression and clinical events. J Am Coll Cardiol 1995;26:1133-39.

26.   Pitt B, Ellis SG, Mancini GBJ, Rosman HS, Mcgovern ME. Design and recruitment in the United States of a multicenter quantitative angiographic trial of pravastatin to limit atherosclerosis in the coronary arteries (PLAC-I). Am J Cardiol 1993;72:31-35.

27.   Pitt B, Mancini GBJ, Ellis SG, Rosman HS, Park JS, McGovern ME. Pravastatin limitation of atherosclerosis in the coronary- arteries (PLAC-I) - reduction in atherosclerosis progression and clinical events. J Am Coll Cardiol 1995;26:1133-39.

28.   Assmann G, Schulte H, von Eckardstein A. Hypertriglyceridemia and elevated levels of lipoprotein (a) are risk factors for major coronary events in middle-aged men. Am J Cardiol 1996;77:1179-84.

29.   Martin MJ, Browner WS, Wentworth D, Hulley SB, Kuller LH. Serum cholesterol, blood-pressure, and mortality - implications from a cohort of 361 662 men. Lancet 1986;2:933-36.

30.   Stamler J, Vaccaro O, Neaton JD, Wentworth D. Diabetes, other risk-factors, and 12-yr cardiovascular mortality for men screened in the Multiple Risk Factor Intervention Trial. Diabetes Care 1993;16:434-44.

31.   Chen Z, Peto R, Collins R, Macmahon S, Lu J, Li W. Serum cholesterol concentration and coronary heart disease in population with low cholesterol concentrations. BMJ 1991;303:276-82.

32.   Williams RR, Sorlie PD, Feinleib M, McNamara PM, Kannel WB, Dawber TR. Cancer incidence by levels of cholesterol. JAMA 1981;245:247-52.

33.   Garcia-Palmieri MR, Sorlie PD, Costas R, Havlik RJ. An apparent inverse relationship between serum cholesterol and cancer mortality in Puerto Rico. Am J Epidemiol 1981;114:29-40.

34.   Kozarevic D, McGee D, Vojvodic N, et al. Serum cholesterol and mortality - the Yugoslavia Cardiovascular Disease Study. Am J Epidemiol 1981;114:21-28.

35.   Salmond CE, Beaglehole R, Prior IAM. Are low cholesterol values associated with excess

mortality? BMJ 1985;290:422-24.

36. Isles CG, Hole DJ, Gillis CR, Hawthorne VM, Lever AF. Plasma cholesterol, coronary heart disease, and cancer in the Renfrew and Paisley survey. BMJ 1989;298:920-24.

37. Kagan A, McGee DL, Yano K, Rhoads GG, Nomura A. Serum cholesterol and mortality in a Japanese American population - the Honolulu Heart Program. Am J Epidemiol 1981;114:11-20.

38. Stemmermann GN, Chyou PH, Kagan A, Nomura AMY, Yano K. Serum cholesterol and mortality among Japanese-American men - the Honolulu (Hawaii) Heart Program. Arch Intern Med 1991;151:969-72.

39. Frank JW, Reed DM, Grove JS, Benfante R. Will lowering population levels of serum-cholesterol affect total mortality -expectations from the Honolulu Heart Program. J Clin Epidemiol 1992;45:333-46.

40. Kark JD, Smith AH, Hames CG. The relationship of serum cholesterol to the incidence of cancer in Evans County, Georgia. J Chron Dis 1980;33:311-22.

41. White AD, Hames CG, Tyroler HA. Serum cholesterol and 20-year mortality in black and white men and women aged 65 and older in the Evans County study. Ann Epidemiol 1992;2:85-91.

42. Higgins M, Keller JB. Cholesterol, coronary heart disease, and total mortality in middle-aged and elderly men and women in Tecumseh. Ann Epidemiol 1992;2:69-76.

43. Harris T, Feldman JJ, Kleinman JC, Ettinger WH, Makuc DM, Schatzkin AG. The low cholesterol mortality association in a national cohort. J Clin Epidemiol 1992;45:595-601.

44. Schatzkin A, Taylor PR, Carter CL, et al. Serum cholesterol and cancer in the NHANES-I epidemiologic follow-up study. Lancet 1987;2:298-301.

45. Schatzkin AS, Hoover RN, Taylor PR, et al. Site-specific analysis of total serum cholesterol and incident cancer in the national health and nutrition examination survey I epidemiologic follow-up study. Cancer Res 1988;48:452-58.

46. Cowan LD, Oconnell DL, Criqui MH, Barrett-Connor E, Bush TL, Wallace RB. Cancer mortality and lipid and lipoprotein levels - the Lipid Research Clinics Program mortality follow-up study. Am J Epidemiol 1990;131:468-82.

47. Iso H, Naito Y, Kitamura A, et al. Serum total cholesterol and mortality in a Japanese population. J Clin Epidemiol 1994;47:961-69.

48. Goldbourt U, Yaari S, Neufeld HN. High density lipoprotein and total cholesterol as predictors of 7-year mortality from coronary heart disease, cancer and all causes. Am J Cardiol 1981;47:486.

49. Smith GD, Shipley MJ, Marmot MG, Rose G. Plasma cholesterol concentration and mortality - the Whitehall study. JAMA 1992;267:70-76.

50. Rose G, Shipley MJ. Plasma lipids and mortality: A source of error. Lancet 1980;I:523-26.

51. Yaari S, Goldbourt U, Evenzohar S, Neufeld HN. Associations of serum high density lipoprotein and total cholesterol with total, cardiovascular, and cancer mortality in a 7-year prospective study of 10,000 men. Lancet 1981;1:1011-15.

52. Dyer AR, Stamler J, Paul O, et al. Serum cholesterol and risk of death from cancer and other causes in three Chicago epidemiological studies. J Chron Dis 1981;34:249-60.

53. Peterson B, Trell E, Sternby NH. Low cholesterol level as risk factor for non-coronary death in middle-aged men. JAMA 1981;245:2056-57.

54. Schuit AJ, Van Dijk CEMJ, Dekker JM, Schouten EG, Kok FJ. Inverse association between serum total cholesterol and cancer mortality in Dutch civil servants. Am J Epidemiol 1993;137:966-76.

55.   Wald NJ, Thompson SG, Law MR, Densem JW, Bailey A. Serum cholesterol and subsequent risk of cancer - results from the BUPA study. Br J Cancer 1989;59:936-38.

56.   Klag MJ, Ford DE, Mead LA, et al. Serum cholesterol in young men and subsequent cardiovascular disease. N Engl J Med 1993;328:313-18.

57.   Stamler J, Dyer AR, Shekelle RB, Neaton J, Stamler R. Relationship of base line major risk factors to coronary and all-cause mortality, and to longevity - findings from long-term follow-up of Chicago cohorts. Cardiology 1993;82:191-222.

58.   Stamler J, Garside D, Dyer A, Stamler R, Liu K, Greenland P. The strong positive relationship of serum cholesterol to risk of death from coronary heart disease (CHD), all cardiovascular diseases (CVD), cancers, other diseases, and all causes in employed young adult men - findings of the Chicago Heart Association study (CHA). Circulation 1993;88:124.

59.   Stamler J, Garside D, Stamler R, et al. Low risk women and men - 19 year mortality data, Chicago Heart Association detection project in industry (CHA). Circulation 1994;89:938.

60.   Heady JA, Morris JN, Oliver MF. WHO clofibrate/cholesterol trial: Clarifications [letter]. Lancet 1992;340:1405-6.

61.   Stamler J, Neaton JD, Wentworth D. Mortality of low risk and other men: 16-year follow-up of 353,340 men screened for the Multiple Risk Factor Intervention Trial (MRFIT). Circulation 1994;89:938 Abstract.

OBESITY AND DIABETES

Jules Hirsch

Introduction

Noninsulin-dependent or adult-onset diabetes (NIDDM) affects nearly 10 million people in the United States, but obesity can be found in 10 times that number. Both diseases have high heritability but are also markedly influenced by the environment. Dietary and other life style changes appear to be responsible for a recent great increase in the expression of the obesity and diabetes genes. This close relationship between obesity and diabetes has been a cause for much investigation and speculation. One might consider obesity as a compensated form of NIDDM, which in some genetic backgrounds is decomposed to florid diabetes by the stress of environmental factors. Both obesity and diabetes show alterations in pancreatic function, carbohydrate intolerance, and hepatic overproduction of glucose. How the action of one or even several genes can produce these three alterations of physiology remains unknown and thus the basic nature of the obesity-diabetes remains a mystery. One guess is that hypothalamic controls mediated by the activity of the autonomic nervous system along with the effects of a variety of peptides, all of which normally act in concert to maintain a given level of fat storage and of blood glucose level, become disordered. Since this control system has many components, the disorders can arise at many different sites. Because of the interest of my laboratory in adipose tissue, I have elected, in this brief essay, to examine those changes in adipose tissue which may play a role in the obesity-diabetes link.

Discussion

It is now abundantly clear that obesity is the major risk factor for NIDDM. This becomes particularly manifest during later life, thus after age 55 nearly one-third of those with a body mass index over 30 will be found to have NIDDM [1]. As is well known, if adipose deposits are in the midportion of the body, the likelihood of diabetes is much greater than those with equal size adipose deposits in gluteal or femoral regions.

For many years it has been recognized that there is a close statistical relationship between fat cell size and insulin levels which is more robust than the relationship between insulin levels and total fat mass [2]. Thus, fat cell hypertrophy, rather than fat cell number or total fat mass, correlates best with high insulin levels, often the harbinger of diabetes. With weight reduction and a reduction in fat cell size, there is almost always a marked

A. M. Gotto, Jr. et al. (eds.), Multiple Risk Factors in Cardiovascular Disease, 229–232.
© 1998 Kluwer Academic Publishers and Fondazione Giovanni Lorenzini. Printed in the Netherlands.

decline in insulin levels. Although fat mass also changes, cell number tends to remain constant. Such shrinkage of fat mass and cell size is highly correlated with clinical improvement when NIDDM coexists with obesity.

There are several animal models which underscore the specific relationship of fat cell size to insulin metabolism. It is possible to produce obesity in a rat in which there is no hypertrophy of adipocytes [3] and in this circumstance insulin levels remain normal [4]. The experimental design is as follows: obesity is first produced by a period of high fat feeding sufficient to enlarge fat cells and increase fat cell number, particularly in perinephric regions. Thereafter, the animal is fed an ordinary chow diet. Over time the animal loses some weight and fat cell size returns to normal size, but the increased fat cell number and an increase in total body fat remains. This model of hyperplastic, nonhypertrophic obesity in the rat is accompanied by normal insulin levels. Thus, an isolated increase in body fat in the absence of an increase in fat cell size does not alter carbohydrate metabolism.

Another example of a special relationship of fat cell size both with carbohydrate metabolism and with food intake is offered by studies of the Osborne-Mendel rat [5]. This animal is extremely responsive to a high fat diet and will become obese when an ordinary diet of rat chow is adulterated by the addition of fat. But the effect of diet on food intake is dependent on the cellularity of adipose tissue. If, early in life, lipectomy is performed, adipose tissue develops with fewer, larger cells and when high fat is fed the expected hyperphagia is restricted in the lipectomized animal. The lipectomized animal with fewer fat cells rapidly achieves a marked degree of adipocyte hypertrophy. The nonlipectomized animal eats more of the high fat diet for a longer period of time before it achieves the same degree of cell hypertrophy as the lipectomized animal. Prior to the high fat diet during normal growth and development on a low fat chow diet, fat cell sizes are different in the lipectomized and nonlipectomized animal and insulin levels correlate with fat cell size. But when marked obesity develops following high fat feeding, although the amount eaten, the total fat mass and also the number of cells are different in the lipectomized and the sham-operated animals, fat cell size in the sham operated and lipectomized become the same. Then plasma insulin levels are equal in the two preparations [4]. Experiments such as these suggested that something specific about fat cell size either by secreted substances or the metabolic activity of the cells, led to increases and decreases in food intake and energy metabolism as well as changes in carbohydrate metabolism.

In recent years, the study of rodent mutants by the methods of molecular genetics has been extremely productive [6]. The ob mouse which becomes both obese and develops carbohydrate intolerance with high insulin levels, is unable to elaborate a specific peptide termed leptin. The db mouse mutant and the Zucker rat develop obesity on the basis of abnormalities of leptin receptors in the central nervous system. It is assumed, therefore, that leptin secretion and its central detection are important factors in the regulation of food intake. This is the case for the ob mouse, since administration of leptin can reverse the obesity and leptin is inactive when receptor abnormality is the mutation as in the db mouse and the Zucker rat.

It is tempting to suggest that leptin, the secreted peptide of the adipocyte, is a factor in the relationship of fat cell size and insulin levels and perhaps NIDDM as well. It is most notable, however, that in the db and in the ob mouse, equal degrees of carbohydrate intolerance can develop with the presence of obesity, but in one situation leptin levels are high and in the other they are low to absent. It is furthermore notable that in man leptin levels are increased as fat cell mass increases and this occurs whether diabetes is present or not [7]. It is unlikely therefore, that leptin levels are the major link between fat cell size and NIDDM.

Another fascinating relationship between adipose tissue and insulin metabolism has been the demonstration that a nuclear hormone receptor PPAR gamma or peroxisome proliferated activated receptor, is expressed in white adipose tissue. The expression of PPAR is related to adipocyte differentiation. Fibroblasts that are not regularly considered precursors of adipocytes can be converted to adipocytes by experimentally inducing the expression of PPAR gamma in these cells [8].

When PPAR gamma is expressed, cells show increased insulin sensitivity. The relationship of this newly uncovered system to the adipocyte insulin relationship in NIDDM remains unknown. However, a class of compounds which induce PPAR activity known as thiazoladinediones are now under careful investigation. One of these, troglitaoxone, has been shown to reduce insulin need when administered to humans with NIDDM.

The specific genetic basis for human obesity remains unknown. It appears unlikely that a single gene defect like that found in the ob mouse will explain human obesity. Humans with obesity have no deficiency of leptin production. Likewise, the loci for the gene defects that lead to the carbohydrate intolerance and other phenomena of NIDDM, remain unknown. The possibility exists however, that an adipose tissue link and in particular the hypertrophic fat cell will be important in our understanding of NIDDM. Thus, the study of adipose tissue remains central in evaluating the obesity-diabetes connection and its genetic as well as environmental determinants.

Whatever pathophysiologic events are found to link adipose tissue to NIDDM, one important piece of information is already at hand and is central to the theme of this conference. Small reduction in adipocyte size can have important beneficial effects in patients with NIDDM. Thus, the treatment of obesity by any means, even if only partially successful, remains an imperative in the treatment of NIDDM. Similarly, the prevention of obesity would remove the most important risk factor for the development of diabetes.

References

1.   Rewers M, Hamman RF. Risk factors for non-insulin dependent diabetes in diabetes in America. 2nd ed. NIH Publication, No. 85-1468. 1994:179-232.

2.   Stern JS, Batchelor PR, Hollander N, Cohn CK, Hirsch J. Adipose cell size and immunoreactive insulin levels in obese and normal weight adults. Lancet 1972;November 4: 948-51.

3.   Faust IM, Johnson PR, Stern JS, Hirsch J. Diet-induced adipocyte number increase in adult rats. A new model of obesity. Am J Physiol 1978;235:E279-86.

4.   Schneider BS, Faust IM, Hemmes R, Hirsch J. Effects of altered adipose tissue morphology on plasma insulin levels in the rat. Am J Physiol 1981;240:E358-62.

5.   Faust IM, Johnson PR, Hirsch J. Surgical removal of adipose tissue alters feeding behavior

and the development of obesity in rats. Science 1977;197:393-96.

6.   Rosenbaum M, Leibel RL, Hirsch J. Medical progress: Obesity. N Engl J Med 1997; in press.

7.   Rosenbaum M, Nicolson M, Hirsch J, Heymsfield SB, Gallagher D, Chu F, Leibel RL. Effects of gender, body composition, and menopause on plasma concentrations of leptin. J Clin Endocrinol Metab 1996;81:3424-27.

8.   Spiegelman BM, Flier JS. Adipogenesis and obesity: Rounding out the big picture. Cell 1996; 870:377-89.

CLUSTERING OF CARDIOVASCULAR RISK FACTORS

Steven M. Haffner

Introduction

Hypertension, diabetes, and dyslipidemia have long been noted as risk factors for the development of coronary heart disease (CHD) [1]. It has also been shown that these cardiovascular risk factors may cluster in the same individual. While earlier studies have suggested this clustering is related to increased overall adiposity, more recent attention has focused in the possible role of insulin resistance.

The Insulin Resistance Syndrome

Reaven [2] in his Banting Lecture has suggested that insulin resistance may underlay a cluster of risk factors including hypertension, dyslipidemia, NIDDM and atherosclerosis. Indeed insulin resistance has been linked to hypertension [3], dyslipidemia (especially high triglyceride [4], and NIDDM [5]. Recently, increased plasminogen activator inhibitor-1 (PAI-1) [6] and a preponderance of small dense low density lipoprotein (LDL) [7] have also been associated with insulin resistance.

Clustering of Cardiovascular Risk Factors in the San Antonio Heart Study

In order to show clustering, it is not enough to show that insulin resistance may be associated with each individual cardiovascular risk factors, but also that multiple cardiovascular risk factors occur more often than expected by chance. A second issue is whether this clustering is related to insulin concentrations.

We have recently examined some of these issues in the 8-year follow-up of the San Antonio Heart Study [8]. We used fasting insulin as a surrogate for insulin resistance. (In nondiabetic subjects, the correlation between fasting insulin and insulin resistance as assessed by the hyperinsulinemic euglycemic clamp is about -0.6 [9].) Fasting insulin significantly predicted the development of hypertension, hypertriglyceridemia, noninsulin dependent diabetes, and low high density lipoprotein (HDL) cholesterol but not the development of high low density lipoprotein (LDL) cholesterol levels (Table 1). After adjustment for body mass index (a marker of overall adiposity) and waist-to-hip ratio (a marker of upper body adiposity), baseline fasting insulin continued to predict the

A. M. Gotto, Jr. et al. (eds.), Multiple Risk Factors in Cardiovascular Disease, 233–237.

development of hypertriglyceridemia, noninsulim dependent diabetes mellitus (NIDDM), and low HDL cholesterol. However, fasting insulin was no longer significantly related to the development of hypertension suggesting that hypertension was perhaps more strongly related to adiposity than to insulin.

Table 1. Eight-Year Incidence of Multiple Metabolic Disorders According to the First and Fourth Quartiles of Fasting Insulin at Baseline

	Baseline Insulin			
Disorder	Low	High	Relative Risk	p-Value
Hypertension	5.5%	11.4%	2.04	.021
Hypertriglyceridemia	2.6%	8.9%	3.46	<.001
Low HDLC	16.2%	26.3%	1.63	.012
High LDLC	16.4%	20.1%	1.23	.223
NIDDM	2.2%	12.3%	5.62	<.001

Abbreviations: HDLC: high density lipoprotein cholesterol; LDLC: low density lipoprotein cholesterol; NIDDM: noninsulin dependent diabetes mellitus
Adapted from [8].

Subjects developed multiple metabolic abnormalities more often than would be predicted from the probability of developing a single disorder. Lastly, subjects who developed multiple metabolic abnormalities had higher baseline fasting insulin than subjects who developed only a single metabolic disorder.

The Prediabetic State

Mykkänen et al. [10] has shown that multiple metabolic disorders (hypertriglyceridemia, low HDL cholesterol, hypertension, and impaired glucose tolerance) cluster with both insulin concentrations and insulin resistance as determined by the frequently sampled intravenous glucose tolerance test. Some of the best data supporting the existence of clustering of cardiovascular risk factors comes from the study of prediabetic subjects. Several studies have shown increased cardiovascular risk factors at baseline prior to the onset of NIDDM [11-13]. Haffner et al. [12] showed that the increased cardiovascular risk factors prior to the onset of NIDDM could be explained by the higher levels of insulin in prediabetic subjects. The latter observation is consistent with both hyperinsulinemia [14] and insulin resistance [15] predicting the development of NIDDM.

Insulin and the Development of CHD

Since insulin resistance is related to multiple cardiovascular risk factors [2] and since cardiovascular factors predict the development of CHD [1], it seems reasonable to assume that hyperinsulinemia (or insulin resistance) would also predict the development of NIDDM. Surprisingly, the data is somewhat mixed. While most studies have suggested that hyperinsulinemia predicted CHD [16-18], a few studies in elderly subjects did not find such an association [19,20]. (The prospective association of insulin resistance to CHD has not yet been examined.) The study of Després et al. [18] provides the strongest evidence that hyperinsulinemia is associated prospectively with the development of CHD. This study had more comprehensive lipid and lipoprotein measurements, including HDL cholesterol and apoprotein B (apo B), at baseline than previous studies. In earlier reports [16,17], HDL cholesterol was not measured at baseline. Furthermore, the investigators in the Quebec study used an insulin assay that did not recognize proinsulin. The authors found that adjustment for other cardiovascular risk factors did not diminish the predictive power of insulin for CHD and that increasing levels of both fasting insulin and apo B predicted CHD strongly.

Insulin Resistance and Atherosclerosis

Only a few cross-sectional studies have found an association of insulin resistance (as determined by the hyperinsulinemic euglycemic clamp) with atherosclerosis as measured by carotid ultrasound [21] or coronary angiography [22]. These studies [21,22], however, were small. The relationship between insulin resistance (by the frequently sampled intravenous glucose tolerance test (FSIGT) and atherosclerosis (by B-mode ultrasound of the carotid) was recently reported in a large multiethnic population (398 African Americans, 457 Mexican Americans, and 542 non-Hispanic whites) [23]. This effect was reduced but not totally explained by adjustment for traditional cardiovascular disease risk factors, glucose tolerance, measures of adiposity and fasting insulin levels. However, there was not significant association between insulin resistance and intima media wall thickness in African Americans.

Factor Analyses of Cardiovascular Risk Factors

Recently, two interesting reports have appeared in the Insulin Resistance Syndrome using factor analyses [24,25]. Wingard et al. used principal component analyses [24] and found in 1,371 elderly subjects that lipids (HDL, LDL, and triglycerides), blood pressure (systolic and diastolic), glucose tolerance (post challenge glucose and insulin, and in women, fasting glucose) and body size (weight, waist circumference, and fasting insulin) loaded into 4 orthogonal factors. Only body weight loaded with fasting insulin suggested that the components of the insulin resistance syndrome are not related to a single underlying metabolic abnormality. Similar analyses have been done with the Framingham data in 3,321 subjects [25]. Four components were identified. Fasting insulin was associated glycemia (component 1) and glycemia (component 2). Body mass index was associated with dyslipidemia (high triglyceride and low HDL) (component 2) and blood pressure (component 3). Total cholesterol and triglyceride comprised a fourth component. These authors also suggested that the insulin resistance might reflect several distinct physiologic domains. However, factor analyses does not reveal causality and fasting insulin is only a surrogate for insulin resistance.

Conclusions

Clustering of cardiovascular risk factors clearly occurs in population although there is uncertainty about its relation to insulin resistance and whether there may be separate underlying etiologies.

References

1.   Assmann G, Schulte H. The Prospective Cardiovascular Munster (PROCAM) Study: Prevalence of hyperlipidemia in persons with hypertension and/or diabetes mellitus and the relationship to coronary heart disease. Am Heart J 1988;116:1713-24.

2.   Reaven GM. 1988 Banting Lecture: Role of insulin resistance in human disease. Diabetes 1988;37:1595-607.

3.   Ferrannini E, Buzzigoli G, Bonadonna R, et al. Insulin resistance in essential hypertension. N Engl J Med 1987;317:350-57.

4.   Garg A, Helderman JH, Koffler M, Ayuso R, Rosenstock J, Raskin P. Relationship between lipoprotein levels and in vivo insulin action in normal young white men. Metab Clin Exp 1988;37:982-87.

5.   DeFronzo RA. Lilly Lecture 1987. The triumvirate: Beta-cell, muscle, liver. A collusion responsible for NIDDM. Diabetes 1988;37:667-87.

6.   Juhan-Vague I, Alessi MC, Vague P. Increased plasma plasminogen activator inhibitor 1 levels. A possible link between insulin resistance and atherothrombosis. Diabetologia 1991; 34:457-62.

7.   Reaven GM, Chen YD, Jeppesen J, Maheux P, Krauss RM. Insulin resistance in individuals with small, dense lipoprotein particles. J Clin Invest 1993;92:141-46.

8.   Haffner SM, Valdez RA, Hazuda HP, Mitchell BD, Morales PA, Stern MP. Prospective analyses of the Insulin Resistance Syndrome (Syndrome X). Diabetes 1992; 41:715-22.

9   Laakso M. How good a marker is insulin level for insulin resistance? Am J Epidemiol 1993; 137:959-65.

10.   Mykkänen L, Haffner SM, Rönnemaa T, Bergman RN, Laakso M. Low insulin sensitivity is associated with a clustering of cardiovascular risk factors. Am J Epidemiol 1997; in press.

11.   Mykkänen L, Kuusisto J, Pyörälä K, Laakso M. Cardiovascular disease risk factors as predictors of type II (non-insulin-dependent) diabetes mellitus in elderly subjects. Diabetologia 1993;36:553-59.

12.   Haffner SM, Stern MP, Hazuda HP, Mitchell BD, Patterson JK. Cardiovascular risk factors in confirmed prediabetic individuals. Does the clock for coronary heart disease start ticking before the onset of clinical diabetes? JAMA 1990a;263:2893-98.

13.   McPhillips JB, Barrett-Connor E, Wingard DL. Cardiovascular disease risk factors prior to

the diagnosis of impaired glucose tolerance and non-insulin dependent diabetes mellitus in a community of older adults. Am J Epidemiol 1975;131:443-53.

14. Haffner SM, Stern MP, Mitchell BD, Hazuda HP, Patterson JK. Incidence of type II diabetes in Mexican Americans predicted by fasting insulin and glucose levels, obesity, and body fat distribution. Diabetes 1990b;39:283-88.

15. Lillioja S, Mott DM, Spraul M, et al. Insulin resistance and insulin secretory dysfunction as precursors of non-insulin dependent diabetes mellitus. Prospective studies of Pima Indians. N Engl J Med 1993;329:1988-92.

16. Pyörälä K, Savolainen E, Kaukola S, Haapakoski J. Plasma insulin as coronary heart disease risk factor: Relationship to other risk factors and predictive during 9 1/2 year follow-up of the Helsinki Policeman Study population. Acta Med Scand 1985; 701(Suppl.):38-52.

17. Eschwege E, Richard JL, Thibult N, et al. Coronary heart disease mortality in relation to diabetes, blood glucose and plasma-insulin levels: The Paris Prospective Study, 10 years later. Horm Metab Res 1985;15:41-46.

18. Després JP, Lamarche B, Mauriége P, et al. Hyperinsulinemia as an independent risk factor for ischemic heart disease. N Engl J Med 1996;334:952-57.

19. Welin L, Eriksson H, Larsson B, Ohlson LO, Svardsudd K, Tibblin G. Hyperinsulinemia is not a major coronary risk factor in elderly men. The study of men born in 1913. Diabetologia 1992;35:766-70.

20. Ferrara A, Barrett-Connor E, Edelstein SL. Hyperinsulinemia does not increase the risk of fatal cardiovascular disease in elderly men or women without diabetes: The Rancho Bernardo Study, 1984-1991. Am J Epidemiol 1994;140:857-69.

21. Laakso M, Sarlund H, Salonen R, et al. Asymptomatic atherosclerosis and insulin resistance. Arterioscler Throm 1991;11:1068-76.

22. Bressler P, Bailey S, Matsuda M, DeFronzo RA. Insulin resistance and coronary artery disease. Diabetologia 1996;39:1345-50.

23. Howard G, O'Leary DH, Zaccaro D, et al. Insulin sensitivity and atherosclerosis. Circulation 1996;93:1809-17.

24. Wingard DL, Von Muhlen D, Barrett-Connor E, Kritz-Silverstein D. Factor analysis of proposed components of the Insulin Resistance Syndrome. Diabetes 1996;45 (Suppl.2):137A.

25. Meigs JB, D'Agostino RJ, Cupples LA, Wilson PW, Nathan DM, Singer DE. Evidence that insulin resistance does not verify metabolic cardiovascular disease risk variable clustering: The Framingham Offspring Study. Diabetes 1996;45(Suppl.2): 137A.

NEUTROPHIL-ENDOTHELIAL CELLS COOPERATION IN THE HANDLING OF LEUKOTRIENES: ROLE IN CORONARY INFLAMMATION

Carola Buccellati, Giuseppe Rossoni, Albino Bonazzi, Simona Zarini, Manlio Bolla, Jacques Maclouf, Giancarlo Folco, and Angelo Sala

Introduction

Sulphido-peptide leukotrienes (cys-LT, LTC_4, D_4, and E_4), are products of the 5-lipoxygenase (5-LO) pathway of arachidonic acid (AA) metabolism and are intimately involved in the genesis of inflammatory responses, due to their vasopermeant properties that cause plasma extravasation and diapedesis of white cells into perivascular tissues [1]. The generation of cys-LT exhibits remarkable cellular specificity; polymorphonuclear leukocytes (PMNL) generate predominantly the unstable epoxide LTA_4 which is then transformed to leukotriene B_4 (LTB_4) [2], whereas mast cells and eosinophils show preferential generation of cys-LT.

Recently another process of biosynthesis of LTs has emerged. It involves the participation of different cell types whereby PMNL (i.e. donor cells) can synthesize LTA_4 which can be metabolized by vicinal cells (i.e. acceptor cells) into leukotriene B_4 or C_4. Such reaction involves the cooperation of PMNL, possessing the 5-LO enzyme, with erythrocytes, platelets, or the endothelial cell, possessing the secondary enzymes LTA_4-hydrolase or LTC_4 synthase [3-5]. This process has been termed "transcellular biosynthesis" and suggests that the cellular environment (i.e. cell-cell interaction) is an important control in the production of eicosanoids [6].

Recently formation of cys-LT due to cell-cell cooperation between PMNL and coronary endothelial cells has been shown in spontaneously beating, perfused heart of the rabbit [7] where conditions are created which facilitate the transfer and further metabolism of PMNL-derived leukotriene A_4 (LTA_4) to cys-LT by the endothelial acceptor cells. These observations emphasize the importance of PMNL adhesion to the vessel wall as a key event for the initiation of microvascular damage, as suggested to occur in a variety of diseases such as myocardial infarction and cardiac reperfusion damage [8,9].

Prostacyclin (PGI_2) and nitric oxide (NO) are potent autacoids which modulate vessel tonus, inhibit platelet aggregation, and may attenuate cardiac damage through mechanisms related to inhibition of neutrophil activation and migration [10,11]. These features give PGI_2 and NO compounds the potential to interfere with the mechanisms of cell-cell cooperation and the generation of substances such as cys-LT which are formed via

A. M. Gotto, Jr. et al. (eds.), Multiple Risk Factors in Cardiovascular Disease, 239–245.

transcellular biosynthesis.

We describe the effectiveness of the PGI$_2$-analogue iloprost [for review see 11], as well as that of l-arginine, in counteracting acute changes of coronary and cardiac contractility triggered by PMNL activation in isolated heart of the rabbit.

Methods

Hearts were isolated and perfused retrogradely at 37°C through the aorta as previously described [12]. Coronary perfusion pressure (CPP) and left ventricular end-diastolic pressure (LVEDP) were monitored continuously.

PMNL were isolated from blood (40 ml) withdrawn from healthy donors who had not taken medications for at least one week, and purified using a discontinuous Percoll density gradient (42% and 51%, v/v, in PPP) as described previously [7].

The PMNL suspension was added at a flow rate of 0.6 ml per minute, in order to avoid mechanical obstruction of coronary vasculature, and left to equilibrate for additional 5 minutes before challenge with A-23187 (0.5 μM). Thirty minutes later, the entire heart reservoir (approximately 45 ml) was withdrawn for storage under argon atmosphere at -20°C until HPLC analysis.

Cell Incubation

PMNL (5×10^6 ml^{-1}) were supplied with Ca^{2+} (2 mM) and Mg^{2+} (0.5 mM), and allowed to equilibrate for 5 minutes at 37°C; after addition of iloprost (3 nM), l-NMMA (10μM) or l-arginine (100 μM), PMNL were equilibrated further for 5 minutes and challenged with A-23187 (0.5 μM). Stimulation was terminated after 30 minutes by addition of 2 ml ice cold methanol, containing 30 ng of PGB$_2$ and the samples stored at -20°C overnight. Incubates were then centrifuged for 15 minutes at 3,500 g, the supernatant diluted to 15 ml with H$_2$O and extracted using a solid phase cartridge (Supelclean LC-18, Supelco, Bellafonte, PA, USA). Ninety percent aqueous methanol eluates were taken to dryness, reconstituted, and analyzed as previously described [12].

Results

When isolated hearts of rabbit were perfused in the presence of human PMNL (5×10^6 cells) under recirculating conditions, no obstruction of the coronary vascular bed due to PMNL clumping or activation took place. On the contrary, challenge of recirculating PMNL with the calcium-ionophore A-23187 (0.5 μM for 30 minutes) brought about a progressive increase in CPP that, after 30 minutes, reached values approximately fivefold higher than in control preparations (Figure 1, left panel). This event was accompanied by formation of cys-LT, measured in the recirculating medium (Figure 1, right panel).

Pretreatment of the rabbit hearts with iloprost (3nM) prevented the rise in CPP and significantly ablated the presence of cys-LT in the perfusate (Figure 1).

In a similar set of experiments, treatment (20 minutes before challenge) of the rabbit hearts with l-NMMA (10 μM) caused a progressive increase in CPP which was slow in onset and unaffected by A-23187 (0.5 μM) (Figure 2). When l-NMMA-treated hearts were challenged in the presence of PMNL, a marked increase in CPP (and LVEDP, not shown) was observed, accompanied by cys-LT release in the perfusion buffer. Functional alterations were fast in onset and so pronounced as to cause cardiac arrest in systole in 5 out of 6 hearts at 20 minutes (Figure 2).

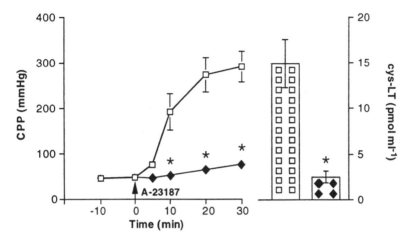

Figure 1. Effect of the prostacyclin mimetic iloprost (3 nM) on coronary perfusion pressure (CPP) and levels of cys-LT of rabbit isolated hearts perfused with polymorphonuclear leukocytes. Open squares: control challenge with A23187 + PMNL; closed diamonds: challenge with A23187 + PMNL in iloprost-pretreated hearts. Reproduced from J Cardiovasc Pharmacol 1996;27:680.

The striking increase in CPP (and LVEDP), as well as the increase in cys-LT formation, observed in the presence of l-NMMA, were significantly prevented by l-arginine (Figure 3).

Cell Incubation Experiments

Challenge of purified human PMNL with A-23187 (0.5 μM for 30 minutes) resulted in the expected generation of LTB_4 as well as of its metabolites, 20-hydroxy- and 20-carboxy-LTB_4. Trivial amounts of cys-LT were also detected, probably due to the presence of eosinophils in the PMNL preparation. Pretreatment of human PMNL with iloprost, l-arginine, l-NMMA or their combination, did not interfere with the neutrophil metabolic pathway of AA.

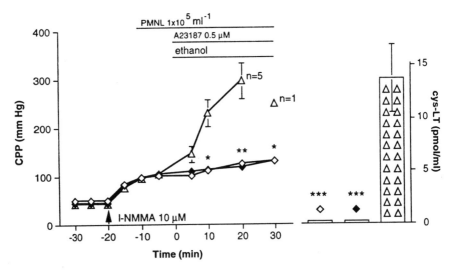

Figure 2. Effect of treatment with l-NMMA (10 μM) on coronary perfusion pressure (CPP) and levels of cys-LT of rabbit isolated hearts perfused with polymorphonuclear leukocytes. Open triangles: challenge (A23187) of l-NMMA-treated hearts in the presence of PMNL; open diamonds: challenge (A23187) of control 1-NMMA-treated heaarts; closed diamonds: challenge (A23187) of control 1-NMMA-treated hearts + blank ethanol. Reproduced from Br J Pharmacol 1997;120:1128

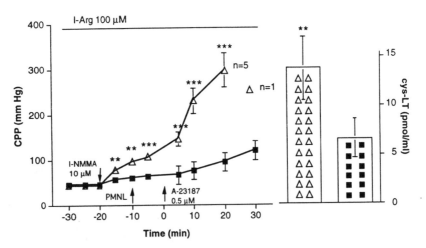

Figure 3. Prevention by l-arginine (l-Arg, 100 μM) of the effect of l-NMMA (10 μM) on coronary perfusion pressure (CPP) and levels of cys-LT of rabbit isolated hearts perfused with polymorphonuclear leukocytes. Open triangles: challenge (A23187) of 1-NMMA-treated hearts in the presence of PMNL; closed squares: challenge (A23187) of 1-NMMA-treated hearts in the presence of PMNL + 1-arginine.

Effect of Nitric Oxide on the Dynamic of Recirculating PMNL in Rabbit Perfused Heart

We evaluated myeloperoxidase enzyme activity (MPO) in aliquots (1 ml) of the recirculating buffer, taken at different time intervals, as an index of PMNL adhesion to the intima of the coronary vascular bed. Pretreatment with l-NMMA (10 μM) before challenge (A-23187, 0.5 μM), caused a rapid disappearance of MPO activity from the recirculating buffer, suggesting intravascular adhesion of PMNL. When hearts were pretreated with l-arginine (100 μM) + l-NMMA, the drop of MPO activity was slower in onset and significantly less pronounced, indicating persisting presence of recirculating PMNL.

Discussion

The results obtained in the present investigation emphasize the importance of activated neutrophils in causing alterations of coronary vasomotion and predisposing the heart towards ischemic damage. In fact, challenge of PMNL which are recirculating within the coronary vascular bed in a spontaneously beating, perfused rabbit heart, causes a progressive and marked increase in coronary resistance to perfusion pressure, indicating: a) constriction of the smooth muscles of this vasculature and b) mechanical pressure exerted by the perivascular edema on the vessel wall, since the increase in coronary tone is partially reversed by the nonspecific vasodilator nitroprusside [7].

In line with our previous findings [7], the increase in coronary perfusion pressure was accompanied by the formation of sulphidopeptide leukotrienes (cys-LT) namely LTD_4, which has been shown to be a potent constrictor of the coronary circulation [13]; LTD_4 may also affect microvascular permeability and therefore contribute significantly to vascular changes in acute inflammation [1].

The functional and biochemical consequences of PMNL activation within the context of spontaneously beating rabbit hearts were almost completely prevented by addition to the preparations of nanomolar concentrations of the PGI_2-analogue iloprost. Its action does not appear to involve a direct inhibition of cys-LT formation at the level of 5-lipoxygenase (5-LO) enzyme, nor can be ascribed to antagonism at the level of cys-LT receptors. The more likely explanation of the present findings could lie in the recognized ability of iloprost (direct action) to provide a defense mechanism/s by attenuating cell-cell interactions. In this respect, iloprost has been shown to reduce infarct size in animal models of experimental ischemia and reperfusion via modulation of PMNL activation and infiltration at the site of tissue injury [14,15].

In a similar fashion, the pharmacological modulation of the NO pathway can markedly affect the cooperation between PMNL and coronary endothelial cells. Endothelial cells possess the constitutive enzyme but are also able to express the inducible form by the action of bacterial products and/or cytokines. Continuous generation of NO has been shown to play an important role in setting the resting tone of systemic as well as coronary resistance vessels; in addition, NO exerts several other effects including inhibition of PMNL activation and adherence [16]. These properties may be of considerable importance in explaining the modulatory role of NO on the transcellular biosynthesis of cys-LT, taking place between PMNL and coronary endothelial cells. Inhibition of NO synthesis resulted in an expected increase in coronary tone, in a marked worsening of the PMNL-dependent and cys-LT-dependent coronary vasoconstriction as well as in enhanced biosynthesis of cys-LT. This was competitively antagonized by pretreatment with exogenous l-arginine, without direct action either on coronary perfusion pressure or on 5-lipoxygenase enzyme activity. This indicates that the cardioprotective effect of NO is not simply restricted to the control of the coronary vascular tone, but may reside in its capacity to modulate the cross-talk between circulating cells and vessel wall.

Increased adhesion of PMNL to the endothelium has been reported following treatment with l-NMMA [17]; moreover the protection observed in the presence of l-arginine, is in line with previous findings, showing significant antiadherence effects and prevention of integrin-induced PMNL adhesion to postischemic venules [18]. The rapid disappearance of MPO enzyme activity that we have observed in the circulating buffer following l-NMMA treatment, compared to its persistence in the presence of l-arginine, confirms the proposed role of nitric oxide as an endogenous modulator of PMNL adhesion. Research directed at the prophylactic use of agents which are able to prevent the adhesion of PMNL to the vascular endothelium and to cut off the biochemical interplay between these two cell populations, may prove effective in reducing the incidence of ischemic heart disease and myocardial infarction.

References

1. Dahlen SE, Bjork J, Hedqvist P, et al. Leukotrienes promote plasma leakage and leukocyte adhesion in postcapillary venules; in vivo effects with relevance to the acute inflammatory response. Proc Natl Acad Sci USA 1981;78:3887-91.
2. Sala A, Bolla M, Zarini S, Muller-Peddinghaus R, Folco GC. Release of LTA_4 versus LTB_4 from human plymorphonuclear leukocytes. J Biol Chem 1996;271:17944-48.
3. Maclouf JA, Murphy RC. Transcellular metabolism of neutrophil-derived leukotriene A_4 by human platelets. J Biol Chem 1988;263:174-81.
4. Feinmark SJ, Cannon PJ. Endothelial cell leukotriene C_4 synthesis results from intracellular transfer of leukotriene A_4 synthesized by polymorphonuclear leukocytes. J Biol Chem 1986; 261:16466-72.
5. McGee JE, Fitzpatrick FA. Erythrocyte-neutrophil interaction: Formation of leukotriene B_4 by transcellular biosynthesis. Proc Natl Acad Sci 1986;83:1349-53.
6. Maclouf J, Murphy RC, Henson P. Transcellular sulfidopeptide leukotriene biosynthetic capacity of vascular cells. Blood 1989;74(2):703-7.
7. Sala A, Rossoni G, Buccellati C, Berti F, Folco GC, Maclouf J. Formation of sulphidopeptide-leukotrienes by cell-cell interaction causes coronary vasoconstriction in isolated, cell-perfused heart of rabbit. Br J Pharmacol 1993;110:1206-12.
8. Kloner RA, Giacomelli F, Alker KJ, Hale SL, Matthews R, Bellows S. Influx of neutrophils into the walls of large epicardial coronary arteries in response to ischemia/reperfusion. Circulation 1991;84:1758-72.
9. Lucchesi BR, Mullane KM. Leukocytes and ischemia-induced myocardial injury. Ann Rev Pharmacol Toxicol 1986;26:201-24.

10. Schror K. Cytoprotective properties of prostacyclin. In: Rubanyi GM, Vane J, editors. Prostacyclin: New perspectives for basic research and novel therapeutic indication. Amsterdam:Elsevier, 1992:157-68.

11. Vane J, Botting R. Prostacyclin in perspective. Crit Ischaemia 1993;3(Suppl.1):4-13.

12. Berti F, Rossoni G, Magni F. Non-steroidal antiinflammatory drugs aggravate acute myocardial schemia in perfused rabbit heart; a role for prostacyclin. J Cardiovasc Pharmacol 1988;12:438-44.

13. Letts LG, Piper PJ. The effects of LTC4 and LTD4 on the guinea-pig isolated heart. J Physiol 1981;317:94-95.

14. Simpson PJ, Mickelson J, Fantone JC, Gallagher KP, Lucchesi BR. Iloprost inhibits neutrophil function in vitro and in vivo and limits experimental infarct size in canine heart. Circulation Res 1987;60:666-73.

15. Smith EF III, Gallenkamper W, Beckman R, Thomsen T, Mannesmann G, Schror K. Early and late administration of PGI2 analogue, ZK 36374: Effects on myocardial preservation, collateral blood flow and infarct size. Cardiovasc Res 1984;18:163-73.

16. McCall TB, Boughton-Smith NK, Palmer RMJ, Whittle BJR, Moncada S. Synthesis of nitric oxide from l-Arginine by neutrophils. Release and interaction with superoxide ion. Biochem J 1989;261:293-96.

17. Kubes P, Suzuki M and Granger DN. Nitric oxide: An endogenous modulator of leukocyte adhesion. Proc Natl Acad Sci USA 1991;88:4651-55.

18. Kubes P, Kurose I, Granger DN. NO donors prevent integrin-induced leukocyte adhesion but not P-selectin-dependent rolling in postischemic venules. Am J Physiol 1994;267:H931-H937.

Integrin Expression and Macrophage Resistance to Apoptosis in Atherosclerosis

Raymond Judware, Jong K. Yun, Thomas S. McCormick, and Eduardo G. Lapetina

Introduction

Development and progression of atherosclerosis is a complex pathologic event involving cells from both the arterial vessel wall and the immune system, including monocyte-derived macrophages. Monocytes are recruited to the atherosclerotic lesion via an elaborate process involving adhesion to and migration through the endothelial cell layer and into the arterial wall. Adhesion and migration of monocytes is accompanied by activation/differentiation to tissue macrophages. Once inside the atheroma, macrophages are exposed to many factors which further stimulate the cells. Cytokines, low density lipoproteins, and low oxygen levels (hypoxia; a product of tissue thickening in the absence of neovascularization [1]) are all factors which have profound effects on the state of differentiation, function, and survival of macrophages within the atheroma.

The precise role of macrophages within an atherosclerotic lesion is not yet well understood. In the course of an inflammatory event (i.e. bacterial infection), macrophages stimulate killing of infected cells and infecting pathogens, then undergo apoptosis, resulting in clearance of the macrophages from the inflammation. In an atheroma, macrophages may behave in a similar manner. However, it has been proposed that some macrophages in the atheroma may fail to undergo apoptosis in a timely manner, thus perpetuating and exacerbating the inflammatory state. Both apoptotic and nonapoptotic macrophages have been identified in human atherosclerotic lesions [2,3], and it has been suggested that apoptosis may clear one population of macrophages from damaged tissue while another population is not cleared [4].

An important survival factor for many adherent cells (including macrophages) is adhesion to an extracellular matrix (ECM). Integrins are heterodimeric cell-surface receptors composed of one α and one β subunit which recognize, attach to, and transmit signals from ECM proteins [5], including collagen, fibronectin, and vitronectin. Engagement of integrins by (with concomitant cell adhesion to) the ECM activates many well-characterized signal transduction systems [6]. Disruption of the integrin-ECM interaction has been demonstrated to promote apoptosis in a number of cell types [7,8], and over-expression of specific integrin subunits can protect cells from apoptosis [9,10].

Our laboratory is interested in conditions which induce macrophage apoptosis and

247

A. M. Gotto, Jr. et al. (eds.), Multiple Risk Factors in Cardiovascular Disease, 247–252.

in mechanisms which may produce apoptosis-resistant macrophages. We have utilized a mouse macrophage-like cell line, RAW264.7 (RAW cells) [11], to generate an apoptosis-resistant derivative cell line (RES cells) [12,13] by chronic stimulation with bacterial lipopolysaccharide and interferon-γ. RAW and RES cells make a highly useful model system to study the mechanisms of apoptosis and resistance to apoptosis in macrophages. We have found that one condition of the atheroma, hypoxia, can promote apoptosis of RAW and RES cells. However, RES cells are somewhat resistant to the effect of hypoxia. Interestingly, one significant difference between RAW and RES is the pattern of expression and function of integrins. We propose that the integrin expression profile may modulate sensitivity or resistance to apoptosis. The potential significance of our results to apoptosis in the atheroma will be discussed.

Results and Discussion

EFFECTS OF HYPOXIA ON CELL GROWTH AND APOPTOSIS

As mentioned above, one condition encountered by macrophages within the atheroma is low oxygen (hypoxia [1]). Experiments were performed to examine the effect of hypoxia on RAW and RES cell apoptosis. Cells were inoculated into culture plates and incubated in normoxia (21% O_2) or hypoxia (2% O_2). The growth kinetics of RAW and RES cells differed in hypoxia. Both cell types grow for a short time in hypoxia, then growth peaks and cell numbers decline concomitantly with the appearance of a population of cells which have detached from culture plates. RES cell growth continued 24 hours longer in hypoxia when compared with RAW cells. In addition, the appearance of detached cells was delayed 12 or more hours in RES when compared with RAW cells. Hypoxia stops cell proliferation and causes detachment from culture plates of both RAW and RES cells. However, both effects are delayed 12 to 24 hours in RES cells.

We next examined the effects of hypoxia on survival of attached or detached RAW and RES cells. At intervals during hypoxic incubation, attached and detached populations of RAW and RES cells were obtained and evaluated for apoptotic cells by staining with propidium iodide followed by flow cytometry. It was observed that with cultures of either RAW or RES, cells which remained attached were not affected by hypoxia; viability of attached cells was high with very low levels of apoptosis in either cell type.

Significantly different results were obtained, however, when detached cell populations were examined. Detached RAW and RES were susceptible to apoptosis. Apoptosis of detached RAW cells peaked at nearly 50% after 36 hours of hypoxic incubation, a time coincident with the peak in number of detached cells. The decline in numbers of apoptotic cells after 36 hours is likely a reflection of the advanced state of cellular degradation which occurs as a consequence of apoptosis. At the time when RAW cells exhibit high levels of apoptosis, the numbers of detached RES cells and the extent of apoptosis of these cells is relatively low. Hypoxic incubation did eventually result in appearance of detached cells and apoptosis in RES cultures; however, both responses were significantly delayed as compared with RAW cells. The numbers of detached and apoptotic

RES cells did not peak until well after RAW cells. Hypoxia induces apoptosis in both RAW and RES, but the effect on RES cells is delayed.

INTEGRIN EXPRESSION AND FUNCTION IN RAW AND RES CELLS

Microscopic examination of cultures of RAW and RES cells revealed an interesting difference in the morphology of the two cell types. RAW cells attach to culture plates but do not adhere tightly or spread, maintaining a rounded cell morphology. RES cells are very different. A substantial proportion of cells resemble the parental RAW cells. However, a significant fraction of RES cells (30% to 50%) not only attach, but adhere tightly to and spread on culture plates. It should be noted here that all culture media used in these studies are supplemented with 10% fetal bovine serum. It has previously been documented that the principle attachment factor in this serum is the ECM protein vitronectin [14], which mediates attachment and spreading of many cell types through the "classic vitronectin receptor", the $\alpha V \beta 3$ integrin complex.

In order to determine whether differences in integrin expression relate to the observed differences between RAW and RES described above, cells were examined to identify their integrin expression patterns. To date, we have been able to conclusively demonstrate three integrin subunits in RAW and RES cells: αV, $\beta 1$, and $\beta 3$; αV can form a heterodimer with either β subunit. Both cell types produce equivalent levels of αV and $\beta 3$. Interestingly, the level of $\beta 1$ is significantly different in RAW and RES; RAW cells produce three- to fourfold higher levels of $\beta 1$ than do RES. This difference in the level of $\beta 1$ is reflected in a threefold higher level of $\beta 1$ on the surface of RAW cells, as compared with RES.

Preliminary analysis of integrin function in RAW and RES has been performed. An important initial event in integrin-mediated signal transduction is recruitment and tyrosine phosphorylation of the focal adhesion kinase pp125^{FAK} (FAK). Adhesion signals initiated by FAK are transduced to the nucleus and culminate in adhesion-dependent gene expression [6]. Western blot analysis has revealed that FAK is produced at similar levels in RAW and RES cells. However, FAK phosphorylation is much greater in RES cells. Immuno-precipitations were performed with an anti-FAK antibody; precipitates were separated by SDS-PAGE and western blot analysis was performed with an antibody against phospho-tyrosine. Persistent FAK phosphorylation (16 hours after plating cells) was observed in both RAW and RES, but was five to tenfold higher (per amount of FAK) in RES than in RAW. RAW and RES cells exhibit at least one significant difference in integrin expression, and this difference is associated with a difference in integrin-mediated signal transduction, which is initiated by FAK.

INTEGRIN EXPRESSION DURING HYPOXIC INCUBATION

Considering the differences in apoptosis during hypoxia and in integrin expression/function between RAW and RES, it was of interest to examine integrin expression during hypoxia. No significant change in the level of the αV integrin subunit occurred in either attached or detached RAW or RES after hypoxic incubation. Levels of β1 and β3 also did not change in either RAW or RES cells that remained attached during hypoxic incubation. Attached RAW and RES either before or after hypoxia maintained a three- to fourfold difference (higher in RAW) in the level of β1 protein and equivalent amounts of β3.

Significant changes in β1 and β3 were observed, however, in detached cells during hypoxia. In both RAW and RES, β1 levels increased three- to fourfold and β3 levels declined during hypoxia. The primary differences in RAW and RES involved the time course of the effect and the final level of integrin observed. Increases in β1 were delayed in RES cells. In RAW cells, β1 levels increased three- to fourfold by 48 hours of hypoxia; at that time, β3 was reduced threefold in the same cell extracts. In RES cells, levels of β1 eventually (by 72 hours) attained levels similar to those observed in RAW cells prior to hypoxia, and levels of β3 were reduced two- to threefold by 48 hours of hypoxia. Interestingly, the kinetics of alterations of integrin levels is similar to the pattern observed for development of apoptosis during hypoxia. Inhibition of proliferation of attached cells, appearance of maximal numbers of detached cells, and maximal apoptosis all correlate with increased β1 and decreased β3 integrin subunit expression during hypoxic incubation.

We have made the following observations in regard to integrin expression and apoptosis in RAW and RES cells during hypoxic incubation: a) RAW and RES cells exhibit a different integrin expression profile, chiefly represented by high levels of β1 in RAW and low levels in RES cells; b) RAW cells exhibit less FAK phosphorylation than do RES cells; c) when confronted by a hypoxic environment, both cell types detach and subsequently undergo apoptosis, however the process occurs more rapidly in RAW and is delayed in RES cells; and d) detachment and apoptosis of RES cells in hypoxia eventually occurs, when the cells have obtained an integrin profile which resembles that observed in RAW cells prior to hypoxia.

We would like to suggest a model to explain our observations (Figure 1). The αV integrin subunit can pair with either β1 or β3. The αVβ3 integrin is the "classic vitronectin receptor"; αVβ1 is a promiscuous receptor for several ECM proteins. In RAW cells (and in detached RES cells at late times of hypoxia), the high level of β1 may favor cell-surface expression of the αVβ1 heterodimer over αVβ3 (αVβ1 > αVβ3), while normoxic RES cells, with lower levels of β1, may produce relatively more αVβ3 than αVβ1 (αVβ3 > αVβ1). In cells maintained on vitronectin (the principle ECM protein in our culture system), αVβ3 may be required to initiate FAK phosphorylation. Initial levels of FAK phosphorylation correlate with rapid or delayed onset of detachment and apoptosis in RAW and RES cells, respectively. Furthermore, detachment and apoptosis of RES cells during hypoxia correlates with the development of an integrin profile similar to that observed in normoxic RAW cells. Integrins can compete for adhesion in neutrophils [15], and adhesion of neutrophils can promote or protect from apoptosis [16]. Similar processes may be at work in RAW and RES cells.

It is accepted that an atheroma is a very complex environment. It is possible that differences in cytokines and/or oxygen levels may produce different subtypes of macrophages [17], which may respond differently to the complex ECM and stress signals within the atheroma. Different macrophages may exhibit different sensitivities to the stress within the atheroma, and may become more or less resistant to apoptosis. It is possible that macrophages which can survive apoptotic signals within the atheroma may perpetuate the inflammation, thus exacerbating atherosclerosis. Our observation, that differences in integrin expression correlate with sensitivity or resistance to apoptosis, provides a starting point for examination of integrin expression profiles in macrophages (and other cell types, i.e. endothelial cells, smooth muscle cells, neutrophils) which are common in the atheroma.

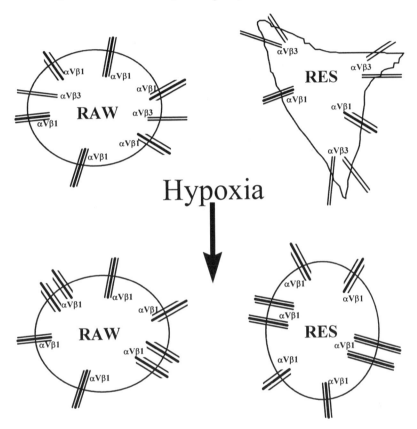

Figure 1. Model for effects of hypoxia on integrin expression in RAW and RES cells. Resting RAW cells produce three- to fourfold more $\beta 1$, and equivalent amounts of $\beta 3$ and αV, as compared with RES cells. This may result in a higher proportion of $\alpha V \beta 1$ on the surface of RAW cells, while RES cells may have a higher proportion of $\alpha V \beta 3$. This difference results in greater adhesion and spreading of, and FAK phosphorylation in, RES cells. Hypoxia increases the level of $\beta 1$, and decreases the level of $\beta 3$, protein. In addition, hypoxia induces rounding and detachment of RES cells. We suggest that alterations in integrin β subunit levels by hypoxia produce cells that resemble normoxic RAW; the predominant cell-surface integrin may be $\alpha V \beta 1$, which does not support adhesion and spreading on vitronectin. Consequently, cells round, detach, and undergo apoptosis.

Acknowledgements

This work was supported by a grant from the Cleveland Foundation and by the Department of Medicine at University Hospitals, Case Western Reserve University, Cleveland, Ohio.

References

1.   Crawford DW, Blankenhorn DH. Arterial wall oxygenation, oxyradicals and atherosclerosis. Atherosclerosis 1991;89:97-108.
2.   Bjorkerud S, Bjorkerud B. Apoptosis is abundant in human atherosclerotic lesions, especially in inflammatory cells (macrophages and T cells), and may contribute to the accumulation of gruel and plaque instability. Am J Pathol 1996;149:367-80.
3.   Geng YJ, Libby P. Evidence for apoptosis in advanced human atheroma: Colocalization with interleukin-1 beta-converting enzyme. Am J Pathol 1995;147: 251-66.
4.   Tidball JG, St. Pierre BA. Apoptosis of macrophages during resolution of muscle inflammation. J Leukoc Biol 1996;59:380-88.
5.   Hynes RO. Integrins: Versatility, modulation, and signaling in cell adhesion. Cell 1992;69:11-25.
6.   Schwartz MA, Schaller MD, Ginsberg MH. Integrins: Emerging paradigms of signal transduction. Annu Rev Cell Dev Biol 1995;11:549-99.
7.   Bates RC, Buret A, van Helden DF, Horton MA, Burns GF. Apoptosis induced by inhibition of cellular contact. J Cell Biol 1994;125:403-15.
8.   Frisch SM, Francis H. Disruption of epithelial cell-matrix interactions induces apoptosis. J Cell Biol 1994;124:619-26.
9.   Montgomery AMP, Reisfeld RA, Cheresh DA. Integrin $\alpha V \beta 3$ rescues melanoma cells from apoptosis in three-dimensional dermal collagen. Proc Natl Acad Sci USA 1994;91:8856-60.
10.   Zhang Z, Vuori K, Reed JC, Ruoslahti E. The $\alpha 5 \beta 1$ integrin supports survival of cells on fibronectin and up-regulates Bcl-2 expression. Proc Natl Acad Sci USA 1995;92:6161-65.
11.   Raschke WC, Baird S, Ralph P, Nakoinz I. Functional macrophage cell lines transformed by Abelson leukemia virus. Cell 1978;15:261-67.
12.   Hirvonen M-R, Brune B, Lapetina EG. Heat shock proteins and macrophage resistance to the toxic effects of nitric oxide. Biochem J 1996;315:845-49.
13.   Brune B, Gotz C, Messmer UK, Sandau K, Hirvonen M-R, Lapetina EG. Superoxide formation and macrophage resistance to nitric oxide-mediated apoptosis. J Biol Chem 1997; 272:7253-58.
14.   Hayman EG, Pierschbacher MD, Suzuki S, Ruoslahti E. Vitronectin - a major cell attachment-promoting protein in fetal bovine serum. Exp Cell Res 1985;160:245-58.
15.   Lub M, van Kooyk Y, Figdor CG. Competition between lymphocyte function-associated antigen-1 (CD11a/CD18) and Mac-1 (CD11b/CD18) for binding to intercellular adhesion molecule-1 (CD54). J Leukoc Biol 1996;59:648-55.
16.   Ginis I, Faller DV. Protection from apoptosis in human neutrophils is determined by the surface of adhesion. Am J Physiol 1997;272:C295-C309.
17.   McLennan IS. Degenerating and regenerating skeletal muscles contain several subpopulations of macrophages with distinct spatial and temporal distributions. J Anat 1996;188:17-28.

EFFECT OF STATINS BEYOND LOWERING CHOLESTEROL: WHERE DO WE STAND?

Pierangelo Quarato, Nicola Ferri, Lorenzo Arnaboldi, Remo Fumagalli, Rodolfo Paoletti, and Alberto Corsini

Introduction

The relation between elevated plasma cholesterol levels and risk for coronary heart disease (CHD) has been established by numerous large-scale epidemiological trials [1]. Several clinical trials have firmly established that aggressive manipulation and normalization of elevated total and low-density lipoprotein (LDL) cholesterol by pharmacological means reduce both the progression of atherosclerosis and the incidence of coronary events [2-4]. A number of cholesterol lowering drugs are currently available for human use [2,5]. In the last decade, a new class of agents which specifically inhibits 3-hydroxy-3-methylglutaryl-coenzyme A (HMG-CoA) reductase, the rate limiting enzyme in cholesterol biosynthesis, has been developed [6]. Six HMG-CoA reductase inhibitors (statins) are available for clinical use: lovastatin, cerivastatin, pravastatin, simvastatin, atorvastatin, and fluvastatin [7-11]. The available clinical data for HMG-CoA reductase inhibitors demonstrate their efficacy and safety in treating hypercholesterolemia and improving long-term morbidity and mortality related to CHD [12]. It has been assumed that, in atherosclerotic patients, any beneficial effect of statins is linked to their hypolipidemic properties, suggesting that this is the main mechanism for preventing the development of atherosclerosis [13,14].

However, mevalonate (MVA) is not only a precursor of cholesterol, but also of a number of nonsteroidal isoprenoid compounds essential for normal cellular activity, such as dolichols, heme A, ubiquinone, and isopentenyladenosine, so that the inhibition of HMG-CoA reductase might have potential pleiotropic effects [15-18]. Indeed this possibility is supported by a variety of experimental evidence indicating that statins can interfere with major events involved in the formation of atherosclerotic lesions, independently of their hypocholesterolemic properties [19-22]. Vascular smooth muscle cell (SMC) proliferation in the arterial wall is a major mechanism for plaque formation as well as a possible determinant of restenosis after angioplasty [23]. MVA and its nonsteroidal isoprenoid derivatives are essential for cell proliferation [16,24] and it has been recently hypothesized that, by inhibiting the MVA pathway, statins may positively influence plaque formation and possibly other pathological processes characterized by increased cell proliferation [25,26]. Based on these findings, the present study investigated the effect of HMG-CoA reductase inhibitors on migration and proliferation of SMC as related to cholesterol biosynthesis. The

253

A. M. Gotto, Jr. et al. (eds.), Multiple Risk Factors in Cardiovascular Disease, 253–265.

role of HMG-CoA reductase inhibitors on other mechanisms involved in the pathogenesis of atherosclerosis has been extensively covered in other reviews and it is not discussed here [25,27,28].

MATERIALS AND METHODS

CHEMICALS

Isoton II was purchased from Coulter Instruments (Milan, Italy). All-*trans* farnesol (F-OH) was from Fluka Chemie AG (Buchs, Switzerland); squalene, all-*trans* geranylgeraniol (GG-OH) and MVA were from Sigma (St. Louis, MD, USA). 2-*cis* GG-OH was prepared as previously described [29]. All reagents were analytical grade.

Simvastatin in its lactone form (Merck Sharp & Dohme Research Laboratories, Woodbridge, NJ, USA) was brought into solution in 0.1 M, NaOH (MSD file) to give the active form and the pH adjusted to 7.4 by adding 0.1 M HCl. Pravastatin, kindly provided by Squibb Pharmaceutical Research Institute (Princeton, NJ, USA) and cerivastatin (Ricerca Bayer Farmacologia, Milan, Italy) were dissolved in saline. Solutions were sterilized by filtration. Racemic fluvastatin (Sandoz Prodotti Farmaceutici, Milan, Italy) and its 2 enantiomers (3R,5S and 3S,5R; Sandoz Research Institute, Hanover, NJ, USA) were dissolved in ethanol.

CELL CULTURES

SMC were cultured according to Ross from the intimal-medial layers of the aortas of male Sprague-Dawley rats (weight 200-250 g) [30]. Cells were grown in monolayers at $37°C$ in a humidified atmosphere of 5% CO_2. Cell viability was assessed by tripan blue exclusion. Human vascular myocytes (A 617 from human femoral artery) were grown in the same culture conditions.

Experimental Protocols

MYOCYTE PROLIFERATION

Myocytes were seeded at a density of $5x10^4$ (human) or $2x10^5$ per 35 mm dish (rat) and incubated with Eagle's Minimum Essential Medium (MEM) supplemented with 10% fetal calf serum (FCS); 24 hours later, the medium was replaced with one containing 0.4% FCS to stop cell growth and the cultures incubated for 72 hours. At this time (time 0), the medium was replaced with one containing 10% FCS plus the compounds under investigation. The incubation was continued for a further 72 hours at $37°C$. After trypsinization of SMC monolayers, proliferation was evaluated using a Coulter Counter (model ZM; Coulter Instruments, Milan, Italy) [18,31].

The concentrations of drugs required to inhibit 50% of cell proliferation (IC_{50}) were computed by linear regression analysis of the logarithm of the concentrations (μM) versus logit [32].

SYNTHESIS OF TOTAL STEROLS

Cholesterol biosynthesis was determined in the same experimental conditions as previously described [18].

RAT SMOOTH MUSCLE CELL MIGRATION

Rat myocytes were seeded at a density of 2×10^5 per 35 mm dish and incubated under conditions identical to those described in the myocyte proliferation experiments. SMC migration was investigated using a modified Boyden chamber (48-well microchemotaxis chamber, Neuro Probe, USA) as previously described [33,34].

RESULTS AND DISCUSSION

EFFECT OF HMG-COA REDUCTASE INHIBITORS ON ARTERIAL MYOCYTE PROLIFERATION AND CHOLESTEROL BIOSYNTHESIS

Fluvastatin, simvastatin, pravastatin, and cerivastatin were investigated on the proliferation of rat aorta and human femoral arterial myocytes. All of them, except pravastatin even at the highest nontoxic concentration (500 µM), decreased the replication of rat aorta myocytes dose-dependently (Figure 1). Similar results were reported when HMG-CoA reductase inhibitors were evaluated in human myocytes (Table 1). The investigated statins also inhibited cholesterol biosynthesis in a dose-dependent manner (Figure 2). The results also indicate that conditions producing a complete inhibition of cholesterol biosynthesis correlate with approximately 50% inhibition of cell growth. The concentrations of drugs required to halve rat and human SMC proliferation and cholesterol biosynthesis are summarized in Table 1.

Fluvastatin is a racemic mixture and the reported IC_{50} values for inhibiting HMG-CoA reductase activity were 0.0024 and 0.08 µM, for the two enantiomers 3R,5S and 3S,5R, respectively [10]. The 3R,5S enantiomer was 33-fold more potent than its counterpart and 2.8-fold more potent than the racemate [10]. The ability of fluvastatin and its enantiomers to inhibit SMC proliferation was related to their potency in suppressing HMG-CoA reductase activity. The 3R,5S enantiomer was 70-fold and 1.6-fold more potent than its counterpart and the racemate, respectively .

To further demonstrate that the interference with SMC growth was due to the inhibition of the HMG-CoA reductase, we investigated the effect of simvastatin, racemic fluvastatin, and cerivastatin on SMC proliferation in presence of MVA or its isoprenoid derivatives. The ability of MVA, all-*trans* F-OH or all-*trans* GG-OH to restore SMC proliferation in a dose-dependent manner (Table 2) indicates that the effect elicited by statins was related to the inhibition of the MVA pathway. 2-*cis* GG-OH, a potential precursor of dolichols [15], did not prevent statin blockade of cell proliferation (Table 2). These results suggest that dolichols are not involved in the regulation of cell growth and support the concept that SMC require MVA or some of its products, such as all-*trans* F-OH or all-*trans* GG-OH, along with an exogenous source of cholesterol (FCS), for proliferation.

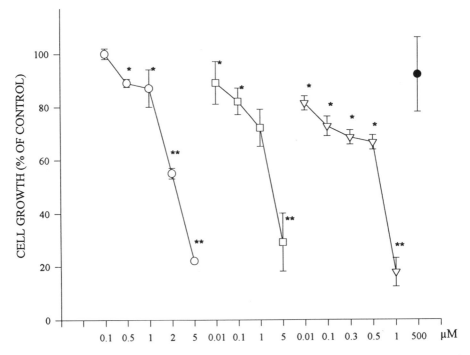

Figure 1. Effect of HMG-CoA reductase inhibitors on the proliferation of rat aortic myocytes. Each point represents the mean ± SD of triplicate dishes. The mean value of control (100%) for cell number was 1286×10^3 ($\pm 41 \times 10^3$) cells per plate. o fluvastatin; □ simvastatin; ∇ cerivastatin; • pravastatin. Drug versus control: * $p < 0.05$; ** $p < 0.01$ (Student's t-test).

EFFECT OF HMG-COA REDUCTASE INHIBITORS ON ARTERIAL MYOCYTE MIGRATION

The effect of statins was investigated on migration of rat aortic myocytes incubated for 5 hours in the presence of fibrinogen as chemotactic factor.

Simvastatin, fluvastatin, and cerivastatin, but not pravastatin, inhibited the fibrinogen-induced migration of arterial myocytes dose-dependently (Table 3). The addition of MVA, all-*trans* F-OH or all-*trans* GG-OH prevented the inhibitory effect of statins (Figure 3), suggesting a specific role of isoprenoid metabolites also in regulating cell migration.

Table 1. Effect of HMG-CoA reductase inhibitors on proliferation and cholesterol biosynthesis in rat and human arterial myocytes.

Drugs	Inhibition (IC_{50} μM)		
	Proliferation	Biosynthesis	Prol/Biosynth
Rat cells			
Fluvastatin (racemate)	2.2	0.15	14.7
Fluvastatin (3R,5S)	1.4	0.12	11.7
Fluvastatin (3S,5R)	104.3	7.26	14.4
Simvastatin	2.8	0.24	11.7
Cerivastatin	0.5	0.03	16.6
Pravastatin	inactive	195	
Human cells			
Fluvastatin	0.3	0.032	9.4
Simvastatin	0.5	0.03	16.7
Cerivastatin	0.046	0.004	11.5
Pravastatin	inactive	15	

IC_{50} = concentration of drug required to inhibit cholesterol biosynthesis and cell proliferation by 50%.

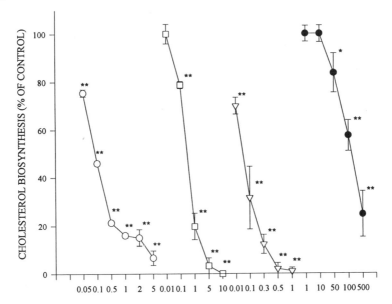

Figure 2. Effect of HMG-CoA reductase inhibitors on the cholesterol biosynthesis of rat aortic myocytes. Each point represents the mean ± SD of triplicate dishes. The mean value of control (100%) for cholesterol biosynthesis was 100.1 (± 15) pmol/mg cell protein per hour. ○ fluvastatin; □ simvastatin; ▽ cerivastatin; • pravastatin. Drug versus control: * p < 0.05; ** p < 0.01 (Student's t-test).

Table 2. Ability of mevalonate and its derivatives to prevent cell growth inhibition by statins.

Addition	µM	Cell Number (% of control)
Simvastatin	3.5	27
Simvastatin plus mevalonate	10	50
"	50	92
"	100	100
Simvastatin plus all-*trans* farnesol	0.1	48
"	1	58
"	5	63
"	10	87
Simvastatin plus all-*trans* geranylgeraniol	0.1	57
"	1	64
"	5	82
Simvastatin plus 2-*cis* geranylgeraniol	5	28
Fluvastatin	3.5	7
" plus mevalonate	100	99
" plus all-*trans* geranylgeraniol	5	73
Cerivastatin	0.5	20
" plus mevalonate	100	97
" plus all-*trans* farnesol	10	77
" plus all-*trans* geranylgeraniol	5	75

Mevalonate or its derivatives were added at time 0 in the presence of simvastatin, fluvastatin, or cerivastatin at the reported concentrations. Each point represents the average of two different experiments that did not differ more than 10%.

The present results show that treatment of cultured arterial myocytes with statins inhibits proliferation in a dose-dependent manner. This effect was overcome by simultaneous exposure of SMC to exogenous MVA (10-100 µM). One critical end-product of MVA is cholesterol, required for cell membrane formation in proliferating cells [16,35]. It is unlikely, however, that inhibition of cholesterol biosynthesis explains the action of fluvastatin, simvastatin, and cerivastatin on SMC proliferation. In fact, cells were stimulated to grow by exposure to a medium containing 10% FCS which provides an exogenous source of cholesterol. Thus, it is likely that the inhibition of cell proliferation by statins resulted from the inhibition of production of one or more isoprenoid intermediates of MVA metabolism. Recently, several proteins involved in growth factor signal transduction have been shown to be lipid-modified by the covalent attachment of MVA-derived isoprenoid groups (prenylation) such as all-*trans* GG-OH or all-*trans* F-OH [16,36,37]. Function and localization of these proteins are dependent on their covalent modification by these specific lipids [14,36,37]. Statins inhibit cell proliferation by reducing the biosynthesis of these two isoprenoids, which are involved in signaling pathways that require prenylated proteins. The fact that all-*trans* GG-OH (0.1-5 µM) can, under these experimental conditions, partially prevent statin-induced inhibition of cell growth in the absence of other prenyl intermediates, suggests that proteins modified by this isoprene (in addition to those undergoing farnesylation) are involved in cell proliferation. The characterization of some of these proteins (such as nuclear lamin B, ras protein and heterotrimeric GTP-binding proteins) provides new insights into the link between the MVA pathway, signal transduction, and cell cycle progression [24,38-40]. Ubiquinone, 2-*cis* GG-OH (a potential precursor of dolichols), and squalene failed to overcome the inhibitory effect of statins, thus ruling out the possibility that the putative regulator(s) of cell proliferation is one of these products of the MVA pathway [29].

Table 3. Effect of HMG-CoA reductase inhibitors on the fibrinogen-induced migration of rat aortic myocytes.

Addition	μM	SMC Migration (cells per HPF) $X \pm SD$
None	—	38.9 ± 4.1
Simvastatin	1	27.8 ± 3.2 *
"	2	23.3 ± 2.6 **
"	3	20.2 ± 1.5 **
"	5	8.0 ± 2.0 **
Fluvastatin	1	23.6 ± 3.0 **
"	2	21.5 ± 4.1 **
"	3	15.2 ± 2.6 **
"	5	6.7 ± 2.0 **
Cerivastatin	0.1	40.8 ± 7.8
"	0.3	47.0 ± 3.5
"	0.5	28.0 ± 5.4 *
"	1	9.7 ± 1.6 **
Pravastatin	500	30.2 ± 5.6

Values are the mean $\pm$ SD of triplicates. 6 HPFs (high power field) were counted per sample and the results averaged. Drug versus control: * $p < 0.05$; ** $p < 0.01$ (Student's t-test).

The failure of pravastatin to inhibit the replication of vascular myocytes may be related to the hydrophilicity of the drug, which impairs diffusion through plasma membrane of peripheral cells and limits its capacity to inhibit cholesterol biosynthesis [41]. On the other hand, pravastatin is internalized via an active transport mechanism into hepatocytes, thus explaining its ability to inhibit cholesterol synthesis to a degree comparable to other statins in these cells [42].

The effects of HMG-CoA reductase inhibitors on fibrinogen-induced SMC migration also suggest a direct relationship between the MVA synthetic pathway and this cellular process.

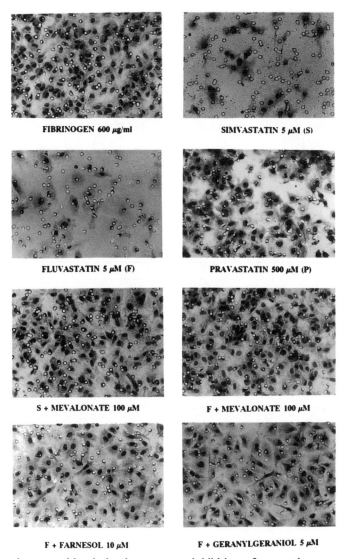

Figure 3. Mevalonate and its derivatives prevent inhibition of rat aortic myocyte migration caused by statins. Cells migrated through the pores appear as black spots.

These *in vitro* studies raise the possibility that the antiatherosclerotic effect of HMG-CoA reductase inhibitors may be mediated, at least in part, by a direct interference with cellular functions. The ability of HMG-CoA reductase inhibitors to interfere with SMC proliferation has been also shown in different models of rapidly proliferating carotid and femoral intimal lesions in rabbits [43,44]. In these models, the effect of statins was not associated to significant changes of serum cholesterol concentrations [19,21,22,43]. The ability of fluvastatin to inhibit SMC proliferation at therapeutic concentrations (0.1-1 μM) [45,46] prompted us to investigate, recently, the pharmacological activity of sera from patients treated with fluvastatin as compared with the more hydrophilic pravastatin, with a lipid-lowering effect similar to fluvastatin but without *in vitro* effects on SMC proliferation. Fluvastatin (40 mg uid) and pravastatin (40 mg uid) given for 6 days to patients with type IIa hypercholesterolemia resulted in a similar decrease of LDL cholesterol levels. Cholesterol biosynthesis and cell proliferation in human SMC exposed to 15% sera from patients treated with either pravastatin or fluvastatin showed striking differences. With pravastatin essentially no changes were seen throughout the 6 hours of exposure, either in cholesterol biosynthesis or SMC proliferation. In contrast, sera from fluvastatin-treated patients 1 hour after drug intake resulted in a 43% inhibition of cholesterol biosynthesis in SMC and in a progressive reduction of cell proliferation, up to 30% after exposure to sera drawn 6 hours after the last dose of fluvastatin [47]. These results suggest its potential use in preventing this process [45,46]. The ongoing clinical trial FLARE, assessing the ability of fluvastatin to prevent postangioplasty restenosis, will provide important information about the potentially beneficial effect of statins in the prevention of lumen renarrowing after percutaneous transluminal coronary angioplasty (PTCA) and on the effective role of SMC proliferation in the pathophysiology of restenosis [47,48]. Recently, it has been reported that statins display other antiatherogenic effects possibly unrelated to the primary action on HMG-CoA reductase. This include the ability of statins to modulate platelet thrombus generation [49], tissue factor activity and expression in human macrophages [50], oxidation of lipoproteins [51,52], natural killer T cell function [53], cholesterol esterification and deposition in macrophages [54], scavenger receptor expression [55], lipoprotein secretion [56], and superoxide generation [57]. Other mechanisms, therefore, may contribute to the beneficial antiatherosclerotic effect of HMG-CoA reductase inhibitors. The important and, as yet, unresolved question is the relative clinical importance of these effects. In the 4S study [3], the observation that the reduction in relative risk produced by simvastatin is partly independent of baseline lipid levels [58], suggests mechanisms other than lowering of plasma cholesterol levels as responsible for the positive outcome in patients under active therapy. In support to this hypothesis, the clinical trial LCAS, investigating the progression and regression of atherosclerotic lesions after fluvastatin treatment, clearly shows that the angiographic benefit of treatment was consistent across all baseline LDL-cholesterol subgroups [59].

In conclusion, HMG-CoA reductase inhibitors exert a direct antiatherosclerotic effect on the arterial wall, independent of their lipid-lowering properties. This activity, which affects major processes involved in the formation of atherosclerotic lesions, is linked to the local modulation of the MVA pathway, and could translate into a more significant prevention of cardiovascular diseases.

Acknowledgements

This research was partially supported by Consiglio Nazionale delle Ricerche - Progetto strategico "Ciclo cellulare e apoptosi". The authors are grateful to Professor Gabbiani (University of Geneva, Switzerland) for providing the human femoral artery cell line A 617. The authors also thank Merck Sharp & Dohme Research Laboratories for providing simvastatin, Bristol-Myers Squibb Pharmaceutical Research Institute for pravastatin, Sandoz Research Institute for the fluvastatin enantiomers, Sandoz Prodotti Farmaceutici for the racemic fluvastatin, and Bayer Ricerca Farmacologica for cerivastatin.

References

1.   Gotto AM Jr. The case for aggressive lipid regulation. Hospital Practice 1997;32(2):145-56.
2.   National Cholesterol Education Program. Second report of the expert panel on detection, evaluation, and treatment of high blood cholesterol in adults (Adult Treatment Panel II). Circulation 1994;89:1329-445.
3.   Scandinavian Simvastatin Survival Study Group. Randomised trial of cholesterol lowering in 4444 patients with coronary heart disease: The Scandinavian Simvastatin Survival Study (4S). Lancet 1994;344:1383-89.
4.   Brown BG, Zhao X-Q, Sacco DE, Albers JJ. Lipid lowering and plaque regression. New insights into prevention of plaque disruption and clinical events in coronary disease. Circulation 1993;87:1781-91.
5.   Havel RJ, Rapaport E. Management of primary hyperlipidemia. New Engl J Med 1995;332:1491-98.
6.   Endo A. The discovery and development of HMG-CoA reductase inhibitors. J Lipid Res 1992;33:1569-82.
7.   Alberts AW, Chen J, Kuron G, et al. Mevinolin: A highly potent competitive inhibitor of 3-hydroxy-3-methylglutaryl coenzyme A reductase and a cholesterol-lowering agent. Proc Natl Acad Sci USA 1980;77:3957-61.
8.   Tsujita Y, Kuroda M, Shimada Y. CS-514, a competitive inhibitor of 3-hydroxy-3-methylglutaryl coenzyme A reductase: Tissue selective inhibition of sterol synthesis and hypolipidemic effect on various animal species. Biochim Biophys Acta 1986;877:50-60.
9.   Stokker GE, Hoffman WF, Alberts AW et al. 3-hydroxy-3-methylglutaryl-coenzyme A reductase inhibitors. 1. Structural modifications of 5-substituted 3,5-dihydroxypentanoic acids and their lactone derivatives. J Med Chem 1985;28:347-58.
10.   Kathawala FG. HMG-CoA reductase inhibitors: An exciting development in the treatment of hyperlipoproteinemia. Med Res Rev 1991;11:121-46.
11.   Bakker-Arkema RG, Davidsen MH, Goldstein RG, et al. Efficacy and safety of a new HMG-CoA reductase inhibitor, atorvastatin, in patients with hypertriglyceridemia. JAMA 1996;275:128-33.
12.   Nash DT. Meeting national cholesterol education goals in clinical practice-A comparison of lovastatin and fluvastatin in primary prevention. Am J Cardiol 1996;78(Suppl 6A):26-31.
13.   Hunninghake DB. HMG-CoA reductase inhibitors. Curr Opin Lipidol 1992;3:22-28.
14.   Feussner G. HMG-CoA reductase inhibitors. Curr Opin Lipidol 1994;5:59-68.
15.   Grunler J, Ericsson J, Dallner G. Branch-point reactions in the biosynthesis of cholesterol, dolichol, ubiquinone and prenylated proteins. Biochim Biophys Acta 1994;1212:259-77.
16.   Goldstein JL, Brown MS. Regulation of the mevalonate pathway. Nature 1990;343:425-30.
17.   Bernini F, Didoni G, Bonfadini G, Bellosta S, Fumagalli R. Requirement for mevalonate in acetylated LDL induction of cholesterol esterification in macrophages. Atherosclerosis 1993;

104:19-26.
18.   Corsini A, Mazzotti M, Raiteri M, et al. Relationship between mevalonate pathway and arterial myocyte proliferation: In vitro studies with inhibitors of HMG-CoA reductase. Atherosclerosis 1993;101:117-25.
19.   Soma MR, Donetti E, Parolini C, et al. HMG-CoA reductase inhibitors: In vivo effects on carotid intimal thickening in normocholesterolemic rabbits. Arterioscl Thromb 1993;13:571-78.
20.   Zhu BQ, Sievers RE, Sun YP, Isenberg WM, Parmley WW. Effect of lovastatin on suppression and regression of atherosclerosis in lipid-fed rabbits. J Cardiovasc Pharmacol 1992;19:246-55.
21.   Gellman J, Ezekowitz MD, Sarembock IJ, et al. Effect of lovastatin on intimal hyperplasia after balloon angioplasty. A study in an atherosclerotic hypercholesterolemic rabbit. J Am Coll Cardiol 1991;17:251-59.
22.   Bocan TMA, Mazur MJ, Mueller SB, et al. Antiatherosclerotic activity of inhibitors of 3-hydroxy-3-methylglutaryl coenzyme A reductase in cholesterol-fed rabbits: A biochemical and morphological evaluation. Atherosclerosis 1994;111:127-42.
23.   Ross R. The pathogenesis of atherosclerosis: A perspective for the 1990s. Nature 1993;362:801-9.
24.   Glomset JA, Farnsworth CC. Role of protein modification reactions in programming interactions between ras-related GTPases and cell membranes. Ann Rev Cell Biol 1994;10:181-205.
25.   Massy ZA, Keane WF, Kasiske BL. Inhibition of the mevalonate pathway: Benefits beyond cholesterol reduction? Lancet 1996;347:102-3.
26.   Soma MR, Baetta R, De Renzis MR, et al. In vivo enhanced antitumor activity of carmustine [N,N'-bis(2-chloroethyl)-N-nitrosourea] by simvastatin. Cancer Res 1995; 55:597-602.
27.   Gotto AM, Jr. Dyslipidemia and atherosclerosis. A forecast of pharmaceutical approaches. Circulation 1993;87(Suppl.III):III-54-III-59.
28.   Corsini A, Bernini F, Quarato P, et al. Non-lipid-related effects of 3-hydroxy-3-methylglutaryl coenzyme A reductase inhibitors. Cardiology 1996;87:458-68.
29.   Raiteri M, Arnaboldi L, McGeady P, et al. Pharmacological control of mevalonate pathway: effect on arterial smooth muscle cell proliferation. J Pharmacol Exp Ther 1997;281:1144-53.
30.   Ross R. The smooth muscle cell. II. Growth of smooth muscle in culture and formation of elastic fibers. J Cell Biol 1971;50:172-86.
31.   Corsini A, Raiteri M, Soma MR, Fumagalli R, Paoletti R. Simvastatin but not pravastatin inhibits the proliferation of rat aorta myocytes. Pharm Res 1991;23:173-80.
32.   Fisher RA, Yates F. Statistical Tables for Biological, Agricultural and Medical Research. 4th Ed. Edinburgh: Oliver and Boyd, 1953:60.
33.   Naito M, Hayashi T, Kuzuya M, Funaki C, Asai K, Kuzuya F. Effects of fibrinogen and fibrin on the migration of vascular smooth muscle cells in vitro. Atherosclerosis 1990;83:9-14.
34.   Corsini A, Quarato P, Raiteri M, et al. Effect of nifedipine-atenolol association on arterial myocyte migration and proliferation. Pharm Res 1993;27:299-307.
35.   Chen HW. Role of cholesterol metabolism in cell growth. Fedn Proc 1984;43:126-30.
36.   Maltese WA. Posttranslational modification of proteins by isoprenoids in mammalian cells. FASEB J 1990;4:3319-28.
37.   Glomset JA, Gelb MH, Farnsworth CC. Prenyl proteins in eukaryotic cells: A new type of membrane anchor. Trends Biochem Sci 1990;15:139-42.
38.   Farnsworth CC, Wolda SL, Gelb MH, Glomset JA. Human lamin B contains a farnesylated

cysteine residue. J Biol Chem 1989;264:20422-29.

39. Casey PJ, Solsky PA, Der CJ, Buss JE. p21ras is modified by a farnesyl isoprenoid. Proc Natl Acad Sci USA 1989;86:8323-27.

40. Hirai A, Nakamura S, Noguchi Y, et al. Geranylgeranylated Rho small GTPase(s) are essential for the degradation of p27^{kip1} and facilitate the progression from G1 to S phase in growth-stimulated rat FRTL-5 cells. J Biol Chem 1997;272:13-16.

41. Scott W. Hydrophilicity and the differential pharmacology of pravastatin. In: Wood C, editor. Lipid management: pravastatin and the differential pharmacology of HMG-CoA reductase inhibitors. London Round Table Series n. 16: Royal Society of Medicine Service. 1989:17-25.

42. Komai T, Shigehara E, Tokui T, et al. Carrier-mediated uptake of pravastatin by rat hepatocytes in primary culture. Biochem Pharmacol 1992;43:667-70.

43. Bandoh T, Mitani H, Niihashi M, et al. Inhibitory effect of fluvastatin at doses insufficient to lower serum lipids on the catheter-induced thickening of intima in rabbit femoral artery. Eur J Pharmacol 1996;315:37-42.

44. Soma MR, Parolini C, Donetti E, Fumagalli R, Paoletti R. Inhibition of isoprenoid biosynthesis and arterial smooth muscle cell proliferation. J Cardiovasc Pharmacol 1995;25: S20-S24.

45. Dain JG, Fu E, Gorski J, Nicoletti J, Scallen TJ. Biotransformation of fluvastatin sodium in humans. Drug Met Disp 1993;21:567-72.

46. Tse FLS, Jaffe JM, Troendle A. Pharmacokinetics of fluvastatin after single and multiple doses of normal volunteers. J Clin Pharmacol 1992;32:630-38.

47. Pentikainen P, Saraheimo M, Schwartz J, et al. Comparative pharmacokinetics of lovastatin, simvastatin and pravastatin in humans. J Clin Pharmacol 1992;32:136-40.

48. Isner JM, Kearney M, Bauters C, et al. Use of human tissue specimens obtained by directional atherectomy to study restenosis. Trends Cardiovasc Med 1994;4:213-21.

49. Sandset PM, Lund H, Abildgaard U, Ose L. Treatment with hydroxymethylglutaryl-coenzyme A reductase inhibitors in hypercholesterolemia induces changes in the components of the extrinsic coagulation system. Arterioscl Thromb 1991;11:138-45.

50. Colli S, Eligini S, Lalli M, Camera M, Paoletti R, Tremoli E. Vastatins inhibit tissue factor in cultured human macrophages. A novel mechanism of protection against atherothrombosis. Arterioscl Thromb Vasc Biol 1997;17:265-72.

51. Kleinveld HA, Demacker PNM, De Haan AFJ, Stalenhoef AFH. Decreased in vitro oxidizability of low-density lipoprotein in hypercholesterolemic patients treated with 3-hydroxy-3-methylglutaryl-CoA reductase inhibitors. Eur J Clin Invest 1993;23:289-95.

52. Hussein O, Schlezinger S, Rosenblat M, Kheidar S, Aviram M. Reduced susceptibility of low density lipoprotein (LDL) to lipid peroxidation after fluvastatin therapy is associated with the hypocholesterolemic effect of the drug and its binding to the LDL. Atherosclerosis 1997;128: 11-18.

53. Kobashigawa JA, Katznelson S, Hillel L, Johnson JA, Yeatman L, Wang XM. Effect of pravastatin on outcomes after cardiac transplantation. New Engl J Med 1995;333:621-27.

54. Bernini F, Scurati N, Bonfadini G, Fumagalli R. HMG-CoA reductase inhibitors reduce acetyl LDL endocytosis in mouse peritoneal macrophages. Arterioscl Thromb Vasc Biol 1996;15: 1352-58.

55. Umetani N, Kanayama Y, Okamura M, Negoro N, Takeda T. Lovastatin inhibits gene expression of type-I scavenger receptor in THP-1 human macrophages. Biochim Biophys Acta 1996;1303:199-206.

56. La Ville A, Moshy R, Turner PR, Miller NE, Lewis B. Inhibition of cholesterol synthesis

reduces low density lipoprotein apoprotein B production without decreasing very low density lipoprotein apoprotein B synthesis in rabbits. Biochem J 1984;218:321-23.

57.   Giroux LM, Davignon J, Naruzewicz M. Simvastatin inhibits the oxidation of low-density lipoproteins by activated human monocyte-derived macrophages. Biochim Biophys Acta 1993;1165:335-38.

58.   Scandinavian Simvastatin Survival Study Group. Baseline serum cholesterol and treatment effect in the Scandinavian Simvastatin Survival Study (4S). Lancet 1995:345:1274-75.

59.   Herd JA, Ballantyne CM, Farmer JA, et al. Effects of fluvastatin on coronary atherosclerosis in patients with mild to moderate cholesterol elevations (Lipoproteins and Coronary Atherosclerosis Study [LCAS]). Am J Cardiol 1997;80:278-86.

LESSONS FROM CLINICAL TRIALS: LCAS AND OTHER STUDIES

J. Alan Herd

Introduction

The levels of lipids and lipoprotein in blood have a causal relation to coronary heart disease (CAD). In particular, high serum levels of low-density lipoprotein cholesterol (LDL-C) and low levels of high-density lipoprotein cholesterol (HDL-C) predispose individuals to myocardial ischemia and acute coronary events. Furthermore, treatment which lowers high levels of LDL-C decreases progression in coronary artery disease and reduces the incidence of acute coronary events.

Many investigators have shown that aggressive lipid-lowering therapy stops progression of coronary artery disease and prevents acute coronary events. Brown et al. [1,2] reported that aggressive lipid-altering therapy in patients at very high risk for CAD halved the expected frequency of progression, tripled the frequency of regression, and reduced clinical events by nearly 75%. Reductions in LDL-C, reductions in systolic blood pressure and increases in HDL-C were significantly related to benefits of treatment with lipid-lowering drugs [1,2].

The profile of risk factors for coronary heart disease includes many factors in addition to the level of cholesterol in blood. Results from the Framingham Heart Study [3] showed that men and women who had high levels of triglycerides in blood and low HDL-C had an increased incidence of coronary heart disease independently of their level of total cholesterol.

Patients who have had signs or symptoms of coronary heart disease have a high likelihood for acute coronary events. Individuals with no history of acute coronary events or myocardial ischemia have a relatively low likelihood. Zhao et al. [4] reported the effects of intensive lipid-lowering therapy on the coronary arteries of asymptomatic subjects with elevated apolipoprotein B levels. At baseline, symptomatic and asymptomatic patients had comparable risk profiles but the symptomatic patients had more severe coronary disease. Patients in both groups treated intensively had less progression and more regression than patients receiving conventional treatment. However, clinical cardiovascular events occurred only in symptomatic patients and occurred less frequently in patients treated intensively compared to patients receiving conventional treatment.

The challenge is to identify and treat individuals who are most likely to have progression of lesions in their coronary arteries. The individuals who would seem most

A. M. Gotto, Jr. et al. (eds.), Multiple Risk Factors in Cardiovascular Disease, 267–274.
© 1998 Kluwer Academic Publishers and Fondazione Giovanni Lorenzini. Printed in the Netherlands.

likely to benefit from lipid-lowering treatment would be those with moderately severe lesions of one or more coronary arteries who also have severely abnormal risk factors. The results of the Lipoprotein and Coronary Atherosclerosis Study (LCAS) and other recent lipid-regulating trials monitored by angiography showed that treatment with an HMG Co-A reductase inhibitor drug reduced rates of progression to less than half.

Methods

The design and methods of the LCAS have been described in previous publications [5,6]. After 10 weeks of treatment on an American Heart Association Step I diet, 429 patients (349 men and 80 women) were randomized into a double-blind, placebo-controlled trial in which they received fluvastatin (20 mg bid), or placebo and were treated and followed for 2.5 years. After 12 weeks of treatment with fluvastatin or placebo, those having LDL-C $\geq$ 160 mg/dl at randomization received a bile acid-binding resin. The design allowed treatment comparisons of fluvastatin with and without resin versus placebo with and without resin as well as pair-wise comparisons of fluvastatin alone versus placebo alone and fluvastatin plus resin versus placebo plus resin on the severity of coronary atherosclerosis.

The primary endpoint was within-patient per-lesion change in minimum lumen diameter (MLD) of qualifying lesions. Dimensions of coronary artery lesions were measured using the Cardiovascular Angiographic Analysis System [7]. Qualifying lesions were defined by MLD $\geq$ 25% of the reference lumen diameter at baseline and MLD > 0.8 mm less than the reference lumen diameter at either baseline or follow up. Lesions with a reference lumen diameter < 1.5 mm at baseline or poorly visualized at either baseline or follow-up were excluded from the analysis. Lesions in arteries with baseline total occlusion or prior angioplasty were excluded from the primary analysis.

The primary endpoint was assessed by hierarchical linear modeling, which allowed the consideration of each qualifying lesion nested within patient while the patient was maintained as the primary unit of analysis.

Results

Mean changes in lipid concentrations between baseline and the end of the trial in patients treated with fluvastatin were total cholesterol -14.7%, LDL-C -23.9%, HDL-C +8.5% and triglycerides -0.1%. Theses changes were all statistically significantly different than changes observed in patients receiving placebo treatment.

Analysis of the primary endpoint, final minus baseline MLD of qualifying lesions within patient adjusted for age and sex, showed significantly less progression in all fluvastatin patients (-0.028 $\pm$ 0.021 mm) compared to placebo patients (-0.100 $\pm$ 0.022 mm) (mean $\pm$ SEM) (p = 0.005) (Figure 1). Although patients in the monotherapy subgroups had lower baseline LDL-C, a similar benefit with treatment was seen. Analysis of change in percent diameter stenosis also showed significantly less progression in all fluvastatin patients (Figure 2).

Primary Endpoint: Change in MLD between Baseline and Final Angiogram for All Subjects

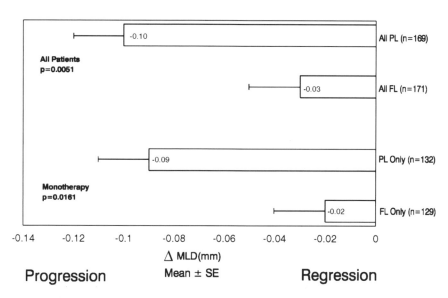

Figure 1. Angiographic change (mean, SEM) in minimum lumen diameter (MLD) adjusted for age and sex, according to prospective treatment group. CME: cholestyramine; FL: fluvastatin; PL: placebo

Lesion severity and the variability of change in lesion severity are shown in Table 1. Of the 429 patients randomized into the clinical trial, there were 340 who had evaluable angiograms both at baseline and following treatment with fluvastatin or placebo for at least 12 months. Among the 340 patients were 1,215 lesions which were analyzed using quantitative coronary angiography. All patients had at least one lesion and one patient had 12 lesions. The average number of lesions analyzed per patient was 3.6. At baseline, the average severity for all lesions was 43.0 ± 12.8 percent diameter stenosis (mean $\pm$ S.D.) and the average range was 4-75 percent diameter stenosis. Patients with greater than 75 percent diameter stenosis were excluded from participation in the clinical trial. At the final angiogram, the lesion severity had increased to 45.9 ± 14.9 percent diameter stenosis and the range of severity was 14-100% diameter stenosis.

The variability of change in percent diameter stenosis is shown in Table 1 as the S.D. of change (final-baseline) among all 1,215 lesions. The range was -37 to +81 percent diameter stenosis and more lesions showed increased severity of stenosis or progression than showed decreased severity or regression.

The Effect of Treatment on Change in Percent Diameter Stenosis between Baseline and Final Angiogram for All Subjects

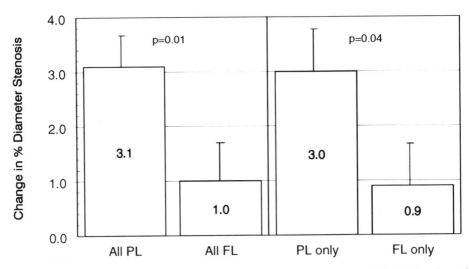

Figure 2. Angiographic change (mean, SEM) in percent diameter stenosis (% DS) adjusted for age and sex, according to prospective treatment group.

Table 1. Lesion Severity (Percent Diameter Stenosis) Among 1,215 Lesions in 340 Patients

	Mean	Standard Deviation	Range
Baseline	43.0	12.8	4 to 70
Final	45.9	14.9	14 to 100
Change (Final-Baseline)	2.9	12.9	-37 to +81

Discussion

Obstructive lesions in coronary arteries tend to progress approximately 1.5% of reference lumen diameter per year without treatment (Figure 3). Results have been reported from several angiographic trials with lipid-lowering treatment. Follow-up angiography was performed at two years in the Canadian Coronary Atherosclerosis Intervention Trial (CCAIT) [8] and the Monitored Atherosclerosis Regression Study (MARS) [9]; 2.5 years in the Familial Atherosclerosis Treatment Study (FATS) [1], the Harvard Atherosclerosis

Reversibility Project (HARP) [10] and the LAS [6]; three years in the Pravastatin Limitation of Atherosclerosis in the Coronary Arteries study (PLAC I) [11]; and four years in the Multicenter Anti-Atheroma Study (MAAS) [12]. All trials tested an HMG Co-A reductase inhibitor, LCAS with or without adjunctive cholestyramine, and HARP with or without nicotinic acid, cholestyramine, and/or gemfibrozil. In most of these trials (except HARP), there was a correlation between severity of progression in coronary atherosclerosis and incidence of clinical cardiac events.

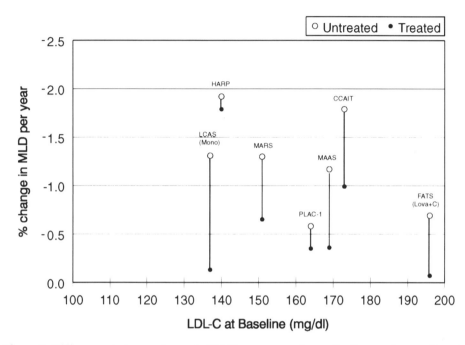

Figure 3. Differences between change in MLD as a percentage of reference lumen diameter per year from angiographic studies. CCAIT: Canadian Coronary Atherosclerosis Intervention Trial. MARS: Monitored Atherosclerosis Regression Study. HARP: Harvard Atherosclerosis Reversibility Project. LCAS: Lipoprotein and Coronary Atherosclerosis Study. FATS: Familial Atherosclerosis Treatment Study. MAAS: Multicentre Anti-Atheroma Study.

The likelihood that patients with coronary artery disease will have acute cardiac events has been studied by several investigators. Harris et al. [13] have followed 1,183 medically treated patients for up to four years after cardiac catheterization and coronary arteriography. They reported data indicating that those patients who had 75 percent diameter stenosis in one coronary artery or 50 percent diameter stenosis in two coronary arteries had a 15% incidence of nonfatal acute cardiac events or death in 2.5 years. In addition, they noted that the number of additional vessels with lesser stenoses did not influence incidence of cardiac events in patients who had a 75 percent stenosis in one or more vessels. They also noted that patients who had only one vessel with a 50 percent stenosis had approximately the same prognosis as patients who did not have 50 percent or greater stenosis in any coronary artery.

Brown et al. [1] reported the incidence of acute cardiac events in the FATS. They observed that treatment which lowered LDL-C by 32% in one group and 46% in another reduced the incidence of acute cardiac events by 73%. Further details were presented by Zhao et al. [4] who reported the association of acute cardiac events with severity of coronary heart disease. Of the 120 men completing the 30-month clinical trial, 91 were symptomatic and 29 were asymptomatic. At baseline, symptomatic and asymptomatic patients had comparable risk profiles but the symptomatic patients had more severe coronary disease. Patients in both groups treated intensively had less progression and more regression than patients receiving conventional treatment. However, clinical cardiovascular events occurred only in symptomatic patients and occurred less frequently in patients treated intensively compared to patients receiving conventional treatment.

Similar results were reported by investigators from the PLAC II and the ACAPS clinical trials. Patients who were enrolled in PLAC II had a history of acute myocardial infarction or coronary artery disease demonstrated by angiography. Crouse et al. [14] reported that treatment which lowered LDL-C by 28% reduced acute cardiac events by 60%. Subjects who were enrolled in ACAPS had ultrasound-demonstrated carotid atherosclerosis but were asymptomatic for coronary heart disease. Furberg et al. [15] reported that treatment which lowered LDL-C by 28% reduced acute cardiovascular events by 64%. The risk for acute events was greater in symptomatic patients but reductions in acute cardiovascular events occurred in both symptomatic and asymptomatic individuals.

The link between progression in lesions and clinical cardiac events probably depends on severity of coronary arterial lesions at baseline and the rapidity of progression in coronary atherosclerosis during the trial. However, the average values reported for change in all lesions do not indicate the severity of change which occurs in a few lesions. Rather it is the variability of change in lesions that is more indicative of risk for clinical cardiac events in relation to progression among individual coronary arteries. For example, an average change of 1.5 percent diameter stenosis per year is not distributed equally among all lesions in all patients. Instead, some lesions in some patients have no change, some have regression, some have mild progression, and some have severe progression. Most clinical cardiac events probably occur because of severe progression in a few coronary arterial lesions in a few patients.

In the LCAS, the average increase in severity of coronary arterial lesions in patients receiving placebo was an increase in percent diameter stenosis of 3.1 and, in patients receiving fluvastatin, the average increase in severity was 1.0 (Figure 2). The average increase in percent diameter stenosis among all lesions in all patients was 2.9 and the standard deviation of change was 12.9 (Table 1). The distribution of change in percent diameter stenosis was approximately normal and those lesions which progressed in severity about one standard deviation from the mean, had an increase in percent diameter stenosis that was greater than 15. Among all lesions in all patients, the lesions with the most severe progression, beyond two standard deviations from the mean, had an increase in percent diameter stenosis that was greater than 25. At the time of final coronary angiography, lesions which progressed beyond two standard deviations from the mean caused a percent diameter stenosis that was greater than 75. The most severe progression was seen among 19 lesions (approximately 1.5% of the total number of lesions) which progressed to total occlusion. Any lesions causing more than 75 percent diameter stenosis might cause symptoms from myocardial ischemia and those which progressed to 100% occlusion would have a high likelihood of causing a clinical cardiac morbid or fatal event.

The bridge from cholesterol to cardiovascular events probably occurs through: 1) cholesterol inhibition of endothelial-mediated vascular reactivity causing arterial constriction; 2) deposition of cholesterol in fibrous caps overlying deposits of macrophages, foam cells, and cholesterol crystals in plaques which are liable to fracture and cause thrombosis; 3) intermediates of cholesterol synthesis causing hypertrophy of vascular smooth muscle, proliferation of fibrocytes, and infiltration of macrophages and inflammatory cells in arterial walls; and 3) accumulation of cholesterol in macrophages, foam cells, and intercellular spaces expanding plaques which obstruct blood flow through arteries. Any or all of these mechanisms can contribute to cardiovascular events.

The effects of cholesterol lowering treatment for patients in the LCAS apparently reduced the progression of plaques. The lowering of LDL-C in blood may have reduced the accumulation of cholesterol in plaques. It also is possible that fluvastatin decreased the hypertrophy of vascular smooth muscle, proliferation of fibrocytes and infiltration of macrophages and inflammatory cells in arterial walls by interfering with the biosynthesis of intermediates in the synthesis of cholesterol. Whatever the mechanism whereby fluvastatin might affect atherosclerosis, patients in the LCAS who received fluvastatin had less progression of lesions than those patients who received placebo. A possible benefit of any reduction in progression among severe lesions would be a reduction in clinical cardiac events.

References

1. Brown G, Albers JJ, Fisher LF. Regression of coronary artery disease as a result of intensive lipid-lowering therapy in men with high levels of apolipoprotein B. N Engl J Med 1990;323:1289-98.
2. Brown BG. Effect of lovastatin or niacin combined with colestipol and regression of coronary atherosclerosis. European Heart J 1992;13(Suppl.B):17-20.
3. Castelli WP. Epidemiology of triglycerides: A view from Framingham Am J Cardiology 1992;70:3H-9H.
4. Zhao XQ, Brown BG, Hillger L, Sacco D, Bisson B, Fisher L, Albers JJ. Effects of intensive lipid-lowering therapy on the coronary arteries of asymptomatic subjects with elevated apolipoprotein B. Circulation 1993;88:2744-53.
5. West MS, Herd JA, Ballantyne CM, Simpson S, Gould KL, Gotto AM Jr. The Lipoprotein and Coronary Atherosclerosis Study (LCAS): Design, methods, and baseline data of a trial of fluvastatin in patients without severe hypercholesterolemia. Control Clin Trials 1996;17:550-83.

6.   Herd JA, Ballantyne CM, Farmer JA, et al. Effects of fluvastatin on coronary atherosclerosis in patients with mild to moderate cholesterol elevations (Lipoprotein and Coronary Atherosclerosis Study [LCAS]). Am J Cardiol 1997; in press.

7.   Reiber JHC, Serruys PW, Kooijman CJ, et al. Assessment of short-, medium-, and long-term variations in arterial dimensions from computer-assisted quantitation of coronary cineangiograms. Circulation 1983;71:280-88.

8.   Waters D, Higginson L, Gladstone P, et al., and the CCAIT Study Group. Effects of monotherapy with an HMG-CoA reductase inhibitor on the progression of coronary atherosclerosis as assessed by serial quantitative arteriography: The Canadian Coronary Atherosclerosis Intervention Trial. Circulation 1994;89:959-68.

9.   Blankenhorn DH, Azen SP, Kramsch DM, et al., and the MARS Research Group. Coronary angiographic changes with lovastatin therapy: The Monitored Atherosclerosis Regression Study (MARS). Ann Intern Med 1993;119:969-76.

10.   Sacks FM, Pasternak RC, Gibson CM, Rosner B, Stone PH, for the Harvard Atherosclerosis Reversibility Project (HARP) Group. Effect on coronary atherosclerosis of decrease in plasma cholesterol concentrations in normocholesterolaemic patients. Lancet 1994;344:1182-86.

11.   Pitt B, Mancini GBJ, Ellis SG, Rosman HS, Park J-S, McGovern ME, for the PLAC I Investigators. Pravastatin Limitation of Atherosclerosis in the Coronary Arteries (PLAC I): Reduction in atherosclerosis progression and clinical events. J Am Coll Cardiol 1995;26:1133-39.

12.   MAAS Investigators. Effect of simvastatin on coronary atheroma: The Multicenter Anti-Atheroma Study (MAAS). Lancet 1994;344:633-38.

13.   Harris PJ, Behar VS, Conley MJ, et al. The prognostic significance of 50% coronary stenosis in medically treated patients with coronary artery disease. Circulation 1980;62:240-48.

14.   Crouse JR III, Byington RP, Bond MG. Pravastatin, lipids, and atherosclerosis in the carotid arteries (PLAC-II). Am J Cardiol 1995;75:455-59.

15.   Furberg CD, Adams HP Jr, Applegate WB, for the Asymptomatic Carotid Artery Progression Study (ACAPS) Research Group. Effects of lovastatin on early carotid atherosclerosis and cardiovascular events. Circulation 1994;90:1679-87.

IMPROVING THE COST EFFECTIVENESS OF LIPID LOWERING THERAPY IN CORONARY HEART DISEASE PREVENTION

Terry A. Jacobson and Kara L. Marchman

Introduction

Despite concerted clinical and public health efforts [1] to improve coronary heart disease (CHD), cardiovascular disease (CVD) remains the number one killer in Western industrialized societies. More than $158 billion in the United States alone is spent on the prevention and treatment of CVD and it continues to impose a formidable burden on both the U.S. and European health-care systems. By one U.S. estimate [2] direct medical expenses in 1997 will approach $47.5 billion for CHD, $26.2 billion for stroke, and $21.8 billion for hypertension. Most of the direct medical expenses are from the costs of hospitalization and revascularization procedures.

Several recent clinical trials with the HMG-CoA reductase inhibitors (statins) clearly demonstrate that lipid lowering therapy with the statins will reduce cardiovascular morbidity and mortality in both secondary and primary prevention. The recent landmark trials include the Scandinavian Simvastatin Survival Study (4S) [3], the Cholesterol and Recurrent Events (CARE) study [4], and the West of Scotland Coronary Primary Prevention Study (WOSCOPS) [5]. Despite all three trials showing clear benefit with lipid lowering therapy, it is estimated that only 25% of CHD patients in the United States are receiving aggressive lipid lowering therapy [6]. With many more patients expected to go on therapy in accordance with the United States and European guidelines, cost-effectiveness analysis offers an important tool to best determine how to allocate inherently limited resources to improve the health of both individual patients as well as society at large.

Clinical-Economics Terminology

Commonly used to determine the value of health-care interventions, cost-effectiveness analysis [7] uses the cost-effectiveness ratio: the difference in cost between two specific interventions divided by the differences in effectiveness (expressed as either years of life saved (YOLS) or quality-adjusted life years (QALY's).

$$CE_{2-1} = \frac{Cost_2 - Cost_1}{YOLS_2 - YOLS_1.}$$

A. M. Gotto, Jr. et al. (eds.), Multiple Risk Factors in Cardiovascular Disease, 275–284.
© 1998 Kluwer Academic Publishers and Fondazione Giovanni Lorenzini. Printed in the Netherlands.

Cost-effectiveness analysis attempts to measure the net cost of providing a service (i.e. the cost of drug treatment minus the savings in reduced CHD morbidity) divided by the additional years of life saved (YOLS) or gained. In the above equation, the denominator may also be expressed using an intermediate outcome such as the cost per 1% low density lipoprotein (LDL) cholesterol reduction.

The cost-effectiveness ratio places equal emphasis on cost and effectiveness and is a useful way in which to express the benefits of a given health-care investment or intervention. By calculating the cost-effectiveness ratio, one can develop clinical strategies that produce the greatest health improvement for a given expenditure. Cost-effectiveness analysis allows health-care planners seeking to achieve the maximum benefit for a specific quantity of money or the lowest cost for a specific health-care improvement.

Historical Context of Medical Economics Concerning Management of Dyslipidemia

Hypercholesterolemia has been extensively studied with respect to cost effectiveness. Early findings indicated that cholesterol reduction as secondary prevention was highly cost effective, at approximately $20,000 per QALY or less. On the other hand, primary prevention showed favorable cost-effectiveness values only in select subgroups at advanced risk, such as smokers or others with multiple CAD risk factors.

Some of the early cost-effectiveness studies used some of the older cholesterol drugs such as the bile acid resins or niacin, which have less potent LDL cholesterol lowering effects and are not optimally tolerated [8] With the advent of the statins, potent lipid lowering could be combined with excellent tolerability, and thus could result in more-favorable cost-effectiveness profiles. In an early cost-effectiveness analysis that assessed the intermediate outcome of cost per percent change in cholesterol [9], Schulman and co-workers demonstrated that treatment with HMG-CoA reductase inhibitors or niacin was superior to therapy with the resins, gemfibrozil, or probucol.

Subsequently, Goldman and co-workers [10] demonstrated that lovastatin (20 mg/day) has a favorable cost-effectiveness profile, particularly among middle-aged men with high total cholesterol (> 250 mg/dL) or with multiple CAD risk factors such as smoking, diabetes, or hypertension. Their findings showed that a 20-mg/day dosage of lovastatin in secondary prevention for moderate or severe hypercholesterolemia exhibited a cost-effectiveness ratio of less than $20,000 per YOLS in middle-aged men and women. As primary prevention, however, lovastatin had favorable cost-effectiveness ratios only in subgroups determined by high pretreatment cholesterol levels and other multiple cardiovascular risk factors.

More recently, Hamilton and colleagues [11] while studying the effects of HMG-CoA reductase inhibitors on both LDL and high density lipoprotein (HDL) cholesterol, reported favorable cost-effectiveness profiles for primary prevention in Canadian men (as low as Can $20,882/YOLS at age 50) and in women (Can $36,627/YOLS at age 60). In their study, the statin-induced rise in HDL cholesterol (typically 7%) translated into a cost-effectiveness ratio that was improved by approximately 40% when compared with previous models that used only total cholesterol. Their model also showed that the cost effectiveness of the statins varied widely with age, sex, and presence of other risk factors, but that treatment of hypercholesterolemia was overall relatively cost effective.

Cost-Effectiveness of Statin Clinical Trials

Many of these previous cost-effectiveness studies were limited because they used simulation models that were based on many clinical and economic assumptions. The impact of a clinical economic analysis can be more readily appreciated by examining the economics of actual clinical trials in secondary and primary prevention.

Prospective clinical trial evidence now gives added support to the predictions of economic models. The costs per YOLS in major statin-based clinical trials are summarized in Table 1. In the 4S trial of 4,444 patients with CAD [3] treatment with simvastatin led to a clinically and statistically significant 30% decline in all-cause mortality (P=.0003) and a 34% decline in major coronary events. In the 4S, the incremental cost effectiveness of statins treatment relative to standard dietary care ranged from $7,800 to $15,000 per YOLS in direct costs, with the variation due to assumptions regarding survival and discounting of benefits and costs [12]. In conclusion, the investigators stated that therapy with an HMG-CoA reductase inhibitor is cost effective among both men and women in the setting of secondary prevention (i.e. postmyocardial infarction (MI) or effort angina). In another publication [13], the authors report that treatment with simvastatin would reduce the effective cost of statin therapy by 88%, to $0.28 per day, principally by reducing expensive hospitalization costs and revascularization procedures.

Table 1. Cost Effectiveness of Major Statin-Based Clinical Trials

	Drug, dosage	$ Cost per YOLS
Secondary-prevention Clinical trials		
• 4S	Simvastatin 20-40 mg/day	5,500 (3,000-12,100) (men) 10,300 (4,500-21,800) (women)
• PLAC I/II (pooled analysis)	Pravastatin 40 mg/day	9,400 (7,124-12,665) (men)
Primary prevention		
• WOSCOPS	Pravastatin 40 mg/day	(16,000-32,000)* (men)

4S: Scandinavian Simvastatin Survival Study; PLAC I: Pravastatin Limitation of Atherosclerosis in the Coronary Arteries; PLAC II: Pravastatin, Lipids and Atherosclerosis in the Carotid Arteries; WOSCOPS: West of Scotland Coronary Prevention Study. *converted to US $ from British Pounds at $1.60/pound.

A number of other studies have demonstrated the cost effectiveness of HMG-CoA reductase inhibitors in the treatment of hypercholesterolemia. The pooled analysis of two angiographic studies also estimated the cost effectiveness of the use of the HMG-CoA reductase inhibitor, pravastatin, in secondary prevention [14] The two angiographic regression studies were the Pravastatin Limitation of Atherosclerosis in the Coronary Arteries (PLAC I) and the Pravastatin, Lipids, and Atherosclerosis in the Carotid Arteries (PLAC II). The pooled PLAC data (n=559) showed a statistically significant (P < .05) difference in the incidence of nonfatal MI in men between the pravastatin and the placebo arm. An analysis of pooled data from the PLAC studies showed that in men with CAD, the cost per YOLS utilizing the average weighted dose of pravastatin (36 mg/day) was $12,665 in patients with one additional risk factor, $9,368 with two additional risk factors, and $7,124 with three additional risk factors [14]

In the WOSCOPS [5] primary prevention trial , pravastatin at 40 mg/day resulted in a 31% decline in the number of nonfatal MIs , a 22% reduction in risk of death (p=0. 051) from any cause, and a 37% reduction in CABG and angioplasty. Although the WOSCOPS trial has yet to be analyzed completely for cost effectiveness, an interim analysis has been presented [15]. Shepherd and colleagues from the WOSCOPS Economic Analysis Group reported that, over 5 years, treatment with pravastatin in 10,000 men similar to the patients in the WOSCOPS would prevent about 300 of them from developing cardiovascular disease. The incremental cost-effectiveness ratios associated with the prevention of these events ranged from £10,000 to £20,000 per YOLS, and the ratio decreased further among high-risk men such as those who smoke, have hypertension, or are older. These cost-effectiveness ratios compare very favorable with already established cardiovascular prevention interventions.

Improving Cost-Effectiveness of Lipid Lowering Therapy

There are several methods to improve the cost-effectiveness of lipid therapy. Table 2 outlines those methods and divides them into several categories: 1) improving CHD risk assessment and targeting higher risk individuals; 2) improving treatment effectiveness; 3) and reducing cost of therapy. Most of the studies point out the need to target those with CHD and those at high risk of CHD. CHD risk assessment can clearly be improved by using equations and calculations from the Framingham study [16] to predict those at highest risk of a CHD event over a 10-year period. In fact, the European Atherosclerosis Society (EAS) [17] has already suggested to target those with an absolute risk of CHD of 20% over a 10-year period (or 2% CHD risk/year) to maximize cardiovascular prevention. This threshold would correspond to greater cost-effectiveness than simply relying on LDL-C levels alone and thus would result in reducing the number of individuals needed to be treated (NNT) with lipid lowering therapy to prevent one CHD event.

Further analysis of the WOSCOPS trial [18] indicate that high risk middle age (55-65) men from could be identified with rates of CHD exceeding 10% over five years (2%/year) with just one of the following additional risk factors: minor ECG abnormalities, pre-existing vascular disease, smoking, HDL less than 35 mg/dl, hypertension, or family history of premature CHD. The use of more refined CHD event prediction rules will improve the cost-effectiveness of treatment. The NNT would decline from about 40 individuals to prevent one event to about 20 individuals to prevent one event if the targeted threshold for treatment was changed from 2% per year to 3% per year [19].

Table 2. Improving Cost-Effectiveness of Lipid Treatment

Target higher-risk patients by improving CHD risk assessment

- Use absolute CHD risk threshold of 2% per year [17]

- Use newer lipid and nonlipid predictors of CHD (molecular and genetic markers)

- Use new technologies: carotid ultrasound, ultrafast CT

Increase treatment effectiveness

- Improve compliance

- Consider agents (niacin, estrogen) that improve other lipids such as HDL-C, Lp(a), or dense LDL

- Increase LDL-C reductions with combination therapies

Reduce cost of lipid therapy

- Maximize diet, exercise, smoking cessation

- Use less expensive drugs (niacin, fluvastatin, estrogen)

In addition to better CHD risk targeting (Table 2), the use of newer lipid and nonlipid tests for CHD such as Lp(a), dense LDL, apolipoprotein B, homocysteine, fibrinogen, or genetic markers may allow better CHD risk prediction. In addition new technologies with high sensitivity and specificity for detecting CHD, such as ultrafast CT, MRI, or carotid ultrasound, may be considered when their predictive values have been validated and their costs have dropped considerably.

Increasing treatment effectiveness would be another way to maximize cost effectiveness. For example any methods that increase medication compliance would increase the amount of benefit. For example, at the end of the WOSCOPS trial, over 30% of the patients had dropped out or stopped their medications over the five-year period of the trial. Examining the benefits of the compliers [20], showed greater reductions in CHD, total mortality, and revascularization procedures. Thus, methods to enhance compliance with dietary and pharmacologic therapy would improve cost effectiveness.

Finally, the most important way to improve cost effectiveness is to use less expensive drugs. Using intermediate endpoints such as $cost/LDL reduction would suggest that of the available statins, that fluvastatin and atorvastatin would be the most cost-effective option (see Table 3). At their entry doses, on the basis of cost per percentage LDL-cholesterol reduction, fluvastatin and atorvastatin are substantially more cost effective than lovastatin, pravastatin, or simvastatin: $18-19 per 1% LDL-C reduction, compared with about $26 to $34 per 1% reduction for the other statins. Clearly, for the moderate (20-30%) LDL-cholesterol reductions typically needed by patients with primary hypercholesterolemia, fluvastatin appears to be the most cost-effective option (Table 3). For more pronounced LDL-cholesterol (30-50%) lowering, atorvastatin may be the most cost-effective alternative due to its greater potency in lowering LDL-cholesterol [22,23]. An algorithm summarizing the most cost-effective management of hypercholesterolemia using the statins has been recently published [24,25]. It suggests that for the majority of patients who require LDL reductions less than 30%, fluvastatin (20 or 40 mg) would be the most cost-effective statin, while atorvastatin (10 mg) would be the most cost effective if reductions greater than 30% were required. With most statins, except fluvastatin, doubling of the dose only adds an additional 6% LDL reduction while increasing cost almost twofold. This illustrates the economic principle of diminishing marginal returns: smaller additional clinical benefits (i.e. LDL-cholesterol reduction) at additional costs. Thus, at higher doses most of the statins are less cost effective.

Table 3. Cost Effectiveness of Treatment with Statins

	Dose (mg/d)	Annual Cost ($/yr)	LDL-C reduction (%)	Cost/LDL-C reduction ($/yr/1% LDL-C reduction)
Fluvastatin	20	439.20	23	19.09
	40	489.60	26	18.83
Lovastatin	20	810.00	24	33.75
	40	1458.00	30	48.60
	80	2916.00	40	72.90
Pravastatin	20	709.20	25	28.37
	40	1195.20	27	44.27
Simvastatin	10	730.80	28	26.10
	20	1274.40	35	36.41
	40	1324.80	40	33.12
Atorvastatin	10	655.20	36	18.20
	20	1015.20	40	25.38
	40	1224.00	47	26.04

Prices from Redbook Update 1997 [21]. Adapted and reproduced with permission from Jacobson [24,25].

The price sensitivity of statin therapy has been demonstrated in most cost-effectiveness analyses. Several cost-effectiveness analyses with the statins support the premise that drug acquisition costs account for the majority of the changes in the cost-effectiveness ratios. In a sensitivity analysis reported by Goldman's group [10] if the cost of lovastatin were reduced by 40% in 1997 as the result of a generic formulation, the cost/YOLS would decrease by 30% in primary prevention. In the more recent analysis by Hamilton and co-workers [11] that incorporated changes in both LDL and HDL cholesterol into their model, a 10% variation in drug cost of lovastatin was associated with changes of 8-9% in the cost per YOLS. Thus, most cost-effectiveness analyses point out the importance of acquisition costs as the dominant determinant of the cost effectiveness of the HMG-CoA reductase inhibitors. With the advent of newer synthetic statins, substantial decreases in acquisition costs could be expected to improve cost effectiveness even more.

The Economic Value of Lipid Lowering Therapy

The value of statin therapy can readily be appreciated when examining the cost-effectiveness of other accepted cardiovascular interventions. Table 4 shows the cost effectiveness of various interventions for patients with CAD and demonstrates the economic value of statin therapy compared to traditionally accepted cardiovascular interventions [26]. Although secondary prevention is very cost effective costing less than $20,000/QALY, primary prevention with a statin is also relatively cost effective.

Table 4. Cost Effectiveness of Cardiovascular Prevention

Intervention	Cost ($/QALY)
Highly cost-effective (<$20,000/QALY)	
• β-blocker post-MI	$3,600
• CABG-left main disease	$9,200
• HMG-CoA therapy-secondary prevention [12]	12,000
Relatively cost-effective ($20,000-$60,000/QALY)	
• Hypertension-hydrochlorothiazide	$25,400
• HMG-CoA therapy-primary prevention [15]	$20,000-$40,000
• Renal dialysis	$40,000
Expensive (> $70,000/QALY)	
• CABG-mild angina, one vessel disease	$72,000
• CCU care-low probability MI	$88,700
• EKG testing-asymptomatic 40-year-old man	$124,000

Adapted and reproduced with permission from Goldman [26]

The value of lipid-lowering therapy is also placed into larger perspective when one considers the costs of CHD and its treatment. Wittels et al. [27] estimate that the average 5-year cost (in 1986 dollars) of acute MI is $51,211, angina $24,980, unstable angina $40,581, while revascularization procedures cost $26,916 for angioplasty and $32,465 for bypass surgery on a per-case basis. Thus the real value of statin therapy is in the CHD events that are averted, as well as the reduction in expensive hospitalization and revascularization procedures.

Treatment decisions concerning patients with hypercholesterolemia are best based on the consideration of not only the LDL cholesterol levels but the absolute CAD risk as established by either the National Cholesterol Education Program (NCEP) Adult Treatment Panel [1] or the European Atherosclerosis Society guidelines [17]. To contain the cost of statin therapy for hypercholesterolemic patients, higher risks patients need to be targeted more aggressively and more cost-effective drugs (niacin, fluvastatin) need to be considered.

Conclusions

In the current medical environment of increasing cost, limited health care resources, and spiraling expenditures for cardiovascular interventions, it becomes increasingly important to make appropriate clinical treatment decisions based on an understanding of the efficacy, safety, and cost effectiveness of pharmacological agents. Treatment interventions that cost less than $40,000 per YOLS are recommended by a number of experts as cost effective. Compared with other generally accepted cardiovascular interventions, treatment with the HMG-CoA reductase inhibitors is very cost effective, especially in patients with CAD or at high risk for CAD (i.e. multiple risk factors). In the management of most patients with primary (i.e. type IIa/IIb) hypercholesterolemia, the synthetic HMG-CoA reductase inhibitor, fluvastatin, appears to be particularly attractive because its clinical efficacy is similar to those of other drugs in its class, but its acquisition costs are substantially lower, resulting in greater cost effectiveness. For the minority of patients who need larger decreases in LDL cholesterol, atorvastatin may represent a major therapeutic advance.

References

1.   Summary of the second report of the National Cholesterol Education Program (NCEP) Expert Panel on Detection, Evaluation, and Treatment of High Blood Cholesterol in Adults (Adult Treatment Panel II). JAMA 1993;269:3015-23.

2.   American Heart Association. Heart and Stroke Facts: 1997 Statistical Supplement. Dallas, Tex: American Heart Association, 1997.

3.   Scandinavian Simvastatin Survival Study Group. Randomised trial of cholesterol lowering in 4444 patients with coronary heart disease: The Scandinavian simvastatin survival study. Lancet 1994;344:1383-89.

4.   Sacks FM, Pfeffer MA, Moye LA, et al. for the Cholesterol and Recurrent Events Trial Investigators. The effect of pravastatin on coronary events after myocardial infarction in patients with average cholesterol levels. N Engl J Med 1996;1001-09.

5.   Shepherd J, Cobbe SM, Ford I, et al. for the West of Scotland Coronary Prevention Study

Group. Prevention of coronary heart disease with pravastatin in men with hypercholesterolemia. N Engl J Med 1995;333:1301-07.

6.   27th Bethesda Conference: Matching the Intensity of Risk Factor Management with the Hazard for Coronary Disease Events; September 14-15, 1995. J Am Coll Cardiol 1996;27: 957-1047.

7.   Eisenberg JM. Clinical economics: A guide to economic analysis of clinical practices. JAMA 1989;262:2879-86.

8.   Kinosian BP, Eisenberg JM. Cutting into cholesterol: Cost-effective alternatives for treating hypercholesterolemia. JAMA 1988;259:2249-54.

9.   Schulman KA, Kinosian B, Jacobson TA, et al. Reducing high blood cholesterol level with drugs: Cost effectiveness of pharmacologic management. JAMA 1990;264:2249-54.

10.   Goldman L, Weinstein MC, Goldman PA, Williams LW. Cost-effectiveness of HMG-CoA reductase inhibition for primary and secondary prevention of coronary heart disease. JAMA 1991;265:1145-51.

11.   Hamilton VH, Racicot F-E, Zowall H, Coupal L, Grover SA. The cost-effectiveness of HMG-CoA reductase inhibitors to prevent coronary heart disease: Estimating the benefits of increasing HDL-C. JAMA 1995;273:1032-38.

12.   Johanneson M, Jonsson B, Kjekshus J, Olsson AG, Pedersen TR, Wedel H, for the Scandinavian Simvastatin Survival Study Group. Cost effectiveness of simvastatin treatment to lower cholesterol levels in patients with coronary heart disease. N Engl J Med 1997;336: 332-36.

13.   Pedersen TR, Kjekshus J, Berg K, et al. Cholesterol lowering and the use of healthcare resources: Results of the Scandinavian Simvastatin Survival Study. Circulation 1996;93:1796-1802.

14.   Ashraf T, Hay JW, Pitt B, et al. Cost-effectiveness of pravastatin in secondary prevention of coronary artery disease. Am J Cardiol 1996;78:409-14.

15.   Shepherd J for the West of Scotland Coronary Prevention Study Economic Analysis Group. The cost-effectiveness of preventing initial coronary events with pravastatin. Results of the West of Scotland Coronary Prevention Study Economic Analysis. J Amer Coll Cardiol 1997; 29(Suppl.A, February):Abstract #968-54 (168A).

16.   Anderson KM, Wilson PWF, Odell PM, Kannel WB. An updated coronary risk profile: A statement for health care professionals. Circulation 1991;83:356-62.

17.   Pyorala K, De Backer G, Graham I, Poole-Wilson P, Wood D on behalf of the Task Force. Prevention of coronary heart disease in clinical practice. Recommendations of the Task Force of the European Society of Cardiology, European Atherosclerosis Society and European Society of Hypertension. Ear Heart J 1994;15:1300-31.

18.   The West of Scotland Coronary Prevention Study Group. West of Scotland Coronary Prevention Study: Identification of high risk groups in comparison with other cardiovascular intervention trials. Lancet 1996;348(9038):1339-42.

19.   Ramsay LE, Haq IU, Jackson PR, Yeo WW, Pickin DM, Payne JN. Targeting lipid lowering drug therapy for primary prevention of coronary disease: An updated Sheffield table. Lancet 1996;348:387-88.

20.   Shepherd J, for the West of Scotland Coronary Prevention Study Group. West of Scotland Coronary Prevention Study: Benefits of Pravastatin in compliant subjects. Circulation 1996; 94(Suppl.1):Abstract 3155.

21.   Red Book Update. Montvale, NJ: Medical Economics Co., January 1997.

22.   Bakker-Arkema RG, Davidson MH, Goldstein RJ, et al. Efficacy and safety of a new HMG-

CoA reductase inhibitor, atorvastatin, in patients with hypertriglyceridemia. JAMA 1996; 275:128-133.

23.   Nawrocki JW, Weiss SR, Davidson MH, et al. Reduction of LDL cholesterol by 25% to 60% in patients with primary hypercholesterolemia by atorvastatin, a new HMG-CoA reductase inhibitor. Arterioscler Thromb Vasc Biol 1995;15:678-82.

24.   Jacobson TA. Cost-effectiveness of 3-hydroxy-3-methylglutary-coenzyme A HMG-CoA reductase inhibitor therapy in the managed care era. Am J Cardiol 1996;78(Suppl.6A):32-41.

25.   Jacobson TA, Orloff SM. Preventing CHD in the managed care era: Improving the cost-effectiveness of lipid lowering therapy. Am J Man Care 1997; in press.

26.   Goldman L, Garber AM, Grover SA, Hlatky MA. Task Force 6. Cost effectiveness of assessment and management of risk factors. J Am Coll Cardiol 1996;27(5):1020-30.

27.   Wittels EH, Hay JW, Gotto AM Jr. Medical costs of coronary artery disease in the United States. Am J Cardiol 1990;65:432-40.

DIET AND CARDIOVASCULAR DISEASE

John C. LaRosa

Introduction

When Ancil Keys demonstrated many years ago that saturated fat intake was related to elevated cholesterol levels and coronary artery disease death rates around the world [1], he ignited a debate which has not yet been fully settled. There is a direct linear relationship between saturated fat intake, cholesterol levels, and coronary artery disease. It is less clear whether changing saturated fat intake changes blood cholesterol levels in adults to a sufficient degree to significantly reduce coronary disease. The implications of these relationships are of great economic as well as health importance in those countries in which saturated fat intake is high. The outcome of this debate is not only of significance to physicians and their patients, but also to farmers, livestock producers, food distributors, and the governments which represent and oversee them.

Epidemiologic Observations

Humans, with their flat, grinding teeth and long intestines, are not ideally suited to be meat eaters. Nevertheless, the caloric density of fat may have been essential to survival in a nomadic lifestyle in which eating was only intermittently possible. It is clear from the Seven Countries and other studies, however, that there is a direct relationship between animal fat intake and the high rate of atherosclerosis which generally characterizes wealthy, meat-eating societies [1].

Population studies demonstrate that changes in animal fat intake are at least temporally associated with changes in coronary disease rates. In the United States, for example, fat intake appeared to reach its peak around 1960 and has been on the decline since [2]. U.S. average cholesterol levels have also fallen during that period of time, from around 225 mg/dl (5.82 mmol/L) to 205 mg/dl (5.5 mmol/L) [3]. In the period since 1960, heart disease rates have fallen almost 50%, as have stroke rates [4].

In contrast, dietary changes in Japan over this same period of time have been in the reverse direction, with an increase in fat intake [5] accompanied by an increase in cholesterol levels [6] and coronary death rates [5]. Japanese migrating from Japan to Hawaii to California adopt diets which increase progressively from about 7 to 26 percent of calories from saturated fat. Those dietary changes are associated with increased serum cholesterol

A. M. Gotto, Jr. et al. (eds.), Multiple Risk Factors in Cardiovascular Disease, 285–296.

levels and increased death rates from coronary heart disease [7,8].

It would be tempting to postulate that all of the effect of diets could be explained through effects on plasma cholesterol. Recent observations in the Seven Countries Study do not support this notion. At similar levels of blood cholesterol, coronary disease rates, for example, are still lower in Japan than they are in the United States or Europe [9]. Since the Japanese migratory studies do not support an inherent genetic resistance to atherosclerosis among Japanese, the explanation is more likely to be in other dietary or cultural factors which distinguish Japanese from Americans and Europeans.

Diet and Circulating Lipids

The relationship between dietary cholesterol and saturated fat intake and blood cholesterol levels was described independently by Keys et al. [10] and Hegsted et al. [11]. In the equations developed by each of these investigators, saturated fat (in dietary triglyceride) was a much stronger determinant of blood cholesterol levels than dietary cholesterol itself. Both of these dietary components inhibit low-density lipoprotein (LDL) receptor activity (although this may not be their only mechanism) [12], thereby raising circulating LDL cholesterol level. Elevation of cholesterol levels, then, is not due primarily to direct accumulation of dietary cholesterol in the blood, which was once supposed, but rather to indirect effects of both dietary cholesterol and saturated fat containing dietary triglyceride on low-density lipoprotein catabolism.

Keys

$$\Delta \text{ serum cholesterol} = 1.26\,(\,2\Delta S - \Delta P\,) + 1.5\,\sqrt{\Delta C}$$

Hegsted

$$\Delta \text{ serum cholesterol} = 2.16\Delta S - 1.65\Delta P + 0.092\,\Delta C$$

S = % total calories from saturated fat
P = total calories from polyunsaturated fat
c = dietary choelsterol in mg/1000 kcal

Figure 1. Equations relating dietary fat to blood cholesterol levels.

The effect of dietary cholesterol on blood cholesterol levels may be modulated by the baseline level of cholesterol in the diet. When baseline dietary cholesterol levels are above 500 mg/day, for example, there is little effect of additional dietary cholesterol [13]. There is considerable individual variation in the responsiveness to dietary cholesterol [14].

Some individuals are quite responsive, while others are quite resistant. Dietary cholesterol may qualitatively affect the atherogenicity of LDL by enhancing the production of a small dense LDL, which is more easily oxidized and more highly atherogenic [15].

As reflected in the Keys and Hegsted equations, dietary saturated fatty acids play an even more important role than cholesterol itself in raising blood cholesterol levels. Individuals who try to control cholesterol simply by eliminating foods that contain high levels of cholesterol but not saturated fat (such as eggs) are likely to fail.

On the other hand, diets high in saturated fat, even without cholesterol, result in increases in LDL. Substituting mono- or polyunsaturated fats lowers LDL, but as demonstrated in a recent meta-analysis, does not result in significant changes in HDL or triglyceride levels. That same analysis did not demonstrate an HDL sparing effect of monounsaturates. If there is such an effect, it is not major [16].

Recently, attention has focused on the practice of hydrogenating polyunsaturated fats, so that they become monounsaturated. This process extends the useful shelf life of commercial cooking fats, but also results in the accumulation of large amounts of elaidic acid, the *trans* isomer of oleic acid. Unlike oleic acid, the *cis* isomer, which has LDL-lowering properties similar to polyunsaturated fats, elaidic acid behaves more like saturated fat, raising LDL cholesterol levels [17]. It also is associated with dramatic increases in the circulating levels of Lp(a), a lipoprotein composed of an LDL molecule linked by a disulfide bond to a plasma analog. Lp(a), particularly in the presence of elevated LDL levels, has shown itself to be an important risk factor in coronary heart disease [18]. Like dietary saturated fat and cholesterol, *trans* fatty acid intake has been strongly associated in the Seven Countries study with increased coronary risk [19].

While the efficacy of lowering dietary cholesterol and saturated fat in promoting lower circulating cholesterol levels has sometimes been questioned, a review of medical data makes it clear that the Keys and Hegsted equation are excellent predictors of the effects of dietary change [20]. The problem is not that dietary change in ineffective, but that it is difficult to achieve, particularly in societies where animal fat is inexpensive and widely available.

A number of issues affect the responsiveness of an individual to dietary changes. As already noted, some individuals appear genetically to be more susceptible to change than others. Recent evidence suggests this may relate to the presence of different alleles for apoprotein E. Individuals with E4 allele are more likely to respond to respond to dietary cholesterol and saturated fat with an increase in total and LDL cholesterol than those with E2 or E3 alleles [21].

Gender also appears to be an important predictor of dietary responsiveness. In premenopausal women, diet appears to have less of an effect either in raising or lowering circulating lipoprotein levels than it does in men of the same age [14]. It is less clear whether this effect is equally strong in postmenopausal women, when the effects of circulating estrogen are lost [22].

Age itself appears to be associated with an increase in circulating LDL levels particularly in women. Even in an elderly cohort followed over a nine-year period, whose saturated fat intake fell during the period of observation, the LDL-to-HDL cholesterol level rose [23]. Whether this is due to a decline in LDL-receptor activity with age or some other effect is unclear. In countries in which habitual animal fat intake is low, however, blood cholesterol levels do not rise with age.

It has been argued that substitution of saturated fat with carbohydrates, as occurs in many vegetarian diets, might be harmful in that high carbohydrate dieting might lead to increased triglyceride and insulin levels. This argument has held that it would be better to use monounsaturated fat such as a the olive oil in the "Mediterranean" diet. The disadvantage to that approach, of course, is that since all fats contain 9 calories per gram, caloric restriction might be more difficult. Counter-arguments have been that the effects of high carbohydrate diets are transient. This is reflected in the fact that long-term vegetarians, such as Seventh Day Adventists, do not have significantly different levels of triglycerides than their neighbors, although their HDL and LDL levels are both significantly lower [24]. Others maintain that HDL and LDL levels are similarly affected, no matter what is substituted for saturated fat [25].

Carbohydrates do raise insulin levels, in the short term, as was demonstrated in a 12-week study of low versus high carbohydrate diets [26]. It should be noted that neither HDL nor triglyceride changes were significantly different on the high or low carbohydrate diets in that study. Nevertheless, an increase in insulin, particularly if persistent, might be itself a risk factor for atherosclerosis. This issue is not a settled one; nevertheless, since there is no particular advantage to high intake of simple carbohydrates, they are best limited in cholesterol-lowering diets.

The effect of body weight and exercise on diet and circulating cholesterol levels are also important to remember. Obese individuals are considerably less likely to demonstrate falls in cholesterol levels with a low fat diet [27]. Exercise, on the other hand, enhances the effects of low fat, low calorie diets on circulating lipoproteins, independent of the degree of weight loss [28].

The Effect of Other Dietary Factors on Circulating Lipoproteins

SOLUBLE FIBER

Dietary soluble fiber derived from oats, psyllium seed, quar gum, and pectin has been demonstrated to consistently lower cholesterol levels 3 to 5 % [29]. This has been explained simply as the effect of substituting calories from saturated fat with calories from complex carbohydrates. It is apparent, however, that the LDL-lowering effect of soluble fiber persists, whether the content of the diet is high or low in fat intake [30]. In a recent study of 22,000 middle-aged Finnish men followed for over six years, soluble fiber intake was associated with a decreased risk of coronary morbidity and mortality, even after controlling for cholesterol and other risk factors [31].

FISH OILS

Fish oils, which contain large amounts of omega-3 fatty acids, have been repeatedly promoted as an important protector against atherosclerosis. Fish oils do have the ability to lower triglycerides and raise HDL levels, although they may, in individuals with hypertriglyceridemia, actually raise LDL levels as well [32]. Specific fish oils may have different effects on lipoproteins. Beneficial changes may, for example, be more pronounced with fish such as tuna, which contains docosahexaenoic acid, than with fish such as pollock, which contains eicosapantaenoic acid [33].

There is little doubt that populations with higher habitual fish intake have lower rates of heart disease [34]. There is also some evidence in clinical trials that fish consumption is associated with lower rates of recurrent coronary disease, lower rates of recurrent restenosis after angioplasty [35]. Once again, the debate about the effects of fish oils is in part related to whether these related effects are specific to fish oil and fatty acids, or simply related to the substitution of saturated fat with fish oils.

Fish oils can have effects beyond alterations of circulating lipoproteins, including inhibition of platelet stickiness which may independently inhibit atherogenesis [36]. On the other hand, such an effect may be responsible for the increased risk of hemorrhagic stroke in populations with high fish intake [37].

ANTIOXIDANTS

Dietary antioxidant vitamins do not appreciably alter levels of circulating lipoproteins. However, the atherogenecity of LDL is thought to be directly related to its level of oxidation. It is oxidized LDL which is taken up by macrophages, converting them to foam cells. On the other hand, preliminary evidence suggests that HDL-mediated enhancement of reverse cholesterol transport, on the other hand, may be enhanced by oxidation [38].

The net effect of antioxidants seems to be the inhibition of atherogenesis. For example, oleic acid from olive oil, when incorporated into LDL, makes it more resistant to oxidation and less likely to be taken up by macrophages [39], thereby contributing to the protective value of the "Mediterranean" diet.

Observational studies of both beta carotene and vitamin E intake, either as dietary constituents or dietary supplements, have shown a trend to lower relative risk of vascular disease, though with wide variation [40]. Trails of beta carotene supplementation, on the other hand, have also demonstrated potential harm in promoting malignancies, particularly in smokers [41,42]. A recent report in over 22,000 male physicians (largely nonsmokers) demonstrated no effect of beta carotene supplementation either on malignant neoplasms, cardiovascular events or death from all causes [43]. A small clinical trial in a subset from that same study, did, however, demonstrate a substantial 44% decline in recurrent coronary events [44].

A recent clinical trial of vitamin E demonstrated a 47% decline in cardiovascular events, although during the period of observation in the study there was a slight excess mortality from cardiovascular disease in the vitamin E group [45]. At this point, the evidence that antioxidants are of benefit in controlling atherogenesis is mixed. It is somewhat better for vitamin E (alpha-tocopherol) than for beta carotene.

ALCOHOL

Like fish oils, alcohol ingestion is associated with a decline in coronary heart disease rates in both men and women. In fact, the "French paradox" in which high levels of saturated fat in the French diet are, paradoxically, not associated with high rates of coronary risk is largely explained by the high alcohol content of the French diet [46]. Alcohol, like estrogen and bile sequestrants, simultaneously raises HDL and triglycerides. In addition, it has other effects which may inhibit atherogenesis, including decreasing LDL oxidation, decreasing platelet stickiness, and decreasing fibrinogen levels [47]. Alcohol, of course, is an addicting drug which has a direct deleterious effect on myocardium, so that only in moderation can it be considered useful for the prevention of atherogenesis.

PLANT STEROLS

Noncholesterol, plant-derived sterols such as sitostanol, have been thought for some time to lower, moderately, circulating cholesterol levels. There have been enthusiastic reports of the cholesterol lowering properties of sitostanol-enriched margarines [48]. While this has led to increased consumption of such margarine, the long-term effects on morbidity and mortality are unknown.

OTHER DIETARY CONSTITUENTS

Other dietary constituents have also been implicated in the prevention of atherosclerosis. Diets high in soy, containing antioxidant flavinoids and phytoestrogens, have been demonstrated in cynomolgus monkeys to raise HDL and lower LDL levels [49]. Similar effects have been reported in humans with soy containing diets, although whether this effect is related to phytoestrogens or some other component of soy, such as antioxidant flavinoids, has not been determined [50]. Estrogens, including (presumably) phytoestrogens, have antiatherogenic effects including favorable changes in circulating lipoproteins, inhibition of arterial wall LDL uptake, inhibition of platelet stickiness, and prevention of paradoxical vascular contraction in response to acetylcholine [51].

Over the years, the effect of coffee on cardiovascular disease has been widely debated. While coffee has no apparent effect on circulating lipoproteins, some studies did indicate excessive coffee intake was associated with the progression of coronary disease. That concern has now been put to rest. In meta-analysis, even coffee consumption of greater than four cups of day did not appear to increase the relative risk of coronary disease [52].

Finally, increased consumption of nuts, particularly walnuts, which contain high levels of polyunsaturated fat, has been associated with reduced risk of coronary heart disease [53]. In similar fashion, meta-analysis of studies of garlic on CAD also indicate a favorable effect on circulating total cholesterol levels [54]. A recent clinical trial, however, did not demonstrate any effect of 300 mg garlic tablets given three times a day on circulating lipoproteins [55].

Clinical Trials of Diet and Coronary Disease

Because dietary changes are difficult to achieve and maintain, and because clinical trials are generally limited in duration, it has been difficult to demonstrate beneficial effects of dietary change on coronary disease. Metanalysis of primary prevention trials have been demonstrated no significant effect of dietary changes on the odds ratio of coronary heart disease, whereas secondary prevention trials have demonstrated borderline benefit [56] (Figure 2). Three angiographic studies of lifestyle change which include diet have demonstrated significant differences in the progression of atherosclerosis on coronary artery disease with nonpharmaceutical interventions including diet and exercise [57]. Similar results with lifestyle change have been demonstrated by repeat positive emission tomography (PET) [58].

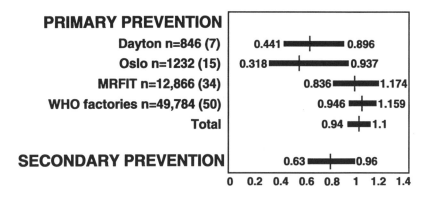

Woodard: Med Clin North Am (1993)77:849

Figure 2. Diet trials in CHD (odds ratio).

Proof of the benefit of diet on coronary artery disease in clinical trials is not definitive, but neither is it absent. Critics of dietary intervention have maintained that clinical trials in which diet has been an included intervention do not demonstrate significant changes in circulating lipids. This, however, is more the result of the fact that baseline diets in many patients are already close to that prescribed in the study. In fact, the Keys/Hegsted equations have, if anything, underestimated the derived cholesterol-lowering effect of diet in clinical trials [20]. Even small dietary changes in large populations can significantly lower coronary artery mortality, and in a cost-effective fashion [59]. Given this, it is reasonable to ask whether current recommendations that total fat intake below 30% of calories from fat and less than 10% from saturated fat should be maintained or whether those targets should be lowered. A recent review by the American Heart Association nutrition committee concluded that current recommendations remained sound although select populations at very high risk would benefit from more intense animal fat restriction [60].

Postprandial Lipoproteins

Most studies of circulating lipoproteins have focused on fasting levels of circulating lipoproteins. There is convincing evidence, however, that individuals with exaggerated postprandial hypertriglyceridemia are at increased risk of atherogenesis, whether the baseline triglycerides are normal or elevated [61] (Figure 3). Increased postprandial hypertriglyceridemia is related to a number of factors, including male sex, age, presence of the apoprotein E2-E3 phenotype (as opposed to phenotypes with the E4 allele which are associated with fasting hypercholesterolemia), elevated fasting triglycerides, diets containing high levels of saturated fats and calories and low levels of dietary fiber, sedentary lifestyle, and diabetes [62,63].

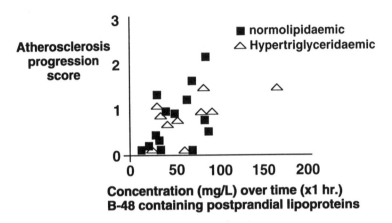

Karpe: Atherosclerosis(1994)106:83

Figure 3. Relationship between postprandial lipoproteins and CAD on angiograms.

The effect of compositional changes in postprandial lipoproteins, including increased cholesterol content on postprandial lipoproteins, is largely unexplored. It is known, however, that dietary cholesterol predicts coronary disease independent of its effects on fasting cholesterol levels. [64] It is tempting to speculate that some of the weakness in the linkages among dietary cholesterol and saturated fat, circulating levels of lipoproteins, and the prevalence of coronary artery disease may be explained by failure to take into account the effects of diet on postprandial lipoproteins.

Conclusions

There is little question that diet is an important determinant both of circulating levels of atherogenic lipoproteins as well as an increased risk of cardiovascular disease. It is also clear that the effect of diet on cardiovascular disease cannot be fully explained by its effect on circulating lipoproteins, particularly fasting lipoproteins. Other characteristics of dietary ingredients, including the antioxidant properties of dietary vitamins, alcohol, flavinoids, and phytoestrogens, and the antiplatelet effects of omega-3 fatty acids, alcohol, and phytoestrogens, are examples of dietary effects which are not dependent on changes in circulating levels of lipoproteins.

Both observational population studies and metabolic studies confirm the profound effect which dietary change can have on both circulating lipoproteins and coronary heart disease. Failure to observe these effects in clinical trials is related to various factors, including the baseline diet, the length of observation of subjects in clinical trials, subject adherence to study diet and the ability to effect dietary change. In the real world, moreover, the ability to effect dietary change may be a function of the availability of animal fat as well as the availability of alternative foods.

It is clear that in societies in which animal fat intake is low, rates of coronary disease are low. It is reasonable to ask whether diets currently proposed for coronary prevention in Western countries are sufficiently low in animal fat. It may be time to reopen the question of the adequacy current dietary population targets in Western countries, even though the resistance of major players in the food economy is likely to be intense.

References

1. Keys A. Seven Countries: A multivariate analysis of death and coronary heart disease. Cambridge, MA: Harvard University Press, 1980.
2. Stephen AM, Wald N. Trends in individual consumption of dietary fat in the United States, 1920-1984. Am J Clin Nutr 1990;52:457-69.
3. Johnson CL, Rifkind BM, Sempos CT, Carroll MD, Bechorik PS, Briefel RR. Declining serum total cholesterol levels among US adults: The National Heath and Nutrition Examination Surveys. JAMA 1993;269:3002-8.
4. Higgins MW, Luepker R, editors. Trends in Coronary Heart Disease Mortality: The Influence of Medical Care. New York: Oxford University Press, 1988:vii-x.
5. Toshima H. Coronary artery disease trends in Japan. Japanese Circulation Journal 1994;58:166-72.
6. Law MR, Wald NJ. An ecological study of serum cholesterol and ischaemic heart disease between 1950 and 1990. Eur J Clin Nutr 1994;48:305-25.
7. Kato H, Tillotson J, Nichaman MZ, Rhoads GG, Hamilton HB. Epidemiologic studies of coronary heart disease and stroke in Japanese men living in Japan, Hawaii and California. Am J Epidemiol 1973;97:372-85.
8. Robertson TL, Kato H, Rhoads GG, et al. Epidemiologic studies of coronary heart disease and stroke in Japanese men living in Japan, Hawaii and California. Incidence of myocardial infarction and death from coronary heart disease. Am J Cardiol 1977;39:239-43.
9. Verschuren WMM, Jacobs DR, Bloemberg BPM, Kromhout D, Menotti A. Serum total cholesterol and long term coronary heart disease mortality in different countries. JAMA 1995; 274:131-36.
10. Keys A, Anderson JR, Grand F. Prediction of serum-cholesterol responses of man to changes in fats in the diet. Lancet 1957;2:955-66.
11. Hegsted DM, McGandy RB, Myers ML, Stare FJ. Quantitative effects of dietary fat on serum cholesterol in man. Am J Clin Nutr 1965;17:281-95.

12. Mustad VA, Ellsworth J, Cooper AD, Kris-Etherton PM, Etherton TD. Dietary linoleic acid increases and palmitic acid decreases hepatic LDL receptor protein and mRNA abundance in young pigs. J Lipid Res 1996;37:2310-23.

13. Hopkins PN. Effects of dietary cholesterol on serum cholesterol: A meta-analysis and review. Am J Clin Nutr 1992;50:1060-70.

14. Ernst N, Bowen P, Fisher M, et al. Changes in plasma lipids and lipoproteins after a modified fat diet. Lancet 1980;1:111.

15. Williams PT, Krauss RM, Kindel-Joyce S, Freon DM, Vranizan KM, Wood PD. Relationship of dietary fat protein, cholesterol, and fiber intake to atherogenic lipoproteins in men. Am J Clin Nutr 1986;44:788-97.

16. Gardner CD, Kraemer HC. Monounsaturated versus polyunsaturated dietary fat and serum lipids: A meta-analysis. Arterioscler Thromb Vasc Biol 1995;15:1917-27.

17. Mensink RP, Katan MB. Effect of dietary trans fatty acids on high density and low-density lipoprotein cholesterol levels in healthy subjects. N Engl J Med 1990;323:439-45.

18. Mensink RP, Zock PL, Katan MB, Honstra G. Effect of dietary cis and trans fatty acids on serum lipoprotein(a) levels in humans. J Lipid Res 1992;33:1493-1501.

19. Kromhout D, Menotti A, Bloemberg B, et al. Dietary saturated and trans fatty acids and cholesterol and 25-year mortality from coronary heart disease: The Seven Countries Study. Preventive Med 1995;24:308-15.

20. Denke MA. Cholesterol-lowering diets: A review of the evidence. Arch Intern Med 1995;155:17-26.

21. Miettinen TA. Impact of apo E phenotype on the regulation of cholesterol metabolism. Ann Med 1991;23:181-86.

22. Barnard RJ. Effects of life-style modification on serum lipids. Arch Intern Med 1991;151:1389.

23. Garry RJ, Hunt WC, Koehler KM, et al. Longitudinal study of dietary intakes and plasma lipids in healthy elderly men and women. Am J Clin Nutr 1992;1:55.

24. Fraser GE, Dysinger W, Best C, Chan R. Ischaemic heart disease risk factors in middle-aged Seventh Day Adventists men and their neighbors. Am J Epi 1987;126:638-46.

25. Kromhout D. Diet-heart issues in a pharmacological era. Lancet 1996;348:S20-S22.

26. Golay A, Eigneheer C, Morel Y, Kujawski P, Lehmann T, de Tonnac N. Weight-loss with low or high carbohydrate diet? Int J Obesity 1996;220:1067-72.

27. Hannah JS, Heiser CC, Jablonski KA, et al. Effects of obesity on the response to a low fat diet. Circulation 1994;90:I-236.

28. Dengel DR, Hagberg JM, Coon PJ, Drinkwater DT, Goldberg AP. Comparable effects of diet and exercise on body composition and lipoproteins in older men. Med Sci Sports 1994;26:1307-15.

29. Van Horn LV, Liu K, Parker D, et al. Serum lipid response to oat product intake with a fat-modified diet. J Am Diet Assoc 1986;86:759-64.

30. Sprecher DL. Efficacy of psyllium in reducing serum cholesterol levels in hypercholesterolemic patients on high- or low-fat diets. Ann Intern Med 1993;119:545-54.

31. Pietinen P, Rimm EB, et al. Intake of dietary fiber and risk of coronary heart disease in a cohort of Finnish men: The Alpha-Tocopherol, Beta-Carotene Cancer Prevention Study. Circulation 1996;94:2720-27.

32. Harris WS. Fish oils and plasma lipid and lipoprotein metabolism in humans: A critical review. J Lipid Res 1989;30:785-807.

33. Childs H, King IB, Knopp RH. Divergent lipoproteins responses to fish oils with various

ratios of eisosapentaenoic acid and docosahexaenoic acid. Am J Clin Nutr 1990;52:632-39.

34. Ascherio A, Rimm EB, Stampfer MJ, Giovannucci EL, Willett WC. Dietary intake of marine n-3 fatty acids, fish intake, and the risk of coronary disease among women. New Eng J Med 1995;332:977-82.

35. Gapinski JP, Van Ruiswyk JV, Heudebert GR, Schectmen GS. Preventing restenosis with fish oils following coronary angioplasty. Arch Intern Med 1993;153:1595-1601.

36. Kinsella JE, Lokesh B, Stone RA. Dietary n-3 polyunsaturated fatty acids and amelioration of cardiovascular disease: Possible mechanisms. Am J Clin Nutr 1990;52:1-28.

37. Goto Y. Serum cholesterol and nutrition in Japan. Nutr Health 1985;3:255-57.

38. Berliner JA, Heinecke JW. The role of oxidized lipoproteins in atherogenesis. Free Radical Biology & Medicine 1996;20:707-27.

39. Parthasarathy S, Khoo JC, Miller E, Barnett J, Witztum JL, Steinberg D. Low-density lipoprotein rich in oleic acid is protected against oxidative modification implications for dietary prevention of atherosclerosis. Proc Nat Acad Sci USA 1990;87:3894-98.

40. Rexrode KM, Manson JE. Antioxidants and coronary heart disease: Observational studies. J Cardiovas Research 1996;3:363-67.

41. Albanes D, Heinonen OP, et al. Alpha-tocoherol and beta-carotene supplements and lung cancer incidence in the Alpha-Tocopherol, Beta-Carotene Cancer Prevention Study: Effects of base-line characteristics and study compliance. J Natl Cancer Inst 1996;88:1560-70.

42. Omenn GS, Goodman GE, Thornquist MD, et al. Effects of a combination of beta-carotene and vitamin A on lung cancer and cardiovascular disease. N Engl J Med 1996;334:1150-55.

43. Hennekens CH, Buring JE, Manson JE, et al. Lack of effect of long term supplementation with beta carotene on the incidence of malignant neoplasms and cardiovascular disease. N Eng J Med 1996;334:1145-49.

44. Gaziano JM, Manson JE, Ridker PM, Buring JE, Hennekens CH. Beta carotene therapy for chronic stable angina. Circulation 1991;82(Suppl.)III;201.

45. Stephens NG, Parsons A, Schofield PM, et al. Randomised controlled trial of vitamin E in patients with coronary disease: Cambridge Heart Antioxidant Study (CHAOS). Lancet 1996; 347:781-86.

46. Hegsted DM, Ausman LM. Diet, alcohol and coronary heart disease. J Nutr 1988;118:1184-89.

47. Suh IL, Shaten J, Cutler JA, Kuller LH for the Multiple Risk Factor Interventional Trial Research Group. Alcohol use and mortality from coronary heart disease: The role of high-density lipoprotein cholesterol. Arch Intern Med 1992;116:881-87.

48. Miettinen TA, Puska P, Gylling H, Vanhanen H, Vartiainnen E. Reduction of serum cholesterol with sitostanol-ester margarine in a mildly hypercholesterolemic population. N Engl J Med 1995;333:1308-12.

49. Anthony MS, Clarkson TB, Bullock BC. Soy protein versus soy phytoestrogens (isoflavones) in the prevention of coronary artery atherosclerosis of cynomolgus monkeys. Abstract. Circulation 1996;94:I-265.

50. Hertog MGL, Kromhout D, Aravanis C, et al. Flavonoid intake and long term risk of coronary heart disease and cancer in the Seven Countries Study. Arch Intern Med 1995;155:381-86.

51. LaRosa JC. Estrogen: Risk versus benefit for the prevention of coronary artery disease. Coronary Artery Disease 1993;4:588-94.

52. Grobbee DE, Rimm EB, Giovannucci E, et al. Coffee, caffeine, and cardiovascular disease in men. N Engl J Med 1990;323:1026-32.

53. Sabate J, Fraser GD. Nuts: A new protective food against coronary heart disease. Curr Opin

Lipidology 1994;5:11-16.

54.   Warshafsky S, Kamer RS, Sivak SL. Effect of garlic on total serum cholesterol. Ann
       Intern Med 1993;119:599-605.

55.   Niel HAW, Cilagy CA, Lancaster T, et al. Garlic powder in the treatment of moderate
       hyperlipidaemia: A controlled trial and meta-analysis. J of the Royal College of Physicians
       1996;30:329-34.

56.   Woodard DA, Limacher MC. The impact of diet on coronary heart disease. Med Clin North
       American 1993;77:849-62.

57.   Superko HR, Krauss RM. Coronary artery disease regression: Convincing evidence for the
       benefit of aggressive lipoprotein management. Circ 1994;90:1056-69.

58.   Gould KL, Ornish D, Scherwitz L, Brown S, Edens P, Hess MJ. Changes in myocardial
       perfusion abnormalities by positron emission tomography after long term, intense risk factor
       modification. JAMA 1995;274:894-901.

59.   Tosteson ANA, Weinstein MC, Hunink MGM, et al. Cost-effectiveness of population-wide
       educational approaches to reduce serum cholesterol levels. Circulation 1997;95:24-30.

60.   Stone MJ, Nicolosi RJ, Kris-Etherton P. Summary of the Scientific Conference on the Efficacy
       of Hypercholesterolemic Dietary Interventions. Circulation 1996;94:3388-91.

61.   Karpe F, Steiner G, Uffelman K, Olivecrona T, Hamsten A. Postprandial lipoproteins and
       progression of coronary atherosclerosis. Atherosclerosis 1994;106:83-97.

62.   Bittner V. Atherogenicity of postprandial lipoproteins and coronary heart disease.
       The Endocrinologist 1994;4:359-72.

63.   Nikkila M, Solakivi T, Lehtimaki T, Koivula T, Laippala P, Astrom B. Postprandial plasma
       lipoprotein changes in relation to apolipoprotein E phenotypes and low density lipoprotein size
       in men with and without coronary artery disease. Atherosclerosis 1994;106:149-57.

64.   Shekelle RB, Shyrock AM, Paul O, et al. Diet, serum cholesterol, and death from coronary
       heart disease: The Western Electric Study. N Engl J Med 1981;304:65-70.

ALCOHOL AND CORONARY HEART DISEASE: A COMPARISON OF ECOLOGIC AND NON-ECOLOGIC STUDIES

Michael H. Criqui

Introduction

Several study designs have been utilized to address the question of the association of alcohol consumption with coronary heart disease (CHD). Study designs have included case-control studies, where cases of CHD are selected retrospectively and their alcohol consumption compared to a control group of persons free of CHD; prospective cohort studies, where alcohol consumption at baseline is determined in a defined cohort and the cohort is followed over time for the development of CHD, and ecologic studies, where overall consumption of alcohol in a group, community, or country is compared with CHD rates in those same groups. A fourth study design, which would allow the strongest causal inference, is a randomized clinical trial — a true experiment. However, it seems unlikely that a clinical trial of alcohol consumption for CHD endpoints will ever be done, since a true placebo is not available and such a trial would raise both operational and ethical issues.

The focus of this paper is to review ecologic studies of alcohol intake and CHD, including a recent effort by our group, and to discuss the strengths and weaknesses of such studies, and the degree to which they are consistent with other study designs addressing the alcohol-CHD question.

Strengths of the Ecologic Study

There are two major strengths to ecologic studies. First, since very large units are typically studied, with an entire country often the unit of analysis, the results, to the extent they are valid, are widely generalizable. Second, ecologic studies often allow study of populations with extreme values, which helps address questions where the slope of the association is not steep or where there is a threshold effect. For example, the relationship between dietary cholesterol and serum cholesterol is stronger across populations with widely divergent cholesterol intakes than it is within populations with homogeneous intakes [1]. Another example is dietary salt intake and blood pressure. While it is difficult to demonstrate an association within populations, the Intersalt study has shown that across many populations with widely varying salt intake, there is a consistent, highly significant association, although the slope of the line is shallow [2].

297

A. M. Gotto, Jr. et al. (eds.), Multiple Risk Factors in Cardiovascular Disease, 297–302.
© 1998 Kluwer Academic Publishers and Fondazione Giovanni Lorenzini. Printed in the Netherlands.

Weaknesses of the Ecologic Study

Perhaps the most important potential weakness of ecological studies is that the unit of analysis is a group (e.g. a country), rather than an individual. Thus, dose-response relationships on an individual level can not be discerned. This can give rise to an ecological fallacy. For example, within most countries, higher levels of HDL cholesterol are associated with lower rates of CHD, an inverse relationship. However, across many countries, the relationship may be flat or even positive since countries with lower overall cholesterol levels tend to have lower HDL levels. Fortunately, for most risk factors such a fallacy does not exist. For example, total cholesterol or LDL cholesterol levels are positively associated with CHD both within and across populations. Within a population, a carefully designed study can collect highly valid, reliable data. In ecological studies, existing data is analyzed and data comparability across populations may be reduced by differing availability, customs, and standards. Finally, confounding may be more difficult to control across compared to within populations. Potential confounding factors are more easily assessed within a given cohort than they are across populations, and in addition, differences in various behaviors, lifestyles, and customs may be greater across than within populations. Such "social confounding" may be an important problem in ecologic studies.

Ecologic Studies of Alcohol and CHD

St. Leger et al. evaluated the association between wine consumption and CHD death in 18 developed countries in 1970 in men aged 55-64 years [3]. They excluded Japan because of possible "genetic factors," which removed the country with the lowest CHD death rate. There was a strong inverse association between wine and CHD. Saturated and monounsaturated fat showed a positive association, and monounsaturated fat an inverse relationship. However, in multiple regression, only wine was significantly related to CHD mortality. They presented only univariate data for beer and spirits, and did not present data on total mortality.

Renaud et al. looked at wine and CHD in 17 developed countries in 1987 [4]. Of these 17 countries, 14 overlapped with the St. Leger paper. Unlike St. Leger et al., they did not evaluate Canada, New Zealand, or the USA. They added Portugal, Spain, and Yugoslavia. They studied both genders combined but did not specify which ages were studied. A positive correlation was found between dietary fat and CHD, r = .73, p < 0.001. However, France and (to a lesser degree) Switzerland, were outliers, with lower CHD rates than predicted by the regression line. Multivariate adjustment for wine consumption moved both France and Switzerland quite close to the regression line, and the correlation increased to r = 0.87, p < 0.0001. Data were not presented for alcoholic beverages other than wine, or for total mortality. Artaud-Wild et al. studied the association between an index of cholesterol and saturated fat intake (CSI) and CHD mortality in men aged 55-64 years in 1977 [5]. Forty countries in varying stages of economic development were studied. The CSI had a strong correlation with CHD (r = .78, p < 0.001), but Finland (higher than expected CHD rate) and France (lower than expected CHD rate) were outliers. These outliers were partially explained by a much high milk intake in Finland than in France, and a much higher vegetable intake in France than in Finland. After adjustment for CSI, alcohol was unrelated to CHD. However, in the 18 countries with a CSI index greater than 20 per 1,000 kcal, wine was strongly and inversely associated with CHD ($r = -.67$, $p = .003$). Total mortality was not evaluated in this study.

We studied 21 developed countries that met a gross domestic product income level of U.S. dollars 9,500 per capita [6]. This cutpoint produced a bimodal separation. Five additional countries met this criteria, but were excluded because of problematic data on one or more variables. Both sexes combined aged 35-74 years were studied in four cross-sectional time periods: 1965, 1970, 1980, and 1988. The independent variables were wine ethanol, beer ethanol, spirits ethanol, animal fat, vegetables, and fruit. Both CHD and total mortality were evaluated as endpoints in multivariate analysis. Table 1 shows of the results of the multivariate analysis of CHD mortality. For p values < .10, the exact p value and sign of the coefficient, positive or inverse, are shown. Wine was the strongest and most consistent correlate of CHD, and showed an inverse relationship. Animal fat tended to be positively correlated, and fruit inversely correlated, with CHD. Beer and spirits showed only weak inverse correlations with CHD.

Table 1. Multivariate Analysis of CHD Mortality*

	1965		1970		1980		1988	
	Coeff	p-value	Coeff	p-value	Coeff	p-value	Coeff	p-value
Wine ethanol	inv	.07	inv	.01	inv	.01	x	x
Beer ethanol	x	x	inv	.09	x	x	x	x
Spirits ethanol	x	x	x	x	x	x	x	x
Animal fat	pos	.02	pos	.03	x	x	x	x
Vegetable fat	x	x	x	x	x	x	x	x
Fruit	pos	.06	x	x	inv	.08	inv	.06

* Adapted from [6]
Pos = positive beta coefficient
Inv = inverse beta coefficient

The multivariate analysis for total mortality shown in Table 2 was strikingly different than that for CHD, despite the significant proportion of total mortality due to CHD. No alcoholic beverage showed any benefit for total mortality, and there was a suggestion of a hazard for beer intake. The only dietary item which appeared to independently promote longevity was fruit intake. The lack of a protective effect of wine or any alcoholic beverage for total mortality, despite a protective effect of wine for CHD, suggests a positive association between alcoholic beverages and non-CHD causes of death. We have confirmed this positive association in a recent analysis [7].

Table 2. Multivariate Analysis of Total Mortality*

	1965		1970		1980		1988	
	Coeff	p-value	Coeff	p-value	Coeff	p-value	Coeff	p-value
Wine ethanol	x	x	x	x	x	x	x	x
Beer ethanol	x	x	x	x	pos	.01	pos	.05
Spirits ethanol	x	x	x	x	x	x	x	x
Animal fat	x	x	x	x	x	x	x	x
Vegetable fat	x	x	x	x	x	x	x	x
Fruit	x	x	x	x	inv	.03	inv	.05

* Adapted from [6]
Pos = positive beta coefficient
Inv = inverse beta coefficient

Concordance of Ecologic and Other Studies

Case-control and prospective studies have consistently reported a protective effect of moderate alcohol consumption for CHD [8]. This effect is similar whether the beverage consumed is wine, beer, or spirits [9]. However, higher intakes of alcohol are associated with increases in non-CHD causes of death, including cardiovascular disease such as stroke, and decreased overall longevity [10]. In addition, higher alcohol intake is sometimes associated with increased CHD death rates as well [10].

All four of the ecologic studies concurred that wine was inversely associated with CHD mortality, at least in the subset of developed countries with a moderate or higher dietary intake of cholesterol and saturated fat. Only the most recent study looked at total mortality and found no relationship for wine or spirits, and a possible hazard for beer consumption [6].

In terms of CHD, the ecologic studies are generally concordant with non-ecologic studies where the unit of analysis is the individual. Presumably, the greater effect for wine in ecologic studies is due to unadjusted other differences in wine drinking cultures. Unlike other study designs, ecologic analyses cannot look at dose-response relationships in individuals. For example, among the 21 countries we studied, France has a very low CHD rate but a high non-CHD rate [6,7]. We don't know the fate of moderate drinkers versus nondrinkers or heavy drinkers in France from these data. However, we do know that France has a low rate of nondrinkers (15%) and a high rate of heavy drinkers (25%) [11]. We can reason that, based on studies of individuals, the very low rate of CHD is largely present in the 60% of the population who drink light to moderately, and who likely enjoy increased longevity. We can also reason that the high non-CHD death rate in France largely occurs in the 25% of the population who are heavy drinkers, since in non-ecologic studies, heavier drinking has been directly linked to non-CHD causes of death such as stroke, cancer, and injury death [12].

Can We Recommend Light to Moderate Drinking?

Given the consistent association between light to moderate alcohol intake and reduced risk of CHD, should we recommend such drinking? For example, should one encourage a group (e.g. community, country) to neither abstain nor drink to excess? Several facts need to be considered.

The distribution of alcohol consumption is remarkably consistent across populations. The mean consumption always exceeds the median, 10-15% of a given population drink more than twice the mean, and this latter group consumes more than half of all the alcohol [13] . Strikingly, these distributional findings are consistent across groups with per capita consumption of 2.4 liters per year all the way to 47.5 liters per year. Similarly, Rose has reported a 0.97 correlation in the Intersalt study between mean population consumption and the proportion of heavy drinkers in a population [14].

The implications of these findings are clear. Despite vast differences in ethnicity, culture, and customs, the extent of abuse in a population is a direct function of average consumption, and widespread enthusiasm for the "health benefits" of alcohol will prove detrimental to overall health.

There are isolated situations where selected persons at elevated risk of CHD with responsible drinking habits should discuss their alcohol intake with their physician. However, in general any separation of "individual" recommendations from "group" recommendations seems a false dichotomy, since it would be difficult to keep such recommendations confidential.

Conclusions

Ecologic studies can detect associations with thresholds or only moderate slopes. Such associations may be difficult to show within relatively homogeneous populations. However, in ecologic studies, dose-response relationships for individuals cannot be determined and the data may be subject to an ecological fallacy. In addition, data may lack comparability, and confounding is more difficult to control. Ecologic studies of the relationship between alcohol and CHD are consistent with the findings in non-ecologic studies. An ecologic study looking at alcohol and total mortality is also consistent with non-ecologic studies in that the countries with the highest alcohol consumption had high mortality from non-CHD causes.

The consistency and concordance of non-ecologic and ecologic studies strongly suggest light to moderate alcohol consumption affords some protection from CHD, but that higher consumption increases non-CHD death and total mortality. The very high correlation in groups between average alcohol intake and alcohol abuse indicates any public health recommendation favoring drinking is contraindicated [15]. Selected persons at elevated risk of CHD who can use alcohol responsibility should discuss their alcohol intake with their physician.

Acknowledgements

I would like to thank Ms. Linda Sridhar for assistance in manuscript preparation.

References

1. Shekelle RB, Shryock AM, Paul O, et al. Diet, serum cholesterol, and death from coronary heart disease. The Western Electric Study. N Engl J Med 1981;304:65-70.
2. Intersalt Cooperative Research Group. Intersalt: An international study of electrolyte excretion and blood pressure. Results for 24 hour urinary sodium and potassium excretion. BMJ 1988; 297:319-28.
3. St. Leger AS, Cochrane AL, Moore F. Factors associated with cardiac mortality in developed countries with particular reference to the consumption of wine. Lancet 1979;i:1017-20.
4. Renaud S, de Lorgeril M. Wine, alcohol, platelets, and the French paradox for coronary heart disease. Lancet 1992;339:1523-26.
5. Artaud-Wild SM, Connor S, Sexton G, Connor W. Differences in coronary mortality can be explained by differences in cholesterol and saturated fat intakes in 40 countries but not in France and Finland: A paradox. Circulation 1993;88:2771-79.
6. Criqui MH, Ringel BL. Does diet or alcohol explain the French paradox? Lancet 1994;344: 1719-23.
7. Criqui MH, Hostettler JL, Denenberg JO. Unpublished manuscript.
8. Marmot M, Brunner E. Alcohol and cardiovascular disease: The status of the U-shaped curve. BMJ 1991;303:565-68.
9. Rimm EB, Klatsky A, Grobee D, Stampfer MJ. Review of moderate alcohol consumption and reduced risk of coronary heart disease: Is the effect due to beer, wine, or spirits. BMJ 1996;312: 731-36.
10. Criqui MH. Alcohol and the heart: Implications of present epidemiologic knowledge. Contemporary Drug Problems 1994;21:125-42.
11. Ministère des Affaire Sociales de la Santé et de la Ville. Haut Comité de la Santé Publique. La santé en France: Rapport général. Documentation Française, Paris, France, 1994.
12. Boffetta P, Garfinkel L. Alcohol drinking and mortality among men enrolled in an American Cancer Society Prospective Study. Epidemiology 1990;1:342-48.
13. Skog OH. The collectivity of drinking cultures: A theory of the distribution of alcohol consumption. Br J Addict 1985; 80:83-99.
14. Rose G. Ancel Keys Lecture. Circulation 1991;84:1405-9.
15. Criqui MH. Moderate drinking: Benefits and risks. In: Sakhari S, Wassef M, editors. Alcohol and the cardiovascular system. NIAAA Research Monograph No. 31: 1996, 117-23.

PREVENTING CARDIOVASCULAR DISEASE: EFFECTIVE SMOKING CESSATION STRATEGIES FOR THE BUSY CLINICIAN

Judith K. Ockene and Ira S. Ockene

Introduction

Cigarette smoking has been strongly established as a major cause of cardiovascular disease (CVD) [1,2]. For example, women smoking as few as 1 to 4 cigarettes per day are at 2.5 times the risk of fatal cardiovascular disease (CVD) and nonfatal myocardial infarction compared to nonsmokers. Elimination of smoking can produce a substantial reduction in premature morbidity and mortality. Estimates indicate that up to 30%, or 170,000, of all coronary heart disease (CHD) deaths in the United States each year are attributable to cigarette smoking, with the risk being strongly dose-related [2]. In addition, smoking acts synergistically with other risk factors, substantially increasing the risk of CVD.

The compelling reason supporting the need for healthcare providers to support cessation efforts is that prospective investigations have demonstrated a substantial decrease in CVD mortality for former smokers compared with continuing smokers. This diminution in risk occurs relatively promptly following cessation of smoking, and increasing intervals since the time one last smoked are associated with progressively lower mortality rates from CVD [1,3-5]. Smoking is the single most alterable risk factor contributing to premature morbidity and morality in the United States, accounting for more than 400,000 deaths annually [6].

The Importance and Effect of Physician-Delivered Smoking Intervention

More than 90% of the smokers who stop smoking in the U.S. do not use an organized program to help them stop, and most smokers who continue to smoke state that they would prefer to stop without the aid of a formal smoking-cessation program [2,7]. It is with this large group of smokers that the physician can have a major impact. Almost 80% of the adult population has at least one contact per year with a physician [8], with the average yearly number of contacts being six per adult. Thus, the physician as educator, facilitator, or counselor has the potential to be a powerful agent for smoking cessation [9,10]. Individuals probably think more seriously about their health and smoking's effect on it when they are in a physician's office or in a hospital than at any other time. This opportunity for health promotion with smokers, ex-smokers, and would-be smokers should not be overlooked.

A. M. Gotto, Jr. et al. (eds.), Multiple Risk Factors in Cardiovascular Disease, 303–312.

Evidence from randomized trials indicates that physicians who intervene with their smoking patients have a significant effect on their cigarette smoking behavior [11]. The recently released Agency for Health Care Policy and Research (AHCPR) Smoking Cessation Guideline [11] noted "it is essential that clinicians determine and document the tobacco use status of every patient treated in a healthcare setting." Summarizing the smoking intervention literature, the AHCPR recommends that simple advice by one's physician to stop smoking is more effective than no advice at all and that as the physician-delivered smoking intervention becomes more extensive, the effects are greater. The guideline also notes that the success of an intervention increases with the number of intervention modalities employed and the number of healthcare professionals involved. Clinical trials also have demonstrated that special training of physicians to deliver brief interventions and the use of general office practice procedures to help cue the physician to intervene with smokers and provide follow up, increase the likelihood that physicians will intervene and that they will have a favorable impact on patients' smoking behavior [12]. To keep the interventions brief and to meet the special needs of patients, physicians also can refer them to special programs or have someone in their office provide intervention and follow up.

A physician's effect on a patient's smoking varies greatly with the context for change. The patient who is symptomatic or already ill, e.g. post-myocardial infarction (MI) or has had recent coronary artery by-pass surgery, is more likely to respond to the physician's advice. The patient may show immediate interest in change when some acute symptoms caused by smoking occur; the smoking pattern of the patient will be least affected when he feels well and has few if any symptoms or abnormal findings [10,13]. Randomized studies have shown high quit rates (50%-63%) at 6 months follow up for patients who are advised to quit smoking by their physician after having an MI or after having been told they have CHD, and significantly higher rates (65%-75%) for patients who receive additional counseling by health educators or nurses by telephone or in person [13,14]. These cessation rates are directly related to the severity of disease [13,15] and fall to 30 to 40% when intervention is directed at those smokers who are at high risk for infarction but are not yet diseased [16]. This relationship between cessation and disease status is consistent with the principles of the health belief model (discussed in the following section), which note that the person who perceives himself to be vulnerable to the actual effects of a particular behavior such as smoking, and perceives that the benefits of change outweigh the costs, will be more motivated to change a behavior.

Determinants of Smoking Behavior and Change

Cigarette smoking is a complex behavior pattern that, like most behaviors, is affected by multiple and interacting factors: physiologic factors, information, personality, demographic factors, environmental influences (social, cultural, and economic), and other behaviors (e.g. drinking a beer triggers taking a cigarette). The behavior goes through a sequence of phases from initiation to regular smoking to possible cessation and eventual maintenance of cessation or relapse. Each phase is affected by a different set of factors.

Theories and models are useful for helping to explain determinants of behavior and behavior change and in turn help to inform us about how to intervene with different behaviors. There are several theories whose principles are applicable to intervention for smoking cessation. These include the Health Belief Model [17], Social Cognitive Theory [18], the Relapse Prevention Model [19], and the Stages of Change Model [20]. Key principles applicable to smoking intervention from these models are:

- To initiate change a smoker must believe that the benefits outweigh the costs.
- Active participation is an important part of the change process.
- To initiate change a smoker must believe he is capable of it; small steps are important.

Model for Physician-Delivered Smoking Intervention

Smoking cessation advice should be regarded as the minimal standard of practice; and where possible, physicians should go beyond providing advice [11]. Intervention delivered by physicians can be accomplished in three to ten minutes, depending on how ready the smoker is to stop smoking and how much assistance the physician is willing to provide.

A patient-centered model for physician involvement with smokers incorporating three different levels of physician intervention has been developed by Ockene and colleagues at the University of Massachusetts Medical School during 15 years of research and development [21-24] as part of their provider-delivered smoking intervention training program (see Figure 1). The model takes into account that: physicians have little time to spend counseling, therefore interventions must be brief; most smokers want to quit; and other healthcare providers can assist the physician with his efforts. The three levels of intervention are: 1) brief physician-delivered counseling; 2) brief physician-delivered counseling plus physician assistance; and 3) brief physician-delivered counseling with referral for comprehensive individual or group intervention (either one session or multiple sessions) [21,23]. An algorithm has been developed to make it easy for the physician to implement the intervention at either of the three intervention levels (Figure 1). This algorithm is similar to, but more extensive than, one that was developed by the National Cancer Institute [25]. The patient-centered model has been tested in several settings and found to be efficacious [26]. That is, when physicians use patient-centered counseling, they have a significantly greater effect on their patients' smoking than physicians who provide advice only. The following overview of what the physician can do in the smoking cessation process must be adapted to the individual physician's needs and situation.

BRIEF COUNSELING (3-5 MINUTES)

The basic steps for brief counseling are: 1) ask/assess smoking; 2) advise cessation; 3) assist (minimal); and 4) arrange for follow up. Step 1, ask/assess includes assessing the patient's interest and reasons for stopping and assessing nicotine dependency (see section below). Step 2, advise cessation, needs to be personalized to the smoker (i.e. based on the patient's reasons for wanting to quit). Step 3, minimal assistance, could include provision of self-help materials and nicotine replacement therapy (NRT) if appropriate. (See sections below on

NRT.) Step 4, arrange for follow up, which can occur either in person or by telephone, is important because it conveys to the patient that, "This is important enough to me that I want to follow up with you." The brief 4-step intervention can be expanded if the physician is willing to further assist the patient with cessation. (See next section, Brief Counseling with Physician Assistance.)

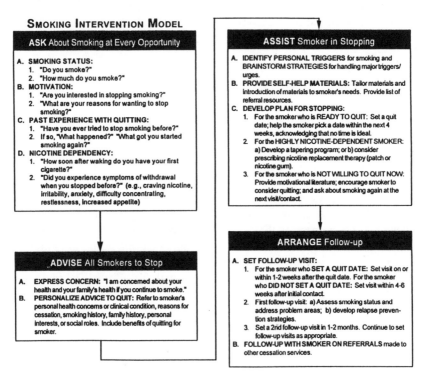

Figure 1. Smoking intervention Model.

BRIEF BEHAVIORAL COUNSELING WITH PHYSICIAN ASSISTANCE (5-10 MINUTES)

Brief patient-centered behavioral counseling with further assistance to help smokers to develop plans for change, and specific strategies for cessation, has been demonstrated to be significantly more efficacious in helping patients to alter smoking than advice alone [26]. The smaller print in Figure 1 indicates what the physician can do if she wishes to go beyond the simple Ask, Advise, Assist (minimal) and Arrange. It emphasizes the importance of the patient's input in developing an effective plan for change and can be accomplished using an additional three to five minutes of the physician's time.

Some of the patient-centered counseling steps presented here to assist the patient to develop cessation strategies and a plan for cessation are similar to the ones used above in brief counseling. However, questioning can be more in-depth. The following steps are interchangeable and should be adapted to the physician's needs and style and the needs of the patient:

- Assess motivation (personalized reasons for wanting to stop smoking);
- Ask about past experiences with cessation;
- Assess nicotine dependency;
- Develop a plan (this could include referral for some intensive assistance); and
- Arrange for follow up.

Assess motivation. It is necessary to determine the patient's reasons for wanting to stop, which may be different from the physician's reasons for wanting her to do so. He/she may be more concerned about the impact of her smoking on his/her children than on the risk for disease.

Ask about past experiences. The second step, exploration of past experiences with cessation, helps patients focus on possible past successes, no matter how small, and helps them to develop a belief that they are capable of cessation. Eighty percent of all smokers have stopped sometime in the past [2]. The physician can help patients focus on the resources and strategies they used and the positive feelings they had about themselves when they were nonsmokers.

Determining past experiences with cessation can reveal problems encountered which need to be prepared for and coping strategies that were used and successful which can be used for the current cessation effort. Once the problem is identified, possible coping strategies can be identified. For example, walking may help reduce anxiety or increased appetite.

Assess nicotine dependency. Determine whether the smoker is physiologically addicted to nicotine. Assessment of the patient's past experiences with cessation can uncover whether he or she had experienced symptoms of nicotine withdrawal. The more intense the withdrawal symptoms were in previous quit attempts, the more likely they are to be a problem again. Assessment of withdrawal and the use of a specially developed scale for measuring addiction, the Fagerstrom Addiction Scale (Figure 2) [27,28], can help the physician to decide whether to suggest the use of pharmacologic therapy in addition to educational and behavioral interventions. (See below for pharmacologic treatment of nicotine addiction.) The smoker should be alerted to the symptoms associated with withdrawal, that these symptoms decrease quickly, and that a variety of approaches, such as tapering nicotine intake before stopping "cold turkey" or use of NRT can be used to handle them.

Develop a plan/arrange follow up. The counseling sequence leads to a plan for change. The plan may focus on immediate goals, e.g. not staying at the table after completing dinner. It also can focus on goals closer to the endpoint (e.g. using NRT or relaxation exercises or exercise in place of cigarettes). Finally, end with an arrangement for follow up.

Figure 2. Fagerstrom Tolerance Questionnaire

---

1. How many cigarettes a day do you smoke?

2. What is the nicotine yield per cigarette of your usual brand?
    0.3-0.8 g   0.9-1.5 g   1.6-2.2 g
    (Low to Medium)   (Medium)   (Medium to high)

3. Do you inhale?
    Never   Sometimes   Always

4. Do you smoke more during the morning than during the rest of the day?
    No   Yes

5. How soon after you wake up do you smoke your first cigarette?
    More than 30 minutes   Less than 30 minutes

6. Of all the cigarettes you smoke during the day, which would you most hate to give up?

7. Do you find it difficult to refrain from smoking in places where it is forbidden (e.g., in church, at the library, in a no-smoking cinema)?

8. Do you smoke even if you are so ill that you are in bed most of the day?
    No   Yes

Scoring: Add up the scores as follows:

1. 0-15, 0; 16-25, 1; 25+, 2
2. Low to medium, 0; Medium, 1; Medium to high, 2
3. Never, 0; Sometimes, 1; Always, 2
4. No, 0; Yes, 1
5. Less than 30 minutes, 1; more than 30 minutes, 0
6. Score one point if you answered: The first cigarette of the day; all others, 0
7. Yes, 1; No, 0
8. Yes, 1; No, 0

This questionnaire measures the degree of physical dependence on the nicotine in cigarettes: 0-3, light dependence; 4-7, medium dependence; 8-11, dependence

Figure 2: Fagerstrom Tolerance Questionnaire) [27] or the revised FTQ [28]. The recommended revisions to the FTQ include dropping items 2 and 3, and adding additional categories to items 1 and 5 [28].

If the physician wants, a patient can be referred for additional assistance to several types of providers including nurses, psychologists, social workers, and health educators. This can be for individual counseling or group intervention. Optimally, physicians should become familiar with referral resources in their own institution or community and develop a list of places or people to whom referrals can be made.

To summarize, physician-delivered intervention is efficacious: the greater the intensity of the intervention, the greater the effect [11]. Whatever intervention is used, the following consistent, brief messages can be delivered by the physician [23]:

- Quitting smoking is a process, not a one-time event. It progresses from becoming aware of the need to stop smoking, to taking action, to stopping and maintaining cessation;
- Quitting smoking often takes several attempts before long-term cessation can occur;
- A return to smoking is not a failure, it can be used as a learning experience to help you prepare for the next time you stop;
- Many methods can help you to stop smoking. The best method is the one you choose for yourself, based on your own experiences;
- Pharmacologic intervention, such as NRT, may be needed for the physiologically-addicted smoker.

Addressing Nicotine Dependency

Persons who smoke more than a pack a day, those who smoke within 30 minutes of waking, those who have had intense withdrawal symptoms in the past with a pattern of relapsing within a few hours or days, those who score high on the FTQ, and those who have difficulty refraining from smoking in public areas, are likely to have the greatest difficulty with withdrawal symptoms, and nicotine dependence probably plays an important role in maintaining the behavior. If the smoker is ready to quit but is highly dependent, either nicotine fading or NRT or an antidepressant should be considered.

NICOTINE FADING

Nicotine fading [29] has two components: brand switching to a lower-nicotine-level cigarette, and gradual reduction of the number of cigarettes (i.e. tapering). When tapering, remind the smoker not to inhale more deeply or smoke more of the cigarette than he or she did in the past, and not to cover the vents in the filter of lower-nicotine cigarettes as that increases nicotine availability.

NICOTINE REPLACEMENT THERAPY

Nicotine replacement therapy (NRT) includes nicotine-containing gum, the transdermal nicotine patch, and nicotine nasal spray. Physicians should be clear on the proper use of each product by reading the insert materials provided. The most common problem is when the smoker perceives NRT as a "magic" solution; a more appropriate way to present it is as an aid to "take the edge off the physical craving" while the person "learns" to become a "nonsmoker." Both the gum and the patch are now available over-the-counter.

Nicotine-containing gum, approved in 1984, has been shown to be effective in aiding cessation when used in combination with behavioral treatment [30]. However, certain side effects and its often improper use which includes chewing it too vigorously, rather than primarily "parking" it (i.e. letting it sit between the cheek and teeth for proper absorption), using too few pieces per day (the recommended number being about half the number of cigarettes smoked), and using it for too short a period of time (the recommended time period being three to six months with tapered use), have limited its effect for smokers who use it.

The transdermal nicotine patch, marketed in slightly different formulations and delivery systems, also has been shown to be effective in aiding cessation of smoking [11]. It provides a more passive delivery system, thereby improving adherence to use; allows for a more continuous delivery of nicotine; and avoids the gastrointestinal and oral side effects of the gum.

Nicotine nasal spray (NNS) has been approved for use in the U.S. and can be offered to patients. One study which tested the safety and efficacy of NNS found that it significantly enhanced success rates (i.e. continuous abstinence) over placebo [31].

ANTIDEPRESSANT

The FDA has recently approved the use of bupropion tablets, an antidepressant, for use as a smoking cessation aide. It has been found to be efficacious when compared to a placebo [32]. However, the effects do not appear to be sustained at three months.

Setting Up the Office Practice to Support Interventions

Learning intervention strategies and developing skills are necessary but not enough if physicians are to do smoking intervention. Office systems need to be set up to screen patients, remind the physician to intervene, and provide the materials needed for intervention. If possible, office staff should assess and document smoking status for every patient at each clinical visit to ensure that all smokers are identified before they see a physician. Smoking status (current, former, never) can be added to the list of other vital signs (blood pressure, pulse, temperature) routinely documented in a patient's chart during an office visit. This alone has been found to increase cessation rates among patients seen by a physician [33].

Summary

Brief advice/counseling delivered by a physician is effective for helping patients to stop smoking. For the physician who wishes to go further, effective strategies are available. More complicated smokers can be referred to other providers.

References

1.   U.S. Department of Health and Human Services. The health consequences of smoking: Cardiovascular disease: A report of the Surgeon General. Rockville, MD: Office on Smoking and Health, 1983. (vol Publication PHS 84-50204).

2.   U.S. Department of Health and Human Services. The health benefits of smoking cessation: A report of the Surgeon General. Washington, DC: U.S. Govt Printing Office, (CDC)90-8416, 1990.

3.   Doll R, Peto R. Mortality in relation to smoking: Twenty years' observations on male British doctors. Br Med J 1976;2:1525-36.

4.   Friedman G, Petitti D, Bawal R, et al. Mortality in cigarette smokers and quitters: Effect of baseline differences. N Engl J Med 1981;304:1407-10.

5.   Ockene J, Kuller L, Svendsen K, Meilahn E. The relationship of smoking cessation to coronary heart disease and lung cancer in the Multiple Risk Factor Intervention Trial (MRFIT). Am J Public Health 1990;80:954-58.

6.   Centers for Disease Control and Prevention. Smoking-attributable mortality and years of potential life lost -- United States, 1990. MMWR 1993;42(33):645-48.

7.   Fiore M, Novotny T, Pierce J, et al. Methods used to quit smoking in the United States: Do cessation programs help? JAMA 1990;263(20):2760-65.

8.   U.S. Department of Health and Human Services. Current estimates from the National Health Interview Survey, 1993 (Series 10: Data from the National Health Survey No. 190). Hyattsville, MD: Public Health Service, Centers for Disease Control, National Center for Health Statistics, 1994.

9.   Ockene J. Physician-delivered interventions for smoking cessation: Strategies for increasing effectiveness. Prev Med 1987;16:723-37.

10.   Ockene I, Ockene J, editors. Prevention of Coronary Heart Disease. Boston: Little, Brown and Company, 1992.

11.   Fiore M, Bailey W, Cohen S, et al. Smoking cessation: Clinical practice guideline No. 18. Rockville, MD: U.S. Department of Public Health and Human Services, Public Health Service, Agency for Health Care Policy and Research, 1996.

12.   Ockene J, McBride P, Sallis J, Bonollo D, Ockene I. Synthesis of lessons learned from cardiopulmonary preventive interventions in healthcare practice settings. Ann Epidemiol In press.

13.   Ockene J, Kristeller J, Goldberg R, et al. Smoking cessation and severity of disease: The Coronary Artery Smoking Intervention Study. Hlth Psychol 1992;11(2):119-26.

14.   DeBusk R, Houston Miller N, Superko H, et al. A case-management system for coronary risk factor modification after acute myocardial infarction. Annals of Intern Med 1994;120:721-29.

15.   Frid D, Ockene I, Ockene J, et al. Severity of angiographically proven coronary artery disease predicts smoking cessation. Am J Prev Med 1991;7(3):131-35.

16.   Rose G, Hamilton P. A randomized controlled trial of the effect of middle-aged men of advice to stop smoking. J Epidemiol Community Health 1982;36:102-8.

17.   Rosenstock I. The Health Belief Model: Explaining health behavior through expectancies. In: Glanz K, Lewis F, Rimer R, editors. Health behavior and health education: Theory, research,

and practice. San Francisco: Jossey Bass, 1990.

18. Bandura A. Self-Efficacy: The exercise of control. New York: WH Freeman and Company, 1997: 604.

19. Marlatt A, Gordon J, McClellan W. Current perspectives: Patient education in medical practice. Patient Ed Couns 1986;8:151-63.

20. Prochaska J, DiClemente C. Stages and processes of self-change of smoking: Toward an integrative model of change. J Consulting and Clinical Psychology 1983;51:390-95.

21. Ockene J. Smoking intervention: A behavioral, educational, and pharmacologic perspective. In: Ockene I, Ockene J, editors. Prevention of coronary heart disease. Boston: Little, Brown and Company, 1992:201-30.

22. Ockene J, Quirk M, Goldberg R, et al. A residents training program for the development of smoking intervention skills. Arch Int Med 1988;148:1039-45.

23. Ockene J, Bonollo D, Adams A. Smoking and coronary artery disease in women: Diagnosis and management in the context of women's lives. In press.

24. Division of Preventive and Behavioral Medicine. Healthcare provider smoking intervention training: Workshop participant manual. In: Massachusetts Tobacco Control Program, Dept. of Public Health. Worcester, MA: University of Massachusetts Medical School, 1994.

25. Glynn T, Manley M. How to help your patients stop smoking. Bethesda: National Institutes of Health, National Cancer Institute, 1993.

26. Ockene J, Kristeller J, Goldberg R, et al. Increasing the efficacy of physician-delivered smoking intervention: A randomized clinical trial. J Gen Intern Med 1991;6:1-8.

27. Fagerstrom K. Measuring degree of physical dependency to tobacco smoking with reference to individualization of treatment. Addict Behav 1978;3:235-41.

28. Heatherton T, Kozlowski L, Frecker R, Fagerstrom K. The Fagerstrom Test for Nicotine Dependence: A revision of the Fagerstrom Tolerance Questionnaire. Brit J Addiction 1991; 86(9):1119-27.

29. Foxx R, Brown R. Nicotine fading and self-monitoring for cigarette abstinence or controlled smoking. J Appl Behav Anal 1979;12:111-25.

30. Lam W, Sze P, Sacks H, Chalmers T. Meta-analysis of randomized controlled trials of nicotine chewing gum. Lancet 1987;2:27-29.

31. Schneider N, Olmstead R, Mody F, et al. Efficacy of a nicotine nasal spray in smoking cessation: A placebo-controlled, double-blind trial. Addiction 1995;90:1671-82.

32. Perry L, Robbins A, Scariati P, et al. Enhancement of smoking cessation using the anti-depressant bupropion hydrochloride. Abstract. Circulation 1992;86:671.

33. Robinson M, Laurent S, Little J. Including smoking status as a new vital sign: It works! J Fam Pract 1995;40(6):556-63.

RISK FACTORS FOR CARDIOVASCULAR DISEASE AND THE ENDOTHELIUM

Hermann Haller

Introduction

Studies on the pathogenesis and the development of hypertension and chronic vascular disease have for a long time concentrated on the disturbed contractility or an increased proliferation propensity of smooth muscle cells [1,2]. More recent work has extended the pathophysiological considerations to other cell systems of the vessel wall which have been recognized to be involved in the pathogenesis of chronic vascular diseases [3,4]. It has become more and more apparent that the endothelium plays a crucial role in the regulation of the vessel wall under physiological and pathological conditions [5]. Endothelial cell functions regulate the homeostasis of the vascular wall. Healthy endothelium is anti-adhesive, regulates the permeability of the endothelial cell layer, and secretes vasorelaxant substances such as NO. Risk factors such a hypertension, hyperglycemia, and hyperlipidemia damage the endothelial cells and increase cell permeability and adhesiveness. They also decrease NO production and may lead to the expression of vasoconstrictive and proliferative substances such as endothelin. In the following text the effects of the risk factors hypertension, hypercholesterolemia, and hyperglycemia on certain aspects of endothelial cell function will be discussed.

Hypertension and Endothelial Cell Function

Hypertension contributes to the enhanced endothelial cell adhesiveness in chronic cardiovascular disease. McCarron et al. have demonstrated that monocyte adhesion to cerebromicrovascular endothelial cells from hypertensive rats is increased and also found that adhesion molecule expression on normotensive and hypertensive rat brain endothelial cells is altered [6,7]. Increased leukocyte binding in hypertension has also been described by others [8,9]. Recently Blann et al. have described increased levels of the soluble adhesion molecule E-selectin in essential hypertension [10]. This finding could indicate that selectins are expressed on the endothelial cells of hypertensive patients and then increasingly sheared off into the blood stream. However, this report has yet to be confirmed. While there is evidence that the adhesive properties of the endothelium can be affected in hypertension, the underlying mechanisms are still unclear. It is obvious that increased shear stress could be an enhancing factor for the stimulation of endothelial cells [11]. However, it is also conceivable

A. M. Gotto, Jr. et al. (eds.), Multiple Risk Factors in Cardiovascular Disease, 313–323.

that circulating factors, such as angiotensin II directly contribute to the enhanced expression of adhesion molecules in hypertension. We have recently investigated the hypothesis that ICAM-1 expression can be induced in two kidney 1 clip hypertension in the rat and that its expression is associated with leukocyte infiltration in the kidney [12]. We could demonstrate that the cell surface adhesion molecule ICAM-1 is expressed along the endothelial surface of small blood vessels in both the clipped and the unclipped kidney. We must speculate on the mechanisms leading to ICAM-1 expression on the walls of blood vessels in the unclipped kidneys. Endothelial cells lining the vessel wall are the first cells exposed to the increase in blood pressure. They respond with functional and structural alterations to the altered conditions. Mechanical factors such as shear stress and the activation of shear sensitive channels on endothelial cells may play a role [13]. Vasoactive substances released from endothelial cells, such as endothelin may contribute to the vasoconstriction observed in these vessels. In addition, endothelin may play a role in the activation of infiltrating macrophages [14].

In hypertension, several authors have found that the permeability of the endothelium is pathologically altered [15]. Nag has demonstrated increased permeability in chronic hypertension in the rat [16]. That albumin transport is increased in rat aorta already in the early phase of hypertension has been shown by Tedgui et al. [17]. It seems that the endothelial cytoskeleton in blood-brain-barrier permeability to protein is altered in hypertension [18]. There is indirect evidence that in patients with essential hypertension the endothelial function is impaired and endothelial permeability increased. Pedrinelli et al. reported a close association between microalbuminuria and endothelial dysfunction in essential hypertension [19]. However, whether endothelial cell dysfunction contributes significantly to the microalbuminuria in hypertension is unlikely, because the glomerular loss of albumin is mostly due to changes in the matrix expression of the basal lamina. However, it is conceivable that the endothelial cell dysfunction in essential hypertension contributes indirectly to the microalbuminuria via altered matrix expression in the damaged endothelium.

Endothelial Permeability

Besides active expression and secretion of growth factors and involvement in the augmented migration of macrophages into the vessel wall, there is a third mechanism by which abnormal endothelial cell function contributes to the increase in smooth muscle cell proliferation and matrix formation. It has already been mentioned that the disturbed permeability of the endothelial layer in patients with diabetes mellitus leads to an increased influx of substances from the circulation into the vessel wall [2,20,21]. These substances also include growth factors, among them insulin, which is a growth factor for smooth muscle cells [22-24]. The majority of studies investigating the effect of insulin on the growth of smooth muscle cells have been performed in cell cultures. But insulin has also been shown to stimulate DNA synthesis in the rat aorta *in vivo*. Although insulin alone has only a weak mitogenic activity and no effect at all on migration, it markedly enhances the mitogenic and migratory action of other factors such as PDGF [25]. The greater endothelial permeability of the vessels in patients with hyperinsulinemia can further increase the influx of insulin into the vessel wall.

It is therefore conceivable that the epidemiological relationship between hyperinsulinemia and the development of atherosclerosis is mediated by the action of insulin as a growth factor [26].

Endothelial cells also have pronounced antithrombotic properties *in vivo*. They can actively contribute to local enhancement of coagulation. The above-described factors such as EDRF and prostacyclin act as inhibitors of thrombocyte activation. Endothelial damage can also affect the role of endothelial cells in fibrinolysis [27]. The expression of plasminogen-activating factors by damaged endothelial cells is markedly reduced [28]. Thus, intact endothelial cells are important not only for the integrity of the vessel wall but also for the interaction with cells in the bloodstream. Endothelial cell dysfunction can lead to accelerated intravasal blood coagulation [29].

Finally, endothelial cells are also able to express and secrete matrix proteins and thus contribute to the sclerotic changes of the vessel wall during the development of atherosclerosis [30]. It has been shown that under conditions of high glucose concentrations the expression of collagen IV and fibronectin in endothelial cells is increased and the activity of enzymes involved in collagen synthesis enhanced. It is interesting to note that the hyperglycemia-induced increase in the gene expression of matrix molecules persists for several weeks after restoration of normoglycemia. The persistence of hyperglycemia-induced changes in cell function has also been observed *in vitro*. Thus, there appears to be not only a brief stimulation of endothelial cells in hyperglycemia but also the occurrence of persistent cell function disturbances due to high glucose concentrations.

From the above-mentioned mechanisms it is evident that the endothelium plays a central role in many of the pathophysiological processes which are involved in the early steps of atherosclerosis. It is therefore of importance to investigate the effects of antiatherosclerotic therapy on endothelial cell function and cell-cell interactions.

Glucose and Endothelial Cell Permeability

The leading cause of morbidity and mortality in patients with diabetes mellitus is accelerated small and large vessel disease [31]. Recent trials have underscored the importance of elevated glucose levels as an independent risk factor [32]. Leakage of serum proteins, particularly albumin, through the endothelium is observed in retinal vessels early in diabetes mellitus [33,34]. Similarly, an increase in endothelial permeability has been implicated in the early diabetic nephropathy [35,36]. Increased endothelial cell permeability in larger vessels leads to interstitial edema and may enhance cell proliferation and matrix production [35]. The mechanisms of increased endothelial permeability in diabetes mellitus are unclear; however, high glucose concentrations have been implicated [37]. The mechanisms by which high glucose concentrations may induce vascular changes in diabetic patients are not well understood; however, several hypothesis have been suggested including direct effects on cellular signaling pathways and diminished Na^+-K^+-ATPase activity [3]. One specific mechanism may involve the activation of protein kinase C (PKC) in vascular cells. PKC is associated with many vascular cell functions that are abnormal in diabetes, including cell contraction, basement membrane production, signal transduction for hormones and growth factors, and cell proliferation [38-41]. PKC activation in endothelial cells leads to an increase in endothelial cell permeability [42,43]. We tested the hypothesis that high glucose increases endothelial cell permeability for albumin via activation of PKC. We investigated the isoforms α, δ, ϵ, ς, and θ, which are all expressed in endothelial cells [44].

High glucose concentration led to a rapid dose-dependent increase in endothelial cell permeability. Further investigations of the glucose effect on endothelial cells showed that repetitive exposure had an additive effect. Different PKC inhibitors reduced the effects of high glucose on endothelial cell permeability. These findings indicate that the effects of glucose are mediated by PKC. High glucose induced changes in intracellular distribution of PKC isoforms α and ϵ. For the specific inhibition of PKC isoforms, we applied an antisense oligodesoxynucleotide (ODN) to specifically suppress expression of PKC α and ϵ. Antisense ODN led to a down regulation of PKC α and ϵ. Endothelial cells were then incubated with lipofectin and antisense ODN, sense ODN, scrambled ODN against PKC isoforms 24 hours before exposure to high glucose concentration (20 mM). Antisense ODN for PKC α almost completely inhibited the increase in glucose-induced endothelial cell permeability. In contrast, antisense ODN for PKC ϵ had only a small effect on glucose-induced endothelial cell permeability.

These experiments demonstrate that PKC α is responsible for the glucose-induced increase in endothelial cell permeability. PKC activation plays a role in the increased endothelial cell permeability induced by hydrogen peroxides [45], lectins [46], thrombin, and endothelins [47]. Thus, in addition to an increase in cytosolic calcium, the activation of PKC appears to be a major determinant of an increase in endothelial cell permeability. However, the exact mechanism of PKC action within endothelial cells is not clear. Exposure to phorbol ester leads to phosphorylation and redistribution of the cytoskeletal proteins caldesmon and vimentin, in concert with agonist-mediated endothelial cell contraction and resultant barrier dysfunction [42]. This observation indicates that PKC activation increases endothelial permeability by an interaction with cytoskeletal proteins. This hypothesis is supported by recent observations in epithelial cells where PKC-dependent actin reorganization leads to modulation of intercellular permeability [48]. Whether activation of PKC α plays a role in glucose-induced endothelial permeability *in vivo* is presently under investigation. A variety of other endothelial functions which are regulated by PKC, are disturbed by hyperglycemia. Endothelium dependent relaxation is impaired by high glucose via the PKC-induced production of vasoconstrictor prostanoids [49]. High glucose impairs the production of prostaglandins in endothelial cells. Several groups have demonstrated that high glucose leads to an increased expression of matrix proteins, such as type IV collagen and fibronectin [50,51]. Cell adhesion, endothelial permeability, endothelium-dependent relaxation, and matrix expression all play a role in the development of diabetic macro- and microvascular changes. Our findings support the hypothesis that PKC activation by high glucose concentration is responsible for the early pathological changes in diabetic vascular disease.

Role of Endothelium in Interaction with Cells in the Flowing Blood

Endothelin and other factors produced by endothelial cells are released not only into the vessel wall but also into the flowing blood, where their chemotactic action can induce white blood cells to migrate to the endothelial wall [52,53]. Near the wall, they slow down and adhere to endothelial cells. This process of cell adhesion to endothelial cells has been known for a long time and its underlying molecular mechanisms have been identified in recent years. Endothelial cells induce adhesion by expressing specific surface adhesion molecules that can interact with ligands on white blood cells and thrombocytes [54]. Many new adhesion molecules have been discovered in recent years and they are subdivided into three groups: the family of selectins (including adhesion molecules such as ELAM and LECCAM), the group of integrins (among them, LFA-1), and a supergene family of immunoglobulins (ICAM-1 and VCAM). These adhesion molecules are expressed upon stimulation of endothelial cells by specific factors such as tumor necrosis factor (TNF-α). Their expression is increased on endothelial cells chronically damaged by risk factors of atherosclerosis such as cigarette smoking and hypercholesterolemia [55,56]. VCAM is expressed on the surface of endothelial cells overlying early "fatty streak" lesions [57]. In rabbits fed cholesterol, the expression of VCAM precedes the subendothelial accumulation of monocytes [58], which suggests a role for VCAM in the early stages of vascular damage [59]. The effect of a high cholesterol diet on VCAM expression *in vivo* suggests that low density lipoproteins (LDL) or LDL modified by oxidation (oLDL), may be responsible for the induction of VCAM [59]. Cultured endothelial cells incubated with LDL [60] or oLDL [61] showed an increased stickiness of monocytes; however, specific adhesion molecules were not studied in these experiments. Kume et al. [62] showed that VCAM expression is enhanced by lysophosphatidylcholine, a component of LDL and we could recently demonstrate a direct effect of LDL on VCAM expression [63].

It has been shown that under pathophysiological conditions, i.e. high glucose concentration and hyperlipidemia, not only the endothelium contributes to the enhanced binding of blood cells but that leukocytes and platelets show increased surface expression of proteins, such as integrins (CD 11/18 etc.), which serve as binding proteins for the adhesion molecules [64]. Binding of blood cells to the endothelium affects the pathogenesis of atherosclerosis in several ways [3,65]. Enhanced binding of leukocytes and platelets leads to changes in the laminar blood flow and to the generation of turbulences. These changes enhance platelet aggregability and thrombosis. The binding of leukocytes to the endothelium affects also production and release of reactive oxygen species from these cells [66]. The adhesion to endothelial cells may possibly affect the release of other substances as well. This has been demonstrated for the binding of monocytes to glycosylated proteins under hyperglycemic conditions. Monocytes have surface receptors for advanced glycosylation end products (AGE) and are activated by binding to glycosylated proteins in the vessel wall [67]. Activation leads to an increased release of cytokines and growth factors including the already mentioned PDGF, interleukins, TNF-α, and transforming growth factor β [68]. The stimulating effects of AGE proteins on macrophages have been demonstrated by several *in vitro* studies (for review see [68]).

Low Density Lipoproteins and Endothelial Cell Adhesion Molecules

Hypercholesterolemia, particularly the low density lipoprotein fraction termed LDL, is an important risk factor for the development of atherosclerosis, a disease process which intimately involves endothelial cells [69]. LDL not only activates endothelial cell signals but also results in endothelial cell responses that eventually lead to vascular injury. For instance, LDL fosters monocyte recruitment within the vascular wall and promotes adhesion to intimal surfaces [56,70]. Monocyte adhesion may involve interaction with adhesion molecules on endothelial cells [71]. The vascular cell adhesion molecule-1 (VCAM) is an inducible receptor that mediates endothelial adhesion of monocytes and lymphocytes [72-74]. VCAM is expressed on the surface of endothelial cells overlying early "fatty streak" lesions [72]. In rabbits fed cholesterol, the expression of VCAM precedes the subendothelial accumulation of monocytes [73], which suggests a role for VCAM in the early stages of vascular damage [74]. The effect of a high cholesterol diet on VCAM expression *in vivo* suggests that low density lipoproteins (LDL) or LDL modified by oxidation (oLDL), may be responsible for the induction of VCAM [15]. Cultured endothelial cells incubated with LDL [75] or oLDL [76,77] showed an increased stickiness of monocytes; however, specific adhesion molecules were not studied in these experiments. Kume et al. [78] showed that VCAM expression is enhanced by lysophosphatidylcholine, a component of LDL. They observed no effect of native LDL or oLDL on VCAM expression in cultured endothelial cells, but suggested instead that the biological properties of modified LDL may be different in living organisms than in *in vitro* studies.

We have investigated the effects of LDL on the expression of VCAM on cultured endothelial cells [79,80]. Incubation of cultured human umbilical vein endothelial cells with LDL resulted in a dose-dependent increase in VCAM expression. We next investigated possible mechanisms of LDL-induced VCAM expression. When endothelial cells were incubated with LDL (100 mg/ml) and the protein kinase C inhibitor staurosporine (10^{-8} M) together for 5 hours, the stimulatory effect of LDL on VCAM expression was abolished completely. While staurosporine completely blocked the LDL effect on VCAM expression, the effect of TNF-α on VCAM surface expression was only partially inhibited. Incubation of the cells with LDL and the calcium antagonist nitrendipine (10^{-7} M) also reduced the VCAM surface expression significantly, but only after 24 hours. To determine whether or not the effect of LDL on VCAM expression was specific for this surface adhesion molecule, we also measured the effect of LDL on the intercellular adhesion molecule-1 (ICAM-1) and on the endothelial leucocyte adhesion molecule (ELAM). LDL (100 mg/ml) induced a slight, but significant increase in endothelial surface expression of ICAM after 2 and 6 hours, while the surface expression of ELAM was not affected by exposure of endothelial cells to LDL. LDL also induced a significant increase in monocyte adhesion to endothelial cells. We demonstrated that LDL leads to a significant increase in VCAM surface expression on human endothelial cells by means of two separate and different techniques [80]. The effect of LDL was small compared to the TNF-α-mediated response. A similar response of ICAM to stimulation with LDL was also observed; however, no effect on ELAM could be demonstrated. This observation suggests that LDL exerts a specific, stimulatory effect on adhesion molecules of the superimmunglobulin family , but not on the selectins. Although the effect is small compared to agonists such as TNF-α, atherogenesis is an interactive process which takes years to develop. We believe that under *in vivo* circumstances, which may include the influence of hypertension [81], cigarette smoking [67], and other concomitant noxious influences, small effects may be clinically significant.

References

1.   Folkow B. Physiological aspects of primary hypertension. Physiol Rev 1982;62:347-504.
2.   Gordon D, Reidy MA, Benditt EP, Schwartz SM. Cell proliferation in human coronary arteries. Proc Natl Acad Sci USA 1990;87:4600-4604.
3.   Schwartz CJ, Valente AJ, Sprague EA. A modern view of atherogenesis. Am J Cardiol 1993; 71(6):21-29.
4.   Ross R. The pathogenesis of atherosclerosis: A perspective for the 1990. Nature 1993;362: 801-9.
5.   Lüscher TF, Vanhoutte PM. The endothelium: Modulator of cardiovascular function. Boca Raton, Florida: CRC Press; 1990.
6.   McCarron RM, Wang L, Siren AL, Spatz M, Hallenbeck JM. Monocyte adhesion to cerebromicrovascular endothelial cells derived from hypertensive and normotensive rats. Am J Physiol 1994;267(6Pt2):H2491-97.
7.   McCarron RM, Wang L, Siren AL, Spatz M, Hallenbeck JM. Adhesion molecules on normotensive and hypertensive rat brain endothelial cells. Proc Soc Exp Biol Med 1994; 205(3):257-62.
8.   Suzuki H, Schmid Schonbein GW, Suematsu M, et al. Impaired leukocyte-endothelial cell interaction in spontaneously hypertensive rats. Hypertension 1994;24(6):719-27.
9.   Kerenyi T, Lehmann R, Voss B, Jellinek H. Changes of DNA-acridine orange binding in monocytes and endothelial cells of hypertensive arteries. Exp Mol Pathol 1991;54(3):230-41.
10. Blann AD, Tse W, Maxwell SJ, Waite MA. Increased levels of the soluble adhesion molecule E-selectin in essential hypertension. J Hypertens 1994;12(8):925-28.
11. Alexander RW. Theodore Cooper Memorial Lecture. Hypertension and the pathogenesis of atherosclerosis. Oxidative stress and the mediation of arterial inflammatory response: A new perspective. Hypertension 1995;25(2):155-61.
12. Haller H, Park JK, Dragun D, Lippoldt A, Luft FC. Leukocyte infiltration and ICAM-1 expression in two-kidney one-clip hypertension. Nephrol Dial Transpl 1997;12:899-903.
13. Haller H, Park JK, Distler A, Luft FC. Increased phorbolester-induced vasoconstriction in SHR is due to endothelial dysfunction. Hypertens Res 1994;17:193-97.
14. Haller H, Schaberg T, Lindschau C, Quass P, Lode H, Distler A. Endothelin increases intracellular free calcium, protein phosphorylation and O_2-production in human alveolar macrophages. Am J Physiol 1991;261:L723-13.
15. Tagami M, Kubota A, Nara Y, Yamori Y. Detailed disease processes of cerebral pericytes and astrocytes in stroke-prone SHR. Clin Exp Hypertens A 1991;13(5):1069-75.
16. Nag S. Cerebral endothelial mechanisms in increased permeability in chronic hypertension. Adv Exp Med Biol 1993;331:263-66.
17. Tedgui A, Merval R, Esposito B. Albumin transport characteristics of rat aorta in early phase of hypertension. Circ Res 1992;71(4):932-42.
18. Nag S. Role of the endothelial cytoskeleton in blood-brain-barrier permeability to protein.

Acta Neuropathol Berl 1995;90(5):454-60.

19. Pedrinelli R, Giampietro O, Carmassi F, et al. Microalbuminuria and endothelial dysfunction in essential hypertension [see comments]. Lancet 1994;344(8914):14-18.

20. Schwartz CJ, Valente AJ, Sprague EA. A modern view of atherogenesis. Am J Cardiol 1993; 71(6):21-29.

21. Esposito C, Gerlach H, Brett J, Stern D, Vlassara H. Endothelial receptor-mediated binding of glucose-modified albumin is associated with increased monolayer permeability and modulation of cell surface coagulant properties. J Exp Med 1989;170:1387-1407.

22. Stout RW, Bierman EL, Ross R. Effect of insulin on the proliferation of cultured primate arterial smooth muscle cells. Circ Res 1975; 36:319-27.

23. King GL, Goodman AD, Buzney S, Moses A, Kahn CR. Receptors and growth-promoting effects of insulin and insulin-like growth factors on cells from bovine retinal capillaries and aorta. J Clin Invest 1985;75:1028-36.

24. Weinstein R, Stemerman MB, Maciag T. Hormonal requirements for growth of arterial smooth muscle cells in vitro: An endocrine approach to atherosclerosis. Science 1981;212: 818-20.

25. Capron L, Jarnet J, Kazandjian S, Housset E. Growth-promoting effects of diabetes and insulin on arteries: An in vivo study of rat aorta. Diabetes 1986;35:973-78.

26. Stout RW. Insulin and atheroma. 20-yr perspective. Diabetes Care 1990;13:631-54.

27. Shultz PJ, Raij L. Endogenously synthesized nitric oxide prevents endotoxin-induced glomerular thrombosis. J Clin Invest 1990;90:1718-25.

28. Lorenzi M, Cagliero E. Pathobiology of endothelial and other vascular cells in diabetes mellitus; Call for data. Diabetes 1991;40:653-59.

29. Steiner G. Diabetes and atherosclerosis: An overview. Diabetes 1981;30(Suppl.2):1-7.

30. Cagliero E, Maiello M, Boeri D, Roy S, Lorenzi M. Increased expression of basement membrane components in human endothelial cells cultured in high glucose. J Clin Invest 1988; 82:735-38.

31. Kannel WB, McGee DL. Diabetes and glucose tolerance as risk factors for cardiovascular disease: The Framingham study. Diabetes Care 1979;241:2035-38.

32. Group, T. D. C. a. C. T. R. The effect of intensive treatment of diabetes on the development and progression of long-term complications in insulin-dependent diabetes mellitus. N Engl J Med 1993;329:599-606.

33. Tooke JE. Microvascular function in human diabetes. A physiological perspective. Diabetes 1995;44:721-26.

34. Wardle EN. Vascular permeability in diabetics and implications for therapy. Diabetes Res Clin Pract 1994;23:135-39.

35. Nannipieri M, Rizzo L, Rapuano A, Pilo A, Penno G, Navalesi R. Increased transcapillary escape rate of albumin in microalbuminuric type II diabetic patients. Diabetes Care 1995; 18(1):1-9.

36. Sander B, Larsen M, Engler C, Lund Andersen H, Parving HH. Early changes in diabetic retinopathy: Capillary loss and blood-retina barrier permeability in relation to metabolic control. Acta Ophthalmol Copenh. 1994;72(5):553-59.

37. Yamashita T, Mimura K, Umeda F, Kobayashi K, Hashimoto T, Nawata H. Increased transendothelial permeation of albumin by high glucose concentration. Metabolism 1995; 44(6):739-44.

38. Williams B. Glucose-induced vascular smooth muscle dysfunction: The role of protein kinase C. J Hypertens 1995;13:477-86.

39. Derubertis FR, Craven PA. Activation of protein kinase C in glomerular cells in diabetes. Mechanisms and potential links to the pathogenesis of diabetic glomerulopathy. Diabetes 1994;43:1-8.

40. Williams B, Tsai P, Schrier RW. Glucose-induced downregulation of angiotensin II and arginine vasopressin receptors in cultured rat aortic vascular smooth muscle cells. Role of protein kinase C. J Clin Invest 1992;90:1992-99.

41. Haller H, Baur E, Quass P. High glucose concentrations and protein kinase C isoforms in vascular smooth muscle cells. Kidney Int 1995;47:1057-67.

42. Lum H, Malik AB. Regulation of vascular endothelial barrier function. Am J Physiol 1994; 267:L223-L241.

43. Lynch JJ, Ferro TJ, Blumenstock FA, Brockenauer AM, Malik AB. Increased endothelial albumin permeability mediated by protein kinase C activation. J Clin Invest 1990;85:1991-98.

44. Haller H, Ziegler W, Lindschau C, Luft FC. Endothelial cell tyrosine kinase receptor and G-protein coupled receptor activation involves distinct protein kinase C isoforms. Arterioscl Thromb Vasc Biol 1996;16:678-86.

45. Johnson A, Phillips P, Hocking D, Tsan MF, Ferro T. Protein kinase inhibitor prevents pulmonary edema in response to H2O2. Am J Physiol 1989;256:H1012-H1022.

46. Siflinger-Birnboim A, Goligorsky MS, del Vecchio PJ, Malik AB. Activation of protein kinase C pathway contributes to hydrogen peroxide induced increase in endothelial cell permeability. Lab Invest 1992;67:24-30.

47. Northover AM, Northover BJ. 1994. Lectin-induced increase in microvascular permeability to colloidal carbon in vitro may involve protein kinase C activation. Agents Actions 1994;41: 136-39.

48. Fassano A, Fiorentini C, Donelli G, et al. Zonula occludens toxin modulates tight junctions through protein kinase C-dependent actin reorganization, in vitro. J. Clin. Invest 195;96:710-20.

49. Tesmafariam B, Brown ML, Cohen RA. Elevated glucose impairs endothelium-dependent relaxation by activating protein kinase C. J Clin Invest 1991;87:1643-48.

50. Studer RK, Craven PA, DeRubertis FR. Role for protein kinase C in the mediation of increased fibronectin accumulation by mesangial cells grown in high-glucose medium. Diabetes 1993;42:118-26.

51. Fumo P, Kuncio GS, Ziyadeh FN. PKC and high glucose stimulate collagen alpha 1(IV) transcriptional activity in a reporter mesangial cell line. Am J Physiol 1994;267:F632-F638.

52. Simionescu M, Simionescu N. Functions of the endothelial cell surface. Annu Rev Physiol 1986; 48:279-304.

53. Schar, RE, Harker LA. Thrombosis and atherosclerosis: Regulatory role of interactions among blood components and endothelium. Blut 1987;55:131.

54. Springer TA. The sensation and regulation of interactions with the extracellular environment: The cell biology of lymphocyte adhesion receptors. Annu Rev Cell Biol 1990;6:359-402.

55. DiCorleto PE, Chisolm GM. Participation of the endothelium in the development of the atherosclerotic plaque. Prog Lipid Res 1986;25:365-374.

56. Gerrity RG. The role of monocyte in atherogenesis. 1. Transition of blood-borne monocytes into foam cells in fatty lesions. Am J Pathol 1981;103:181-90.

57. Cybulsky MI, Gimbrone MJ. Endothelial expression of a mononuclear leukocyte adhesion molecule during atherogenesis. Science 1991;251(4995):788-91.

58. Li H, Cybulsky MI, Gimbrone MJ, Libby P. An atherogenic diet rapidly induces VCAM-1, a cytokine-regulatable mononuclear leukocyte adhesion molecule, in rabbit aortic endothelium.

Arterioscler Thromb 1993;13(2):197-204.

59.   Libby P, Hansson GK. Involvement of the immune system in human atherogenesis: Current
       knowledge and unanswered questions. Lab Invest 1991;64:5-15.
60.   Alderson LM, Endemann G, Lindsey S, Pronczuk A, Hoover RI, Hayes KC. LDL enhances
       monocyte adhesion to endothelial cells in vitro. Am J Pathol 1986;123:334-41.
61.   Frostegard J, Haegerstrand A, Gidlund M, Nilsson J. Biologically modified LDL increases the
       adhesive properties of endothelial cells. Atherosclerosis 1991;90:119-26.
62.   Kume N, Cybulsky MI, Gimbrone MJ. Lysophosphatidylcholine, a component of atherogenic
       lipoproteins, induces mononuclear leukocyte adhesion molecules in cultured human and rabbit
       arterial endothelial cells. J Clin Invest 1992;90(3):1138-44.
63.   Haller H, Schaper D, Philipp S, Distler A. LDL induces surface expression of adhesion
       molecules ICAM-1 and VCAM on endothelial cells via the activation of protein kinase C. J
       Am Soc Nephrol 1992;3:456.
64.   Gilcrease MZ, Hoover RL. Examination of monocyte adherence to endothelium under
       hyperglycemic conditions. Am J Pathol 1991;139:1089-97.
65.   DiCorleto PE. Cellular mechanisms of atherogenesis. Am J Hypertens 1993;6:314S-318S.
66.   Schaberg T, Rau M, Kaiser D, Fassbender M, Lode H, Haller H. Increased number of alveolar
       macrophages expressing adhesion molecules of the leukocyte adhesion molecule family in
       smoking subjects: Association with cell-binding ability and superoxide anion production. Am
       Rev Respir Dis 1992;146:1287-93.
67.   Vlassara H, Brownlee M, Monogue K, Dinarello CA, Pasagian A. Cachectin/TNF and IL-1
       induced by glucose-modified proteins: Role in normal tissue remodeling. Science 1988;240:
       1546-48.
68.   Brownlee M, Cerami A, Vlassara H. Advanced glycosylation end products in tissue and the
       biochemical basis of diabetic complications. N Engl J Med 1988;318:1315-21.
69.   Steinberg D, Parthasarathy S, Carew TE, Khoo JC, Witztum JL. Beyond cholesterol:
       Modifications of low-density lipoprotein that increase its atherogenicity. N Engl J Med 1989;
       320:915-24.
70.   Gerrity RG. The role of monocyte in atherogenesis. 1. Transition of blood-borne monocytes
       into foam cells in fatty lesions. Am J Pathol 1981;103:181-90.
71.   Schwartz CJ, Valente AJ, Sprague EA. A modern view of atherogenesis. Am J Cardiol 1993;
       71(6):21-29.
72.   Cybulsky MI, Gimbrone MJ. Endothelial expression of a mononuclear leukocyte adhesion
       molecule during atherogenesis. Science 1991;251(4995):788-91.
73.   Li H, Cybulsky MI, Gimbrone MJ, Libby P. An atherogenic diet rapidly induces VCAM-1,
       a cytokine-regulatable mononuclear leukocyte adhesion molecule, in rabbit aortic endothelium.
       Arterioscler Thromb 1993;13(2):197-204.
74.   Libby P, Hansson GK. Involvement of the immune system in human atherogenesis: current
       knowledge and unanswered questions. Lab Invest 1991;64:5-15.
75.   Alderson LM, Endemann G, Lindsey S, Pronczuk A, Hoover RI, Hayes KC. LDL enhances
       monocyte adhesion to endothelial cells in vitro. Am J Pathol 1986;123:334-41.
76.   Berliner JA, Territo MC, Sevanian A, et al. Minimally modified LDL stimulates monocyte
       endothelial interactions. J Clin Invest 1990;85:1260-67.
77.   Rostegard J, Haegerstrand A, Gidlund M, Nilsson J. Biologically modified LDL increases the
       adhesive properties of endothelial cells. Atherosclerosis 1991;90:119-26.
78.   Kume N, Cybulsky MI, Gimbrone MJ. Lysophosphatidylcholine, a component of atherogenic
       lipoproteins, induces mononuclear leukocyte adhesion molecules in cultured human and rabbit

arterial endothelial cells. J Clin Invest 1992;90(3):1138-44.

79.   Haller H, Rieger M, Kuhlmann M, Philipp S, Distler A, Luft FC. LDL increases $(Ca^{++})_i$ in human endothelial cells and augments thrombin-induced cell signalling. J Lab Clin Med 1994; 124:708-14.

80.   Haller H, Schaper D, Ziegler W, Kuhlmann M, Distler A, Luft FC. LDL induces surface expression of vascular adhesion molecule (VCAM) on endothelial cells via activation of protein kinase C. Hypertension 1995;25:511-16.

81.   Mai M, Geiger H, Hilgers KF, Veelken R, Mann JFE, Luft FC. Early interstitial changes in hypertension-induced renal injury. Hypertension 1993;22:754-65.

EPIDEMIOLOGY OF RISK FACTOR CLUSTERING IN ELEVATED BLOOD PRESSURE

William B. Kannel, Peter W. F. Wilson, Halit Silbershatz, and Ralph B. D'Agostino

Introduction

A tendency for hypertension to cluster with other risk factors has long been noted in the Framingham Heart Study and elsewhere [1,2]. A metabolic or physiologic basis for this clustering has been postulated [3-5]. Many of the risk factors that tend to cluster with elevated blood pressure also predict its occurrence and greatly influence its impact on the occurrence of atherosclerotic cardiovascular sequelae [1,2]. The population prevalence of risk factor clustering in the presence of hypertension has not been determined. Nor has it been estimated how often coronary events result from hypertension occurring in conjunction with such risk factor clusters.

The purpose of this report is to determine the prevalence of occurrence of clusters of one or more risk factors in persons with elevated blood pressure and to compare this with that expected by chance. We also examine the influence of weight and weight change on the tendency for risk factors to cluster in hypertensive persons. Further, the influence of the extent of risk factor clustering on the hypertensive risk of coronary heart disease and the population burden of this disease is evaluated.

Methods

The Framingham Heart Study began in 1948 with the enrollment of 5,209 men and women who were examined biennially and in 1971 another cohort of 5,124 men and women who were the children or the spouses of the offspring of the original cohort, was enrolled [6]. The population sample under consideration is the Framingham Offspring sample of 2,489 men and 2,646 women ages 18-65 years at the time of the initial examination in 1971-1974. Only subjects ages 30-65 years and free of coronary heart disease at baseline were used in the population considered at risk for initial coronary events in relation to their blood pressure status and burden of risk factors. Each examination included an extensive cardiovascular history and physical examination, blood pressure determination, and measurement of other physiological and biochemical variables. Morbidity and mortality were monitored with clinical examinations, hospital surveillance, and communication with personal physicians and relatives of study participants. All new cardiovascular events were reviewed by a panel of three experienced investigators who had to agree that the suspected

A. M. Gotto, Jr. et al. (eds.), Multiple Risk Factors in Cardiovascular Disease, 325–333.
© 1998 Kluwer Academic Publishers and Fondazione Giovanni Lorenzini. Printed in the Netherlands.

event met criteria. Detailed descriptions of the sampling methods, examination procedures, and the criteria for the various cardiovascular endpoints have been reported elsewhere [6-8].

The risk factors under consideration included total and high density lipoprotein cholesterol (HDL-C), body mass index (BMI), glucose, and systolic blood pressure. Body mass index was calculated as weight in kilogram divided by height in meters squared. Blood pressure measurements were taken from the left arm with a mercury sphygmomanometer with the subject seated. A large cuff was used when required and readings were recorded to the nearest even number. Fasting plasma was used for determination of HDL-C, which was measured after precipitation with dextran-magnesium according to established protocols [9].

Values in the upper quintiles of each variable except HDL-C, where the lowest quintile was used, were considered a "risk factor." The actual values considered as risk factors are displayed in Table 1 for men and women. The value chosen to designate "elevated" blood pressure was a systolic blood pressure ≥ 138 mm Hg in men and ≥ 130 mm Hg in women.

Table 1. Risk Factor Quintile Criteria. Framingham Offspring Exam 1, Ages 18-65 Years, 1971-1974.

Risk Factor (units)	Men (n=2,406)	Women (n=2,569)
Low HDL-C (mg/dl)	< 35	< 44
High cholesterol (mg/dl)	≥ 231	≥ 222
High body mass index (kg/m²)	≥ 29.5	≥ 26.8
High systolic blood pressure (mm Hg)	≥ 138	≥ 130
High triglycerides (mg/dl)	≥ 155	≥ 103
High glucose (mg/dl)	≥ 112	≥ 105

Expected probabilities of clusters of risk factors were calculated from the binomial equation considering the probability of 0, 1, 2, 3, 4, or 5 specified risk factors. Multivariate logistic regression analysis and Cox proportional hazards statistical methods were used to examine the impact of the various risk factors individually and in combination, adjusting for age and other relevant factors. Subjects in the cohort remained at risk as long as they were free of coronary disease at subsequent examinations.

Results

PREVALENCE

The distribution of the number of coexistent risk factors in the subgroup of 530 men and 545 women with elevated blood pressure (upper quintile of systolic pressure) and who had all five additional risk factors measured is displayed in Figure 1. The observed distribution of other risk factors in persons with elevated blood pressure is significantly shifted to the right of the expected distribution, with an excess beginning with a cluster of two additional risk factors (Table 2). The observed-to-expected ratio increases sharply with the extent of clustering. Clusters of three or more of the specified risk factors occurred at 4.5 times the expected rate in men and 5.4 times expected in women. Clusters of three or more risk factors occurred in 22% of men and 27% of women with elevated blood pressure. Only 24% of men and 19% of women had elevated blood pressure in isolation of other risk factors. Thus 75 to 80% of hypertension occurred in association with other major risk factors (Table 2).

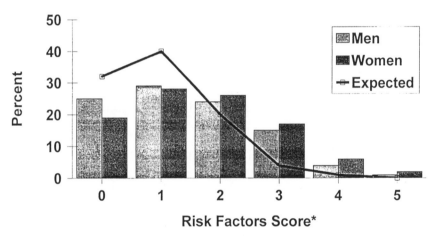

Figure 1. Distribution of risk factor scores. Framingham offspring, age 18-74 years. Persons in the top quintile--systolic blood pressure. Risk variables include bottom quintile for HDL-C and top quintile for BMI, cholesterol, triglyceride, and glucose.

DETERMINANTS

The possible determinants of risk factor clustering in hypertension include insulin resistance, abdominal obesity, and autonomic imbalance [3-5]. It was possible only to examine the influence of obesity and weight gain on the occurrence of risk factor clustering in the general population and in persons with an elevated blood pressure. Obesity and weight gain were the most important identified determinants of hypertension in the Framingham Heart Study [10]. It was also the most highly associated with a predisposition to clustering. However, each of the risk factors found to cluster with hypertension also predisposed to its subsequent appearance in normotensive persons.

Table 2. Number of Other Risk Factors, Framingham Heart Study Offspring with Elevated Blood Pressure, Ages 18-65 Years.

Number of Risk Factors	Percent with Specified Number of Risk Factors		Observed/Expected Ratio	
	Men	Women	Men	Women
0	24.4%	19.5%	0.74	0.59
1	29.1%	28.1%	0.71	0.69
≥ 2	46.5%	52.4%	1.8	2.01

Elevated blood pressure defined as systolic pressure ≥ 138 mm Hg (men) and ≥ 130 mm Hg (women). Other risk factors included the top quintiles of other factors (total cholesterol, body mass index, triglycerides, glucose) and bottom quintile for HDL-C.

The tendency for risk factors to cluster in persons with increased blood pressure varied according to baseline obesity and weight change over the 16-year follow-up interval. The extent of risk factor clustering increased stepwise with the degree of obesity (Table 3). A 5-pound weight increase imposed about a 30% increase in the extent of clustering (not shown).

Risk of coronary heart disease in persons with elevated blood pressure varied widely and increased stepwise with the extent of risk factor clustering (Table 4). Among persons with elevated blood pressure it is estimated that about 40% of coronary events in men and 68% of coronary events in women are attributable to clusters of two or more risk factors (Table 4). Of all the coronary heart disease events that occurred in men with elevated blood pressure over the 16 years of follow up, only 29% had one of these major risk factors, 49% had two or more additional risk factors. In women only 28% had only one other risk factor, whereas 54% had two or more (Table 4).

Discussion

Hypertension or elevated blood pressure is a well-established risk factor for the development of atherosclerotic cardiovascular disease [1,2]. It has become increasingly apparent that the hazard imposed is related to the level of the blood pressure, even within the range of blood pressures formerly considered nonhypertensive. It has also been established that the magnitude of the risk of cardiovascular sequelae in essential hypertension depends on the associated burden of other risk factors [1,2]. Hypertension seldom occurs in isolation; elevated blood pressure tends to cluster with other risk factors, suggesting that such pressure elevations may reflect a more fundamental metabolic or physiologic process that accelerates atherogenesis. Abdominal obesity promoting insulin resistance and abnormal sympathoadrenal activity have been implicated as possible mechanisms [11,12].

Table 3. Risk Factor Clustering in Framingham Study Offspring with Elevated Blood Pressure According to Body Mass Index, Subjects Ages 18-74 Years.

Men		Women	
Body Mass Index (kg/m^2)	Average Number of Risk Factors	Body Mass Index (kg/m^2)	Average Number of Risk Factors
< 23.7	1.68 ± 0.91	< 20.8	1.80 ± 0.87
23.7 to 25.5	1.85 ± 0.95	20.8 to 22.3	2.00 ± 1.02
25.6 to 27.2	2.06 ± 1.05	22.4 to 23.9	2.22 ± 1.06
27.3 to 29.5	2.28 ± 1.09	24.0 to 26.8	2.20 ± 0.99
≥ 29.5	2.35 ± 1.08	≥ 26.8	2.66 ± 1.09

Elevated blood pressure defined as systolic pressure ≥ 138 mm Hg (men) and ≥ 130 mm Hg (women). Other risk factors included the top quintiles of other factors (total cholesterol, body mass index, triglycerides, glucose) and bottom quintile for HDL-C.

Abnormalities of lipoprotein metabolism, insulin resistance, and glucose tolerance are common in persons with essential hypertension and their normotensive first degree relatives [4]. Such metabolic abnormalities appear to have a role in the pathogenesis of essential hypertension and do not cluster with most causes of secondary hypertension. Hyperinsulinemia and insulin resistance are found in obese and nonobese persons with hypertension, and may persist despite antihypertensive therapy [13,14]. Patients with elevated blood pressure also tend to have dyslipidemia characterized by elevated triglyceride and reduced HDL cholesterol concentrations [13,14]. It is not clear what percentage of patients have the insulin resistance syndrome as resistance to insulin-mediated uptake of glucose and compensatory hyperinsulinemia are related to hypertension in a continuous, graded fashion [16]. It has been estimated that approximately half of hypertensive persons have insulin resistance [4,17].

Multiple abnormalities are frequently associated with hypertension and help to account for an increased risk of coronary heart disease. Dyslipidemia, characterized by elevated triglycerides and reduced HDL-C appear to be an important feature of the connection between hypertension and CHD [4,18]. Such persons also tend to have atherogenic small dense LDL particles [19,20].

Insulin resistance and hyperinsulinemia are more severe and more closely associated

Table 4. 16-Year Coronary Heart Disease Incidence by Number of Other Risk Factors. Framingham Heart Study Offspring with Elevated Blood Pressure, Ages 30-65 Years at Baseline.

Number of Other Risk Factors	Relative Risk (95% C.I.)	Prevalence	CHD Events Number (%)	Population Attributable Risk (Multivariate)
Men				
0	1.0 (referent)	22%	10 (14%)	--
1	1.33 (0.57,3.06)	29%	17 (24%)	0.09
≥ 2	2.28 (1.09,4.78)	49%	45 (63%)	0.39
Total			72 (100%)	
Women				
0	1.0 (referent)	18%	2 (5%)	--
1	2.05 (0.41,10.18)	28%	7 (18%)	0.23
≥ 2	4.93 (1.14,21.27)	54%	31 (78%)	0.68
Total			40 (100%)	

High blood pressure defined as systolic pressure ≥ 138 mm Hg (men) and ≥ 130 mm Hg (women). Other risk factors included the top quintiles of other factors (total cholesterol, body mass index, triglycerides, glucose) and bottom quintile for HDL-C.

with hypertension in obese than nonobese persons [4,21,22]. Abdominal obesity appears to promote insulin resistance and hyperinsulinemia, which in turn is associated with lipoprotein lipase abnormality, leading to raised triglyceride and reduced HDL-C. Hyperinsulinemia is also associated with glucose intolerance and hypertension that also accelerate atherogenesis. Reaven and coworkers have postulated that hyperinsulinemia, resulting from insulin resistance, stimulates the sympathetic nervous system, increasing sympathetically mediated thermogenesis to reestablish energy balance. However, this increase in sympathetic activity also stimulates the heart, the vasculature, and kidneys, contributing to hypertension [4]. Thus, obesity-related hypertension may be an unwanted byproduct of mechanisms to restore energy balance and stabilize body weight. However, weight gain worsens all the elements of the insulin resistance syndrome and weight loss improves them. Increased abdominal adiposity may particularly account for insulin resistance and hyperinsulinemia among obese persons [23]. Although a predisposition to insulin resistance may be inherited, evidence also suggests that saturated fat intake may be involved in its pathogenesis [24]. Consistent with a causal role of insulin resistance and sympathetic nervous activity in the pathogenesis of hypertension, calorie restriction [25], weight loss [26], and exercise [27] all decrease insulin resistance, and along with it, reduce the activity of the sympathetic nervous system [28].

The reported prevalence of insulin resistance in the general population varies from 25% to 80% [3,4,29]. Accurate estimates are not available because of the technical difficulty in measuring insulin resistance. The prevalence of the insulin resistance syndrome in either the general population or hypertensive persons is likewise unknown because the syndrome lacks a precise definition. However, it is clear from this investigation in the Framingham Heart Study, that if three or more of the ingredients would quality for a diagnosis, the prevalence could be as high as 22% in men and 27% in women.

Whatever the cause of risk factor clustering in the segment of the population with an elevated blood pressure, it is clear that it is the rule and that when confronted with a subject with hypertension, screening for the presence of the other metabolically linked risk factors would appear mandatory. At present, it seems reasonable to suspect that the insulin resistance syndrome is present in persons with elevated blood pressure when two or more of the other markers are present. Coronary heart disease is the most prevalent and lethal hazard of elevated blood pressure. Coronary heart disease risk in persons with hypertension is concentrated among those who have a high total-cholesterol-to-HDL-cholesterol ratio, impaired glucose tolerance, and elevated triglycerides. These associated risk factors determine the need for treatment. Weight control, exercise, and fat-modified diets have great potential for control of mild-to-moderate hypertension. Obesity, glucose intolerance, dyslipidemia, and hypertension are evidently metabolically linked and jointly atherogenic. Drug therapies that improve insulin resistance along with the blood pressure should have enhanced antiatherogenic potential. Reduction of blood pressure as the sole treatment goal of antihypertensive therapy is no longer acceptable, and hypertensive persons can be more appropriately targeted for therapy after considering the extent of risk factor clustering.

Acknowledgements

From the National Heart, Lung, and Blood Institute's Framingham Study, National Institutes of Health (NIH/NHLBI Contract N01-HC-38038) and partially supported by Astra USA, Visiting Scientist Program.

References

1.   Kannel WB. Implications of Framingham Study data for treatment of hypertension: Impact of other risk factors. In: Laragh JH, Buhler FR, Seldin DW, editors. Frontiers in hypertension research. New York: Springer-Verlag, 1981:17-21.
2.   Kannel WB. Potency of vascular risk factors as the basis for antihypertensive therapy. Eur Heart J 1992;13(Suppl.G):34-42.
3.   Julius S, Gudbrandsson T, Jamerson K, Andersson O. The interconnection between sympathetics, microcirculation, and insulin resistance in hypertension. Blood Press 1992;1: 9-19.

4.   Reaven GM, Chen YD. Insulin resistance, its consequences, and coronary heart disease. Must we choose one culprit? [editorial; comment]. Circulation 1996;93:1780-83.

5.   Weber MA, Smith DH, Neutel JM, Graettinger WF. Cardiovascular and metabolic characteristics of hypertension. Am J Med 1991;91:4S-10S.

6.   Kannel WB, Feinleib M, McNamara PM, Garrison RJ, Castelli WP. An investigation of coronary heart disease in families: The Framingham Offspring Study. Am J Epidemiol 1979; 110:281-90.

7.   Dawber TR, Kannel WB, Lyell LP. An approach to longitudinal studies in a community: the Framingham Study. Ann N Y Acad Sci 1963;107:539-56.

8.   Kannel WB, Wolf PA, Garrison RJ. Section 34: Some risk factors related to the annual incidence of cardiovascular disease and death using pooled repeated biennial measurements: Framingham Heart Study, 30-year followup. Springfield: National Technical Information Service, 1987:1-459.

9.   Lipid Research Clinics Program. Manual of Laboratory Operation. Bethesda: NIH, 1974:NIH 75-628

10.   Garrison RJ, Kannel WB, Stokes J, III, Castelli WP. Incidence and precursors of hypertension in young adults: The Framingham Offspring Study. Prev Med 1987;16:234-51.

11.   Despres JP. Abdominal obesity as important component of insulin-resistance syndrome. Nutrition 1993;9:452-59.

12.   Gray RJ, Matloff JM, Conklin CM, et al. Perioperative myocardial infarction: late clinical course after coronary artery bypass surgery. Circulation 1982;66:1185-89.

13.   Reaven GM. Insulin resistance, hyperinsulinemia, and hypertriglyceridemia in the etiology and clinical course of hypertension. Am J Med 1991;90:7S-12S.

14.   Shen DC, Shieh SM, Fuh MM, Wu DA, Chen YD, Reaven GM. Resistance to insulin-stimulated-glucose uptake in patients with hypertension. J Clin Endocrinol Metab 1988;66:580-83.

15.   Shieh SM, Shen MD, Fuh MM, Chen YD, Reaven GM. Plasma lipid and lipoprotein concentrations in Chinese males with coronary artery disease, with and without hypertension. Atherosclerosis 1987;67:49-55.

16.   Zavaroni I, Bonora E, Pagliara M, et al. Risk factors for coronary artery disease in healthy persons with hyperinsulinemia and normal glucose tolerance. N Engl J Med 1989;320: 702-706.

17.   Pollare T, Lithell H, Berne C. A comparison of the effects of hydrochlorothiazide and captopril on glucose and lipid metabolism in patients with hypertension. N Engl J Med 1989; 321:868-73.

18.   Reaven GM. Are triglycerides important as a risk factor for coronary disease? Heart Dis Stroke 1993;2:44-48.

19.   Austin MA, Breslow JL, Hennekens CH, Buring JE, Willett WC, Krauss RM. Low density lipoprotein subclass patterns and risk of myocardial infarction. JAMA 1988;260:1917-21.

20.   Siegel RD, Cupples A, Schaefer EJ, Wilson PW. Lipoproteins, apolipoproteins, and low-density lipoprotein size among diabetics in the Framingham offspring study. Metabolism 1996;45:1267-72.

21.   Christlieb AR, Krolewski AS, Warram JH, Soeldner JS. Is insulin the link between hypertension and obesity? Hypertension 1985;7:II54-7.

22.   Manicardi V, Camellini L, Bellodi G, Coscelli C, Ferrannini E. Evidence for an association of high blood pressure and hyperinsulinemia in obese man. J Clin Endocrinol Metab 1986; 62:1302-1304.

23.   Johnson D, Prud'homme D, Despres JP, Nadeau A, Tremblay A, Bouchard C. Relation of abdominal obesity to hyperinsulinemia and high blood pressure in men. Int J Obes Relat Metab Disord 1992;16:881-90.

24.   Parker DR, Weiss ST, Troisi R, Cassano PA, Vokonas PS, Landsberg L. Relationship of dietary saturated fatty acids and body habitus to serum insulin concentrations: The Normative Aging Study. Am J Clin Nutr 1993;58:129-36.

25.   Jung RT, Shetty PS, James WP, Barrand MA, Callingham BA. Caffeine: Its effect on catecholamines and metabolism in lean and obese humans. Clin Sci 1981;60:527-35.

26.   Stamler R, Stamler J, Grimm R, et al. Nutritional therapy for high blood pressure. Final report of a four- year randomized controlled trial--the Hypertension Control Program. JAMA 1987; 257:1484-91.

27.   Krotkiewski M, Mandroukas K, Sjostrom L, Sullivan L, Wetterqvist H, Bjorntorp P. Effects of long-term physical training on body fat, metabolism, and blood pressure in obesity. Metabolism 1979;28:650-58.

28.   Tuck ML. Obesity, the sympathetic nervous system, and essential hypertension. Hypertension 1992;19:167-77.

29.   Modan M, Halkin H, Almog S, et al. Hyperinsulinemia. A link between hypertension obesity and glucose intolerance. J Clin Invest 1985;75:809-17.

HYPERTENSION AND CORONARY HEART DISEASE RISK FACTOR MANAGEMENT

Mark C. Houston

Introduction

Chronic hypertension is associated with an increased morbidity and mortality due to target organ damage (heart, brain, kidneys). In particular, cardiac complications including coronary heart disease (CHD), angina, myocardial infarction (MI), systolic and diastolic congestive heart failure (CHF), and left ventricular hypertrophy (LVH) are increased in all degrees of hypertension. The drug treatment of mild to moderate hypertension (diastolic blood pressure [DBP] ≤ 110 mmHg) has not reduced CHD or other atherosclerotic complications associated with hypertension [1]. Trials that included patients with DBP ≥ 110 mmHg have had reductions in CHD. Although CHD has declined in the United States, this is due primarily to reduction in other risk factors such as hypercholesterolemia, smoking, and severe hypertension (DBP ≥ 115 mmHg) as well as reduction in deaths related to acute MI, but not specifically to the drug treatment of mild hypertension [2].

Maximal reduction in CHD can only be achieved if drug therapy has a favorable impact on all CHD risk factors. Reduction in blood pressure alone cannot be considered adequate therapy in view of newer concepts and present understanding of the effects of antihypertensive drugs on CHD risk factors.

Hypertensive Syndrome

Hypertension is a syndrome of genetic and acquired metabolic and structural abnormalities characterized by dyslipidemia, insulin resistance, glucose intolerance, central obesity, renal defects on sodium and water balance, structural abnormalities of vascular and cardiac smooth muscle, and abnormal cellular cation transport or membranopathy [3,4]. Treatment should be directed toward improvement in these abnormalities in addition to reduction in intra-arterial pressure.

Epidemiologic Prospective Observational Studies and CHD

MacMahon et al. [5] reviewed nine studies of 420,000 patients followed a mean of 10 years noting 4,856 CHD events in the DBP range of 70-110 mmHg. Differences in DBP of 5.0, 7.5, and 10 mmHg were respectively associated with a 21%, 29%, and 37% reduction in

A. M. Gotto, Jr. et al. (eds.), Multiple Risk Factors in Cardiovascular Disease, 335–348.

CHD. These studies imply that a lower blood pressure will reduce CHD.

Therapeutic Intervention Trials and CHD

The most accurate meta-analysis by Cutler et al. [1] of nine prospective clinical trials of mild hypertension in 43,000 patients demonstrated that CHD (fatal and nonfatal MI) was reduced by 8%, a nonsignificant difference between control and treatment groups. There are now 19 clinical prospective trials in mild hypertension that have been published [3,6-8] (Table 1). In two trials, the treated group had a higher death rate from CHD than the untreated group. In two trials, sudden death was greater in the aggressively treated group. Four trials showed a reduction in CHD mortality in the treated patients, but the results differed in beta blocker versus diuretic-treated patients. In the remaining 11 studies, there was no significant difference in CHD mortality between placebo versus control patients. All of these studies used diuretics and beta blockers as primary drug therapy. The adverse effects of diuretics and beta blockers on CHD risk factors (Table 2) may account in part for the lack of reduction in CHD as predicted by the decrease in BP.

Therapeutic Intervention

A more pathophysiologic and tailored approach to the treatment of hypertension is recommended in place of the traditional stepped care (diuretic and beta blocker based). This approach addresses the hypertensive syndrome as well as other important concepts. This new approach is "Subsets of Hypertension" which is based on eight parameters (or subsets) of hypertensive treatment:

1. Pathophysiology: Membranopathy, ion transport defects, structural factors, smooth muscle hypertrophy (vascular, cardiac, cerebral, and renal) functional factors, and vasoconstrictive forces;
2. Hemodynamics: Systemic vascular resistance (SVR), cardiac output (CO), arterial compliance, organ perfusion, and BP;
3. End-organ damage: Reduce risk factors for all end-organ damage;
4. Concomitant medical diseases and problems: Favorable effect by drugs;
5. Demographics: Race, sex, and age;
6. Adverse effects of drugs and quality of life (QOL);
7. Compliance with medical regimen; and
8. Total health care costs: Direct and indirect costs.

Pathophysiology

Various abnormalities in membrane ion transport [9-11] and structural abnormalities in vascular smooth muscle [12] are genetically transmitted in essential hypertension. The calcium channel blockers (CCB), angiotensin converting enzyme inhibitors (ACEI), A-II receptor antagonists, central alpha agonists (CAA), and alpha blockers (AB) improve the membranopathy and structural abnormalities [3,13]. Diuretics, beta blockers, and direct

Table 1. Clinical Trials in Mild to Moderate Hypertension and Coronary Heart Disease: Summary 19 Trials

CHD Mortality Increased		
Oslo	1980	
MPPCD	1985	
Sudden Death Increased (Abnormal Electrocardiogram [ECG])		
MRFIT	1982	
HDF	1979	
CHD Mortality Decreased		
HDFP	1979	
SHEP	1991	SBP>160
MRC #2	1992	Diuretic group only, not beta-blocker group
MAPHY	1988	Beta-blocker better than diuretic; no placebo

No Difference in CHD Mortality Between Control versus Treatment or Aggressive versus Less Aggressive Treatment

VA Cooperative	1970
USPHS	1977
VA-NHLBI	1978
Australian	1980
MRC	1984
MRFIT	1982
EWPHE	1985
IPPPSH	1972
HEP	1986
HAPPHY	1987
STOP	1991

Legend: VA-NHLBI, Veterans Administration-National Heart, Lung, and Blood Institute; HDFP, Hypertension Detection and Follow-up Program; IPPPSH, International Prospective Primary Prevention Study in Hypertension; EWPHE, European Working Party on Hypertension in the Elderly; HAPPHY, Heart Attack Primary Prevention in Hypertension; HEP, Hypertension in Elderly Patients; MRFIT, Multiple Risk Factor Intervention Trial: MPPCD, Multifactorial Primary Prevention of Cardiovascular Diseases; MAPHY, Metoprolol Atherosclerosis Prevention in Hypertension trial; USPHS, United States Public Health Service trial; MRC, Medical Research Council trial; SHEP, Systolic Hypertension in Elderly Program; STOP, Swedish Trial in Old Patients.

Table 2. Coronary Heart Disease Risk Factors: Influence of Diuretic and Beta Blocker Therapy

	Diuretic (Thiazide and Thiazide-like)	Beta Blocker (Without ISA)
1. Hypokalemia	Yes	No
2. Hypomagnesemia	Yes	No
3. Dyslipidemia	Yes	Yes
A. Hypercholesterolemia	Yes	Yes or No Change
B. Hypertriglyceridemia	Yes	Yes
C. Elevated LDL-C	Yes	Yes or No Change
D. Lowered HDL-C	Yes or No Change	Yes
E. Elevated Apolipoprotein B	Yes	Yes
F. Lowered Apolopoprotein A	Yes	Yes
G. Elevated Lipoprotein A (Lpa)	Yes	Yes
4. Glucose Intolerance (Hyperglycemia)	Yes	Yes
5. Insulin Resistance	Yes	Yes
6. Hyperuricemia	Yes	Yes
7. Impaired Aerobic Exercise	No to Minimal	Yes
8. LVH Regression	No (No Change or Increase LVH)	(Inconsistent)
9. Diastolic Dysfunction Improved	No	(Inconsistent)
10. Increase Blood Viscosity	Yes	No
11. Increase Catecholamines	Yes	Yes
12. Increase Angiotensin II	Yes	No
13. Potentiate Arrhythmias	Yes	No
14. Acid Base Abnormalities and Other Electrolyte Disorders	Yes	No
15. Blood Velocity and Arterial Turbulence Abnormalities	Yes	No
16. Hyperfibrinogenemia	Yes	No
17. Abnormal Platelet Function (Aggregation and Adhesion)	Yes	No
18. Increased Thrombeogenic Potential	Yes	No

ISA=intrinsic sympathomimetic activity; LDLC=low density lipoprotein cholesterol; HDLC=high density lipoprotein cholesterol; LVH=left ventricular hypertrophy vasodilators either do not change or worsen the membranopathy and structural abnormalities [3,13]. CCB decreases intracellular calcium and ACEI increases intracellular magnesium which may reverse some of the metabolic and structural abnormalities present in the hypertension syndrome.

Hemodynamics

Antihypertensive therapy should reverse and improve the hemodynamic dysregulation of essential hypertension. The optimal effect would be as follows:

1. Reduce systemic vascular resistance (SVR);
2. Improve cardiac output (CO);
3. Improve arterial compliance (AC); and
4. Improve perfusion and blood flow (BF).

The effects of each class of antihypertensive drug is shown in Table 3. The CCB, ACEI, angiotensin II receptor antagonists, CAA, and AB have the best hemodynamic profile, diuretics are in between and beta blockers without intrinsic sympathomimetic activity (ISA) have the worst hemodynamic profile, by adversely affecting all the hemodynamic parameters [3,13].

Table 3. Hemodynamic Effects of Antihypertensive Therapy

---

1. Reduce SVR, preserve CO, improve AC and BF

   - Calcium channel blockers

   - ACE inhibitors

   - Angiotensin II receptor antagonists

2. Reduce SVR, preserve CO, improve BF, effects on AC unknown

   - Central alpha agonists

   - Alpha blockers

3. Reduce SVR, CO, BF, worsen AC

   - Diuretics

4. Increase SVR, decrease CO, BF, worsen AC

   - Beta blockers without ISA

Antihypertensive Therapy and CHD Risk Factors

There are 18 CHD risk factors which can be altered by antihypertensive therapy [3,14].

These effects are summarized in Table 4, which shows that diuretics have the most adverse effects, beta blockers are in between, and CCB, ACEI, angiotensin II receptor antagonists, CAA, and AB have the best CHD risk factor profile. Theoretically, these latter five classes of drugs with the 0/18 CHD risk factor profile index should reduce CHD better than diuretics (especially high doses) and beta blockers assuming an equal reduction in arterial pressure [3].

Concomitant Diseases, Quality of Life, and Cost

The CCB, CAA, ACEI, angiotensin II receptor antagonists, and AB have few contraindications and can be used as initial monotherapy in numerous concomitant diseases and problems in hypertension with a good quality of life, acceptable or equal adverse effects compared to diuretic and beta blocker therapy, and certainly better than methyldopa or reserpine and a competitive total health care cost if one considers the numerous hidden cost factors. A detailed analysis of these issues is reviewed in several recent articles [3,14-16] (Table 5 and 6).

Table 5. Total Cost of Antihypertensive Therapy

1. Acquisition cost.
2. Coprescription of secondary drugs.
3. Office visits.
4. Ancillary laboratory costs (electrolytes, glucose, lipids, ECG).
5. Costs to patient's lifestyle: quality of life and adverse effects.
6. Cost of increasing end-organ damage.
7. Mean costs per drug cost category -- 1-year use

	Acquisition Cost	Suppl. Drug Cost	Laboratory Cost	Clinic Visit Cost	Side Effect Cost	Total Cost
Diuretics	$133	$232	$117	$298	$263	$1043
β-Blockers	$334	$115	$ 56	$187	$203	$895
α-Blockers	$401	$290	$114	$227	$256	$1288
Centrally acting α-agonists	$285	$295	$125	$267	$193	$1165
ACE inhibitors+ A-II receptor antagonists	$444	$291	$ 95	$218	$195	$1243
Calcium entry blockers	$540	$278	$ 87	$214	$306	$1425

Table 4. Effects of Antihypertensive Drugs on Coronary Heart Disease Risk Factors

	Diuretics	Indapamide	Beta-Blockers without ISA	Beta-Blockers with ISA	Labetalol	Guane-thidine, Guanadrel	Central Alpha-Agonists	Methyl-dopa	Direct Vasodilators	Alpha-Blockers	A-II Inhibitors + ACE Inhibitors	Calcium Blockers	Reserpine
Hypertension	↗	↗	↗	↗	↗	↗	↗	↗	↗	↗	↗	↗	↗
Dyslipidemia	↘	↑	↘	↑	↑	↑	↗	↘	↑	↘	↑	↗	↘
Glucose intolerance	↘	↑	↘	↘	↘	↑	↗	↑	↑	↗	↗	↗	↑
Insulin resistance	↘	↑	↘	↘	?	?	↗	↑	↑	↗	↗	↑/↗	?
LVH	↘/↗	↗	↑	↘	↗	↗	↗	↗	↘	↗	↗	↗	↗
Exercise	↑/↘	↑	↗	↗	↑/↗	↗	↑	↑	↑	↑	↑	↑	↗
Potassium	↗	↘*	↑/↗	↑	↑	↑	↑	↑	↑	↑	↘	↑	↑
Magnesium	↗	↘*	↑	↑	↑	↑	↑	↑	↑	↑	↑/↗	↗	↑
Uric acid	↘	↘*	↘	↘	↘	↑	↑/↗	↑/↗	↑	↑	↗	↑/↗	↑
Blood viscosity	↘	↑	↑	↑	↑	↑	↑	↑/↗	↗	↗	↗	?	?
Blood velocity	↑/↗	↑	↘	↑	↑	↑	↗	↘	↘	↑/↗	↑	↗	↗
Catecholamines	↘	↗	↘	↘	↑	↗	↗	↗	↘	↑/↗	↗	↗	↗
Angiotensin II	↘	↑	↗	↑	↗	↑	↗	↗	↘	↑	↗	↗	↘
Arrhythmia potential	↘	↑	↗	↑/↘	↑	↑	↗	↗	↘	↑	↗	↗	↘
Fibrinogen	↘	↑	?	?	?	?	?	?	?	↗	?	?	?
Platelet function	↘	↗	↑/↗	?	?	?	↗	↑	?	?	↗	↗	?
Thrombogenic potential	↘	↗	?	?	?	?	?	?	?	?	?	↗	?
Antiatherogenic	↑	↑	↘↑	?	?	?	?	?	?	?	↘↑	↘↑	↘↑
CHD relative risk ratio	16:18	3:18	6:18	7:18	3:18	3:18	0:18	2:18	5:18	0:18	0:18	0:18	3:18

*Minimal.?
†Animal studies.
‡Animal and human studies.
↘, Reduced; ↗, increased; →, no change; ?, unknown.

Table 6. Selection of Therapy Based on Subsets of Hypertension

Selection of antihypertensive therapy based on the subsets of hypertension approach allows for the categorization of drugs into three groups: drugs of choice, alternatives, and contraindicated drugs. Diseases in the left-hand column are often associated with hypertension. A drug should be selected considering all disease factors. Drugs are listed in *alphabetical order*, not by preference, in each column.

Table 6A.

Concomitant Condition	Drug(s) of Choice	Alternatives	Relative or Absolute Contraindication
Addictive Syndromes: withdrawal from tobacco, alcohol, opiates	Central alpha-agonist (clonidine)		
Angina: mixed	Beta-blocker without ISA, Calcium channel blocker	A-II antagonist, ACE inhibitor, Alpha-blocker, Central alpha-Agonist, Diuretic, Alpha-and beta-Blocker	Beta-blocker With ISA, Direct vasodilators, Neuronal inhiBitors, Reserpine
Angina: Obstructive	Beta-blocker without ISA, Calcium channel blocker	A-II antagonist, ACE inhibitor, Alpha-blocker, Central alpha-agonist, Diuretic, Alpha-and beta-blocker	Beta-blocker With ISA, Direct Vasodilators, Neuronal Inhibitors, Reserpine
Agina: Vasospastic	Calcium Channel Blocker	A-II antagonist, ACE inhibitor, Alpha-blocker, Agonist, Diuretic	Beta-blocker Without ISA, Beta-blocker With ISA, Direct vasodilator, Alpha-and beta-Blocker, Neuronal Inhibitor, Reserpine
Anxiety/ Stress	Central alpha-agonist, Beta-blocker without ISA		

Table 6C.

Concomitant Condition	Drug(s) of Choice	Alternatives	Relative or Absolute Contraindication
Depression	A-II antagonist ACE inhibitor Alpha-blocker Calcium channel blocker	Central alpha-agonist Diuretic Direct vaso-dilator	Beta-blocker without ISA Beta-blocker with ISA Alpha- and beta-blocker Methyldopa Neuronal inhibitor Reserpine
Diabetes mellitus	A-II antagonist ACE inhibitor Alpha-blocker Calcium channel blocker Central alpha-agonist	Beta-blocker With ISA Direct Vasodilator Indapamide Alpha- and Beta-blocker	Beta-blocker Without ISA Diuretic Methyldopa Neuronal inhibitor Reserpine
Diabetic diarrhea and gustatory sweating	Central alpha-agonist (clonidine)		
Diastolic Dysfunction or Failure	Calcium channel blocker		Beta-blocker with ISA Direct vasodilator Neuronal inhibitor Reserpine
Dyslipidemia	Alpha-blocker Calcium channel blocker Central alpha-agonist	A-II antagonist ACE inhibitor Beta-blocker with ISA Alpha- and beta-blocker Direct Vasodilator Indapamide	Beta-blocker without ISA Diuretic Methyldopa Neuronal inhibitor Reserpine

Table 6B.

Concomitant Condition	Drug(s) of Choice	Alternatives	Relative or Absolute Contraindication
Supraventricular tachy-Cardia	Central alpha-Agonist Diltiazem Verapamil	ACE inhibitor Alpha-blocker Amlodipine Diuretic Felodipine Alpha-and beta-blocker Nicardipine Nifedipine Nisoldipine Reserpine	Direct vasodilator Neuronal inhibitor
Cerebrovascular disease	ACE inhibitor Calcium channel blocker A-II antagonist	Alpha-blocker Central alpha-Agonist Direct vasodilator Alpha- and beta-blocker	Beta-blocker without ISA Beta-blocker with ISA Diuretic Neuronal inhibitor Reserpine
Chronic liver disease	Alpha-blocker Calcium Channel Blocker Central alpha-Agonist	ACE inhibitor Direct vasodilator Diuretic Alpha- and beta-blocker	Beta-blocker Methyldopa Neuronal inhibitor Reserpine
CHF (systolic failure)	A-II Antagonist? ACE inhibitor Direct Vasodilator Diuretic	Alpha-blocker Central alpha-agonist Diltiazem (caution) Calcium channel Blocker Amlodipine Isradipine Nicardipine Nifedipine Nisoldipine	Beta-blocker without ISA Beta-blocker with ISA Alpha- and beta-blocker Neuronal inhibitor Reserpine Verapamil

Table 6E.

Concomitant Condition	Drug(s) of Choice	Alternatives	Relative or Absolute Contraindication
Microvascular Angina	Calcium channel blocker	A-II antagonist ACE inhibitor Alpha-blocker Central alpha-agonist	Beta-blocker without ISA Beta-blocker with ISA Direct vasodilator Diuretic Alpha- and beta-blocker Neuronal inhibitor Reserpine
Migraine headache (Prophylaxis)	Beta-blocker without ISA Calcium channel blocker Central alpha-agonist	A-II antagonist ACE inhibitor Alpha-blocker Beta-blocker with ISA Diuretic Alpha- and beta-blocker	Direct vasodilator Neuronal inhibitor Reserpine
Mitral valve prolapse	Beta-blocker without ISA Calcium channel blocker Central alpha-agonist	A-II antagonist ACE inhibitor Alpha-blocker Alpha- and beta-blocker	Beta-blocker without ISA Beta-blocker with ISA Neuronal inhibitor Reserpine
Obesity	ACE inhibitor A-II antagonist Alpha-blocker Calcium channel blocker Central alpha-agonist	Direct vasodilator Diuretic Alpha- and beta-blocker	Beta-blocker without ISA Beta-blocker with ISA Neuronal inhibitor Reserpine
Obstructive airway disease	Alpha-blocker Calcium channel blocker Central alpha-agonist	A-II antagonist ACE inhibitor Direct vasodilator Diuretic	Beta-blocker without ISA Beta-blocker with ISA Alpha- and beta-blocker Neuronal inhibitor Reserpine

Table 6D.

Concomitant Condition	Drug(s) of Choice	Alternatives	Relative or Absolute Contraindication
Essential tremor	Central alpha-agonist Beta-blocker without ISA		
Glaucoma	Beta-blocker Central alpha-agonist Diuretic		
Hyperuricemia	A-II antagonist ACE inhibitor Alpha-blocker Calcium channel blocker Central alpha agonist	Direct vasodilator Alpha- and beta-blocker Neuronal inhibitor Reserpine	Beta-blocker without ISA Beta-blocker with ISA Diuretic
Exercise	A-II antagonist ACE inhibitor Alpha-blocker Calcium channel blocker Central alpha-agonist	Beta-blocker with ISA Diuretic Direct vasodilator Alpha- and beta-blocker Methyldopa	Beta-blocker without ISA Neuronal inhibitor Reserpine
LVH	A-II antagonist ACE inhibitor Alpha-blocker Calcium channel blocker Central alpha-agonist Indapamide Alpha- and beta-blocker	Beta-blocker without ISA Reserpine Diuretic	Beta-blocker with ISA Direct vasodilator Neuronal inhibitor
Menopausal Symptoms	Central alpha-agonist (clonidine)		Direct vasodilator

Table 6G.

Concomitant Condition	Drug(s) of Choice	Alternatives	Relative or Absolute Contraindication
Post-MI: Q-wave Normal left ventricular function	Beta-blocker without ISA	Calcium channel blocker, Central alpha-agonist, Alpha- and beta-blocker	Beta-blocker with ISA, Direct vasodilator, Diuretic, Neuronal inhibitor, Reserpine
Abnormal left ventricular function	A-II antagonist? ACE inhibitor Diuretic		A-II antagonist, ACE inhibitor, Beta-blocker without ISA, Beta-blocker with ISA, Diuretic, Alpha- and beta-blocker, Neuronal inhibitor, Reserpine
Pregnancy (first and second trimester)	Hydralazine Methyldopa Central alpha-agonist	Possibly alpha-blocker, calcium channel blocker*	
Premature ventricular contractions	Beta-blocker without ISA, Calcium channel blocker, Verapamil	A-II antagonist, ACE inhibitor, Alpha-blocker, Central alpha-agonist, Alpha- and beta-blocker, Diltiazem, Nifedipine	Beta-blocker with ISA, Direct vasodilator, Diuretic, Neuronal inhibitor, Reserpine
Pulmonary hypertension	Calcium channel blocker, Direct vasodilator	A-II antagonist, ACE inhibitor, Alpha-blocker, Central alpha-agonist, Diuretic, Alpha- and beta-blocker	Beta-blocker

Table 6F.

Concomitant Condition	Drug(s) of Choice	Alternatives	Relative or Absolute Contraindication
Peptic ulcer disease	Calcium channel blocker, Central alpha-agonist	A-II antagonist, ACE inhibitor, Beta-blocker, Direct vaso-dilator, Diuretic, Alpha- and beta-blocker	Neuronal inhibitor, Reserpine
Peripheral vascular disease	Calcium channel blocker	A-II antagonist, ACE inhibitor, Alpha-blocker, Central alpha-agonist, Direct vaso-dilator, Diuretic	Beta-blocker without ISA, Beta-blocker with ISA, Alpha- and beta-blocker, Neuronal inhibitor, Reserpine
Post-MI: non-Q-wave Normal left-ven-tricular function	Diltiazem? Verapamil? ACE inhibitor A-II antagonist?	Alpha-blocker, Beta-blocker without ISA, Central alpha-agonist, Calcium channel blocker, Amlodipine, Isradipine, Nicardipine, Nifedipine, Nisoldipine, Alpha- and beta-blocker	Beta-blocker with ISA, Direct vasodilator, Diuretic, Neuronal inhibitor, Reserpine
Abnormal left ventricular function	A-II antagonist? ACE inhibitor Diuretic		

Table 6I.

Concomitant Condition	Drug(s) of Choice	Alternatives	Relative or Absolute Contraindication
Sinusitis/rhinitis	Central alpha-agonist	A-II antagonist, ACE inhibitor, Alpha-blocker, Calcium channel blocker, Direct vaso-dilator, Diuretic	Beta-blocker, Alpha- and beta-blocker, Neuronal inhibitor, Reserpine
Toxemia of pregnancy (eclampsia)	Central alpha-agonist, Calcium channel blocker*, Hydralazine, Methyldopa	Alpha-blocker*	ACE inhibitor, Beta-blocker without ISA, Beta-blocker with ISA, Diuretic, Alpha- and beta-blocker, Neuronal inhibitor, Reserpine
Use of NSAIDs	Calcium channel blocker	Alpha-blocker, Central alpha-agonist	A-II antagonists, ACE inhibitor, Beta-blocker with ISA, Beta-blocker without ISA, Direct vasodilator, Diuretic, Alpha- and beta-blocker, Neuronal inhibitor, Reserpine
Volume overload	A-II antagonist, ACE inhibitor, Calcium channel blocker, Diuretic	Alpha-blocker, Central alpha-agonist, Alpha- and beta-blocker	Beta-blocker, Direct vasodilator, Neuronal inhibitor, Reserpine

Table 6H.

Concomitant Condition	Drug(s) of Choice	Alternatives	Relative or Absolute Contraindication
Raynaud's phenomenon	Calcium channel blocker	A-II antagonist, ACE inhibitor, Alpha-blocker, Central alpha-agonist, Direct vaso-dilator, Neuronal inhibitor, Reserpine	Beta-blocker without ISA, Beta-blocker with ISA, Alpha- and beta-blocker
Renal insufficiency	Alpha-blocker, Calcium channel blocker, Central alpha-agonist	ACE inhibitor, Direct vaso-dilator, Diuretic†, Alpha- and beta-blocker, A-II antagonist	Beta-blocker without ISA, Beta-blocker with ISA, Neuronal inhibitor, Reserpine
Sexual dysfunction	A-II antagonist, ACE inhibitor, Alpha-blocker, Calcium channel blocker	Central alpha-agonist, Direct vaso-dilator, Diuretic	Beta-blocker without ISA, Beta-blocker with ISA, Alpha- and beta-blocker, Methyldopa, Neuronal inhibitor, Reserpine
Sick sinus syndrome or atrio-ventricular (AV) block	A-II antagonist, ACE inhibitor, Alpha-blocker	Calcium channel blocker, Amlodipine, Isradipine, Nicardipine, Nifedipine, Nisoldipine, Direct vaso-dilator, Diuretic	Beta-blocker without ISA, Beta-blocker with ISA, Central alpha-agonist, Calcium channel blocker, Diltiazem, Verapamil, Alpha- and beta-blocker, Neuronal inhibitor, Reserpine

*These products are not approved for use during pregnancy.
†Use caution in renal artery stenosis (bilateral) and severe chronic renal impairment; monitor K + levels.

Table 6J. Demographics and Antihypertensive Drugs

Demographic Profile	Drug(s) of Choice	Alternatives	Relative or Absolute Contraindication

Young patient	A-II antagonist
	ACE inhibitor
	Alpha-blocker
	Calcium channel
	  blocker
	Central alpha-agonist
		Beta-blocker
		  with ISA
		Direct vaso-
		  dilator
		Alpha- and beta-
		  blocker
			Beta-blocker
			  without ISA
			Diuretic
			Neuronal inhibitor
			Reserpine

Elderly patient	Alpha-blocker
	Calcium channel
	  blocker
	Central alpha-agonist
		A-II antagonist
		ACE inhibitor
		Beta-blocker
		  without ISA
		Beta-blocker
		  with ISA
		Diuretic
		Alpha- and beta-
		  blocker
			Direct vasodilator
			Neuronal inhibitor
			Reserpine

African-American patient	Alpha-blocker
	Calcium channel
	  blocker
	Central alpha-
	  agonist
		A-II antagonist
		ACE inhibitor
		Direct vaso-
		  dilator
			Beta-blocker with
			  ISA
			Beta-blocker with-
			  out ISA
			Alpha- and beta-
			  blocker
			Neuronal inhibitor
			Reserpine

White patient	A-II antagonist
	ACE inhibitor
	Alpha-blocker
	Calcium channel
	  blocker
	Central alpha-agonist
		Direct vaso-
		  dilator
		Alpha- and beta-
		  blocker
		Diuretic
			Beta-blocker with
			  ISA
			Beta-blocker with-
			  out ISA
			Neuronal inhibitor
			Reserpine

Summary and Conclusion

Long-term, prospective, controlled, clinical trials are desperately needed to compare traditional diuretic and beta blocker therapy with CCB, ACEI, angiotensin II receptor antagonists, and AB to determine which drug class(es) most effectively reduce CHD morbidity and mortality. However, until such studies are available, one must rely on the large body of clinical and research data as well as theoretical concepts that suggest that reduction in a CHD risk factor(s) will reduce CHD. It would appear that CCB, ACEI, angiotensin II receptor antagonists, CAA, and AB would achieve a better reduction in CHD than diuretics (particularly high doses) and beta blockers, but this remains unproven to date.

References

1. Cutler JA, MacMahon SW, Furberg CD. Controlled clinical trials of drug treatment for hypertension: A review. Hypertension 1989;13(Suppl.I):I36-I44.
2. Goldberg RJ, Gore JM, Alpert JS, et al. Recent changes in attack and survival rates of acute myocardial infarction (1975 through 1981). The Worcester Heart Attack Study. JAMA 1986;255:2774-79.

3. Houston MC. Hypertension strategies for therapeutic intervention and prevention of end organ damage. Primary Care 1991;18(3):713-53.

4. Nilsson P, Lindholm L, Schersten B. Hyperinsulinemia and other metabolic disturbances in well-controlled hypertensive men and women. An epidemiological study of the Dalby population. J Hypertens 1990;8:953-59.

5. MacMahon S, Peto R, Cutler J, et al. Blood pressure, stroke and coronary heart disease. Part I. Prolonged differences in blood pressure Prospective observational studies corrected for the regression dilution bias. Lancet 1990;335:765-74.

6. SHEP Cooperative Research Group. Prevention of stroke by antihypertensive drug treatment in older persons with isolated systolic hypertension. Final results of the Systolic Hypertension in the Elderly Program (SHEP). JAMA 1991;265:3255-64.

7. Medical Research Council Trial of Treatment of Hypertension in Older Adults: Principal results. Br Med J 1992;304:405-12.

8. Dahlof B, Lindholm LH, Hansson L, Schersten B, Ekbom T, Webster P. Morbidity and mortality in the Swedish Trial in Old Patients with Hypertension (STOP-Hypertension). Lancet 1991;338:1281-85.

9. Carr SJ, Thomas TH, Laker M, et al. Elevated sodium-lithium countertransport: A familial marker of hyperlipidemia and hypertension? J Hypertens 1990;8:139-46.

10. Postnov YV. An approach to the explanation of cell membrane alteration in primary hypertension. Hypertension 1990;15(3):332-37.

11. Ives HE. Ion transport defects and hypertension-where is the link? Hypertension 1989;14:590-97.

12. Folkow BP. "Structural Factor" in primary and secondary hypertension. Hypertension 1990;16:89-101.

13. Safar ME, Bouthier JA, Levenson JA, et al. Peripheral large arteries and the response to antihypertensive treatment. Hypertension 1983;5(Suppl. III):III63-III68.

14. Houston, MC. New insights and approaches to reduce end organ damage in the treatment of hypertension: Subjects of hypertension approach. Am Heart J 1992;123:1337-67.

15. Houston, MC. New insights and approaches for the treatment of essential hypertension: Selection of therapy based on coronary heart disease risk factor analysis, hemodynamic profiles, quality of life, and subsets of hypertension. Heart J 1989;117(4):911-51.

16. Hilleman DE, Mohiuddin SM, Lucas D Jr, et al. Cost minimization analysis of initial antihypertensive therapy in patients with mild to moderate essential diastolic hypertension. Abstract. Circulation 1992:88(Part2):263.

GLOBAL RISK MANAGEMENT: NEW STRATEGIES FOR IMPLEMENTATION

Sidney C. Smith, Jr.

Global risk management refers to both a problem in comprehensive therapy as well as a worldwide concern. Seventy years ago the agenda for the first scientific sessions of the American Heart Association (AHA) revealed striking similarities to problems that are of concern today. Only 200 scientists attended those first sessions to hear ten papers presented; at the most recent AHA meeting, nearly 36,000 physicians, researchers, and other health care professionals attended the sessions and more than 3,600 abstracts were presented. Interestingly, the first four presentations in 1925 dealt with 1) "An official method for lessening heart disease": primary prevention; 2) "The care of adults with moderate heart disorders": secondary prevention; 3) "The economic aspects of heart disease"; and 4) "What can the American Heart Association Accomplish." It is possible to take the agenda from the first AHA meeting and apply it to what is now understood to be a contemporary global problem. The issues and problems have not changed in the intervening years. What has changed is the toll of cardiovascular disease, both in the United States and worldwide. For both American men and women, cardiovascular diseases (CVD) are the leading cause of death and mortality, and in women CVD mortality now exceeds that for men [1]. In fact, for the past decade the in the United States more women than men have died from CVD annually. Throughout the world, one sees a staggering mortality from ischemic heart disease and stroke in both the developed and the developing nations. By the year 2020, heart disease is predicted to be the leading cause of total disease burden for the entire world [2]. Thus a virtual CVD epidemic is occurring on a global basis, while the issue and threat of infectious diseases and nutrition are being resolved.

Treatment strategies to date for coronary artery disease have focused primarily on treating symptomatic manifestations of fixed obstructions. Currently in the United States there are nearly a million admissions yearly for myocardial infarction (MI) and unstable angina and more than 3/4 million revascularization procedures performed [1]. While the procedures are excellent and technically sophisticated, the cost and total burden of treating cardiovascular disease using the present strategies is substantial. In the United States total 1996 expenditure for treating CVD reached an estimated $150 billion in direct cost and close to $250 billion if indirect costs are included [1]. If no change occurs, the direct cost of treating CVD will exceed $200 billion by the year 2000. Additionally, the American population is aging, as are most societies around the world. In the United States, Medicare, which is responsible for funding the medical care of the population older than age 65, is predicted to be out of funds by the year 2001; at the same time, it is also predicted that the projected direct costs for treating CVD will exceed $200 billion. In 1995 two-thirds of the health care dollar was spent on hospital and related services [1]. It is apparent that it has

A. M. Gotto, Jr. et al. (eds.), Multiple Risk Factors in Cardiovascular Disease, 349–355.

become necessary to find ways to extend treatment strategies into the outpatient arena. Drugs and modification of lifestyle occupy only six cents of every health care dollar. Therapies must be extended beyond the treatment of severe fixed obstructions and their symptomatic manifestations to a broader treatment of atherosclerotic disease.

Over the past decade a number of risk reduction treatment strategies have been identified which if broadly implemented can lead to a profound improvement in outcome for patients with CVD. Among the most effective of these risk reduction efforts is smoking cessation, which can reduce total mortality by nearly 50%. A number of other strategies (such as lipid lowering, aspirin therapy, ACE inhibitors, beta blockers, control of hypertension) have all been shown to reduce both cardiovascular events and total mortality. In fact, the recent studies in patients with coronary artery disease (CAD), particularly those conducted with ACE inhibitors (ACEI) and statin pharmacotherapy, reveal a reduction in total mortality and subsequent cardiovascular events, a decrease in the need for revascularization procedures, hospital days and costs, and an improvement in the quality of life [3]. These findings have been so significant that they moved the two Nobel laureates, Brown and Goldstein to speculate in their recent editorial in *Science* that heart attacks might be eliminated as a major health problem by the end of the twentieth century [4]. If such is to be the case, a major effort is needed to implement risk reduction strategies.

Global risk reduction strategies which can significantly reduce morbidity and mortality from CHD are not widely applied. Pilot data from the Cooperative Cardiovascular Project (CCP) study involving Medicare patients hospitalized for MI reveal that only 28% of smokers received documented smoking cessation counseling, less than half who would have benefited from beta-blockers actually received beta-blocker therapy, less than two-thirds who were candidates for ACE inhibitors received the medication, and nearly one out of four who might have benefited aspirin actually received the therapy [5]. Thus, global risk strategies vary in implementation and generally are not widely prescribed.

The data for cholesterol lowering therapies are similar. In a study of cardiologists admitting patients for coronary angiograms with documented hyperlipidemia, on admission before cardiac catheterization, only 18% of the patients who were candidates for therapy were treated, and two years after cardiac catheterization, of those demonstrating coronary artery disease, less than one-third received lipid lowering therapy [6]. As these data were gathered in 1991, prior to the 4-S Trial presented in 1994 and the CARE Trial of 1996, it may be perceived that less than optimal implementation of lipid lowering might have occurred because the dramatic results of the more recent trials were not available. However, the recently published Bypass Angioplasty Revascularization Investigation (BARI) study comparing the results of coronary angioplasty with bypass surgery [7] revealed that five years after being enrolled, only 35-40% of patients with CAD severe enough to warrant coronary artery bypass grafting (CABG) or percutaneous transluminal coronary angioplasty (PTCA) were being treated with lipid lowering medication. Thus, most of the data would suggest that lipid lowering therapy must be included among the list of global risk reduction strategies which are not widely implemented at this time.

There are four reasons for the failure to implement global risk reduction strategies. The first is lack of physician agreement on strategies to prevent CVD. Secondly, physicians do not adhere to established risk reduction guidelines. Thirdly, patient compliance with risk reduction strategies is not good. Fourth, there is a lack of economic reimbursement for risk reduction therapies. All of these issues must be corrected. To reach physician consensus on strategies, the AHA, the American College of Cardiology (ACC), and three European societies (the European Society of Cardiology, the European Atherosclerosis Society, and the European Society of Hypertension) have each published recommendations about global risk reduction [8,9]. The AHA and ACC consensus statement lists nine specific strategies to be considered for all patients with CAD (Figure 1). First on the list is smoking cessation. The CASS trial [10] reports that the leading cause of mortality after coronary bypass surgery is not that the patient had emergency surgery nor that the patient was diabetic nor that incomplete revascularization was performed. The leading cause of mortality after bypass surgery is continuation of smoking. Globally, although expensive medications may not be afforded by all, surely an international effort on smoking cessation is possible. This must be merged with primary efforts at smoking prevention. In the United States, the average age that children start to smoke is 13-14 years; three thousand teenagers start smoking every day of which one thousand will die with a cigarette- or tobacco-related disease [1]. The tobacco industry is spending an estimated $6 billion a year in advertising tobacco products. There are several recent papers addressing cigarette smoking at a global level and the type of international involvement the cardiovascular societies might have to implement in order to reverse this trend. During a visit to Amsterdam two summers ago, the author was impressed by the Vincent Van Gogh painting "Skull with a Burning Cigarette" [11]. Van Gogh was not a molecular biologist. But more than a hundred years ago, he portrayed the hazards of tobacco use in his striking image. It is imperative that smoking cessation programs be promoted on a global basis.

In addition, a low-cholesterol and low-fat diet and exercise should be the foundation for all efforts in treating CAD patients, with additional medical therapies prescribed as necessary. The recently published data using a Mediterranean diet for post-MI patients revealed significant reduction in cardiovascular events for those on the Mediterranean diet [12]. This preliminary, small study clearly calls for confirmation in a larger group of patients. The value and importance of dietary changes and exercise in improving the outlook for patients with atherosclerotic disease should be emphasized. Unfortunately, dietary measures alone do not reduce lipids to goal in many patients. In these cases patient compliance with medical therapies becomes important. More research on the reasons for lack of compliance with medical therapies is needed. As noted earlier in this symposium by Dr. Antonio M. Gotto, Jr., nearly 50% of patients on lipid lowering agents may discontinue therapy within 12 months. The data for estrogen replacement therapy (ERT) are strikingly similar. More than half of women stop ERT after one year [13]. Physicians need to understand how to assist patients adhere to the risk reduction therapies which can improve their outlook.

Another aspect of the overall problem relates to the fact that results seen in randomized secondary prevention trials are produced by support systems not available to most health care providers. The trials have nurses and protocols in addition to medications. Thus patients receive different types of care. It is known, for instance, in at least five areas (hypertension, diabetes, smoking cessation, lipid lowering medication, and post-MI risks)

Risk Intervention	Recommendation
Smoking: Goal: Complete Cessation	Strongly encourage patient and family to stop smoking. Provide counseling, nicotine replacement, and formal cessation programs as appropriate.

Lipid Management:
Primary Goal:
  LDL < 100 mg/dL
Secondary Goal:
  HDL > 35 mg/dL;
  TG < 200 mg/dL
	Start AHA Step II Diet in all patients: ≤ 30% fat, < 7% saturated fat, < 200 mg/d cholesterol.
	
	Assess fasting lipid profile. In post-MI patients, lipid profile may take 4 to 6 weeks to stabilize. Add drug therapy according to the following guide:

LDL < 100 mg/dL No drug therapy	LDL 100 to 130 mg/dL Consider adding drug therapy to diet, as follows:	LDL > 130 mg/dl Add drug therapy to diet, as follows:	HDL < 35 mg/dL Emphasize weight management and physical activity. Advise smoking cessation. If needed to achieve LDL goals, consider niacin, statin, fibrate.
	Suggested drug therapy		
TG < 200 mg/dL Statin Resin Niacin	TG 200 to 400 mg/dL Statin Niacin	TG > 400 mg/dL Consider combined drug therapy (niacin, fibrate, statin)	

If LDL goal is not achieved consider combination therapy.

Risk Intervention	Recommendation

Physical activity:
Minimum Goal:
  30 minutes 3 to 4 times
  per week
	Assess risk, preferably with exercise test, to guide prescription.
	Encourage minimum of 30 to 60 minutes of moderate-intensity activity 3 to 4 times weekly (walking, jogging, cycling, or other aerobic activity) supplemented by an increase in daily lifestyle activities (eg, walking breaks at work, using stairs, gardening, household work). Maximum benefit 5 to 6 hours a week.
	Advise medically supervised programs for moderate- to high-risk patients.

Weight management:	Start intensive diet and appropriate physical activity intervention, as outlined above, in patients > 120% of ideal weight for height. Particularly emphasize need for weight loss in patients with hypertension, elevated triglycerides, or elevated glucose levels.
Antiplatelet agents/ anticoagulants:	Start aspirin 80 to 325 mg/dl if not contraindicated. Manage wafarin to international normalized ratio = 2 to 3.5 for post-MI patients not able to take aspirin.
ACE inhibitors post-MI:	Start early post-MI in stable high-risk patients (anterior MI, previous MI, Killip class II [S₃ gallop, rates, radiographic CHF]). Continue indefinitely for all with LV dysfunction (ejection fraction ≤ 40%) or symptoms of failure. Use as needed to manage blood pressure or symptoms in all other patients.
Beta-blockers:	Start in high-risk post-MI patients (arrhythmia, LV dysfunction, inducible ischemia) at 5 to 28 days. Continue 6 months minimum. Observe usual contraindications. Use as needed to manage angina, rhythm, or blood pressure in all other patients.
Estrogens:	Consider estrogen replacement in all postmenopausal women. Individualize recommendation consistent with other health risks.
Blood pressure control: Goal: ≤ 140/90 mm Hg	Initiate lifestyle modification--weight control, physical activity, alcohol moderation, and moderate sodium restriction--in all patients with blood pressure > 140 mm Hg systolic or 90 mm Hg diastolic. Add blood pressure medication, individualized to other patient requirements and characteristics (ie, age, race, need for drugs with specific benefits) if blood pressure is not less than 140 mm Hg systolic or 90 mm Hg diastolic in 3 months or if *initial* blood pressure is > 160 mm Hg systolic or 100 mm Hg diastolic.

ACE indicates angiotensin-converting enzyme; MI, myocardial infarction; TG, triglycerides; and LV, left ventricular.

Figure 1. AHA Guide to comprehensive risk reduction for patients with coronary and other vascular disease [8].

that nurse case management can enhance the implementation of medical therapies [14]. By working together as a health care team, nurses and physicians can achieve better outcomes for their patients with CVD. In the Stanford MULTIFIT Study [15], with nurse case management, compliance with medication was 98% at six months and 90% at 12 months. The results with lipid lowering therapy were better with nurse case management. In MULTIFIT patients received medications from a health care system similar to the systems involved in large trials.

An additional problem is that most academic centers have not developed models for health care delivery which integrate primary care, general medicine, and subspecialty services. There is disagreement among cardiologists, internists, and family practitioners about responsibility for implementing and following up on risk reduction therapies. The roles of various health care providers must be clarified to insure optimal patient care. Complex multihospital systems have become common. In the United States the number of hospital mergers dramatically increased in 1994 [16]. The result has been the creation of large systems, with as many as six hospitals and four convalescence centers coordinating with three independent multispecialty clinics. Thus, the issue becomes how to coordinate care when a patient enters the system at one point with symptoms of angina, is transferred to another facility for bypass surgery, then transferred again for convalescent care, and finally returns to a clinic for outpatient care. Effective complex care systems need to be developed. Over the last three years at the University of North Carolina, the length of stay on the cardiology ward has decreased from 7.3 days to 3.7 days. In addition, the patient volume has doubled, giving physicians half the time to see twice as many patients. Hospital profits recognized through these changes need to be reinvested in the infrastructure in which physicians practice and to develop outpatient care systems which further risk reduction therapies initiated during hospitalization. Increased profits should be directed towards prevention.

The AHA has recently initiated discussions with representatives of managed care companies regarding the value of global prevention strategies. Two conferences have been held with ten major managed care groups during which the representatives from the managed care groups have indicated interest in supporting broader efforts in secondary prevention. Because the annual percent change in cost of care has flattened out after increasing in the late 1980s and early 1990s, third-party payers find themselves competing on quality of care measures rather than cost of care. They are interested in how the introduction of global risk reduction strategies might make a difference in quality of care outcomes. Economic analyses derived from the 4-S study have shown favorable results for lipid lowering treatments in both direct and indirect costs [17]. With regard to direct costs, this study (which compared men and women, young and old) indicated that the most expensive post-MI individual to treat would be a young woman with a total cholesterol of 213, with an acceptable cost of $27,400 per year, less than the $40,000 cutoff point. In the elderly, the direct cost of treatment is very acceptable. Many managed care companies have indicated a movement towards broader support of prevention efforts due to the results of these large trials.

The National Committee on Quality Assurance (NCQA) using the Health Employer Data and Information Set (HEDIS) criteria affords an opportunity to influence health care delivery [18]. In 1995, using HEDIS criteria, 25% of the managed care programs evaluated either failed or were placed on provisional status. During the past year, the AHA has worked to influence the HEDIS criteria and increased the number of outcome measures specific for cardiovascular disease. In the new HEDIS testing set measures, 8 out of 24 pertain to patients with cardiovascular disease. Thus in the United States, one-third of the performance measures by which managed care will soon be evaluated, relate to cardiovascular disease and the delivery of global risk reduction strategies. Outpatient management of congestive heart failure, control of diabetes, reducing the number of people who smoke, decreasing stroke in those with atrial fibrillation, cholesterol management after diagnosis of coronary disease, treatment of high blood pressure, and aspirin therapy for those with CVD are some of the criteria to be used as testing set measures.

The United States now has a major opportunity to increase preventive therapies. To do so will involve change in at least four areas. First, there must be increased resource allocation for preventive care, in terms of both secondary and primary preventive strategies. Second, the use of health care provider teams can efficiently improve the delivery of these measures. Third, integrated health care delivery systems must be evaluated and implemented as a method for improving health care delivery. Patients will benefit from strategies that address the broadly integrated systems seen in contemporary medicine, instead of single hospital systems. Finally, educational emphasis on prevention must be increased. Concepts of cardiovascular prevention must be taught to medical students, cardiology fellows, and residents. In some cardiology and internal medicine programs, less than 10% of the time is devoted to teaching preventive strategies. Educational efforts in prevention must increase to effect significant changes in the current health care delivery system. John Kenneth Galbraith reminds us that faced with a choice between changing one's mind and proving that there is no need to do so, almost everybody gets busy on the proof. Our health care system must change to emphasize and implement important global risk reduction strategies.

We are now at an exciting and challenging time in the field of cardiovascular disease. In 1957, some 40 years ago, Paul Dudley White, a clinician, teamed with Ancel Keys, an epidemiologist, to jointly explore the importance of global risk factors in cardiovascular disease [19]. Now as we approach the new millennium our vascular biology, our research, and many large clinical trials support the idea that the time has come for broad, global preventive efforts. Our success in addressing the global, expanding epidemic in CVD depends upon broadly based efforts in primary and secondary prevention.

References

1.   American Heart Association. Heart and stroke facts: 1996 statistical supplement. Dallas, Texas: American Heart Association, 1996.
2.   Murray CJL, Lopez AD. The global burden of disease. Cambridge, Massachusetts: Harvard University Press, 1996.
3.   Miller DB. Secondary prevention for ischemic heart disease. Arch Intern Med 1997;157:2045-

52.

4. Brown MS, Goldstein JL. Heart attacks-Gone with the century? (Editorial). Science 1996;272: 629.

5. Ellerbeck EF, Jencks SF, Radford MJ, et al. Quality of care for Medicare patients with acute myocardial infarction: A four-state pilot study from the Cooperative Cardiovascular Project. JAMA 1995;273:1509-14.

6. Cohen MV, Byrne MJ, Levine B, et al. Low rate of treatment of hypercholesterolemia by cardiologists in patients with suspected and proven coronary artery disease. Circulation 1991; 83:1294-1304.

7. The Writing Group for the Bypass Angioplasty Revascularization Investigation (BARI) Investigators. Five-year clinical and functional outcomes comparing bypass surgery and angioplasty in patients with multivessel coronary disease. JAMA 1997;277:715-21.

8. Smith SC Jr., Blair SN, Criqui MH, et al. Preventing heart attack and death in patients with coronary disease. Circulation 1995;92:2-4.

9. Pyrola K, DeBacker G, Graham I, et al. Prevention of coronary heart disease in clinical practice: Recommendations of the Task Force of the European Society of Cardiology, European Atherosclerosis Society and European Society of Hypertension. Eur Heart J 1994; 15:1300-31.

10. Cameron A, Davis K, Rogers W. Recurrence of angina after coronary artery bypass surgery: Predictors and prognosis (CASS Registry). J Am Coll Cardiol 1995;26:895-99.

11. Van Gogh V. Skull with a Burning Cigarette. 1885. Amsterdam, van Gogh Museum.

12. Lorgeril M, Salen P, Martin JL, et al. Effect of a Mediterranean type of diet on the rate of cardiovascular complications in patients with coronary artery disease. J Am Coll Cardiol 1996;28:1103-8.

13. Sullivan JM. Estrogen replacement. Circulation 1996;94:2699-2702.

14. Hill MN, Houston-Miller N. Compliance enhancement: A call for multidisciplinary team approaches. Circulation 1996;93:4-6.

15. De Busk RF, Houston-Miller N, Superko R, et al. A case-management system for coronary risk factor modification after acute myocardial infarction. Ann Int Med 1994;120:721-29.

16. Kassirer J. Mergers and acquisitions - who benefits? Who loses? N Engl J Med 1996;334: 722-23.

17. Johannesson M, Jonsson B, Kjekshus J, et al. Cost effectiveness of Simvastatin treatment to lower cholesterol levels in patients with coronary heart disease. N Engl J Med 1997;336:332-36.

18. Iglehart JK. The National Committee for Quality Assurance. N Engl J Med 1996;335:995-99.

19. Keys A. Coronary heart disease in seven countries. Circulation 1970;41(Suppl.I):1-211.

Eduardo Marban and Gordon F. Tomaselli

Introduction

Over two million Americans suffer from congestive heart failure (CHF) and 200,000 or more die annually [1]. The majority of patients with chronic heart failure have not suffered a myocardial infarction [2], suggesting that classical reentrant ventricular tachycardia (VT) may not be the principal mechanism of sudden cardiac death. Despite therapeutic advances that improve exercise tolerance and survival in these patients, heart failure remains a highly lethal disease with annual mortality rates as high as 50% [3-7]. Of the patients with heart failure that die, 35-50% of the deaths are sudden and unexpected [2,8]. Furthermore, the percentage of deaths which are sudden tends to be highest early in the course of symptomatic heart failure, presumably in patients with the least severe disease [9]. Even if the progression of pump failure were to remain unaltered, effective prevention of sudden cardiac death in the existing heart failure population would extend life in the U.S. population by as much as one million person-years. Large multicenter trials of heart failure therapy have demonstrated the efficacy of vasodilators in delaying overall mortality, yet few therapeutic interventions have decreased the sudden death rate [4] and none has done so selectively. Despite intensive evaluation, the mechanism of sudden death in heart failure remains ill defined [8]. Likewise, there are no reliable strategies to evaluate patients at risk, and therapeutic interventions remain ineffective.

In this article we will explore the evidence for the following hypothesis: Human heart failure is characterized by abnormalities of cardiac repolarization, and these abnormalities increase the risk of sudden cardiac death by predisposing the heart to polymorphic ventricular tachycardia. We focus our attention on patients with heart failure without a prior myocardial infarction, which would produce a scar that could serve as a substrate for classical reentrant tachycardia. The present chapter is adapted from a previously published review from our group [10] to which the reader is referred for additional detail.

The Action Potential Is Prolonged and Repolarization Is Delayed in Heart Failure

An elementary and distinctive signature of any given excitable tissue is its action potential profile. Myocardial cells possess a characteristically long action potential: Figure 1 (left panels) shows examples from normal (top) and failing (bottom) human ventricular myocytes. The ventricular action potential underlies the QT interval of the electrocardiogram, and

A. M. Gotto, Jr. et al. (eds.), Multiple Risk Factors in Cardiovascular Disease, 357–367.

prolongation of the action potential produces delays in cardiac repolarization manifested as prolongation of the QT interval. Cells isolated from failing animal and human hearts consistently reveal a significant prolongation of action potentials compared to those in normal hearts, independent of the mechanism of CHF [11-14]. Figure 1 illustrates the prolongation of action potentials in human heart failure described by Beuckelmann et al. [13]. The importance of this simple finding is difficult to overstate. The plateau and terminal repolarization phases of the action potential are quite labile: this is a time of high membrane resistance, during which small changes in current can easily tip the balance either towards repolarization or towards maintained (or secondary) depolarization. As a rule, the longer the action potential, the more labile is the repolarization process [15]. This lability may be manifest as variability in duration and/or secondary depolarizations that interrupt action potential repolarization, often called "early afterdepolarizations" (EADs) that can initiate triggered arrhythmias including torsades des pointes ventricular tachycardia. A variety of conditions common in patients with heart failure can affect either outward (repolarizing) or inward (depolarizing) currents resulting in action potential prolongation and the propensity for EADs. Such factors include hypokalemia, hypocalcemia, hypomagnesemia [16], acidosis [17], and exposure to a variety of antiarrhythmic drugs. Animal models of cardiac hypertrophy exhibit an increased propensity to EADs [11,15], possibly due to suppression of K^+ currents [18]. Increasing inward current will also favor the production of afterdepolarization-mediated triggered activity, as might occur with β-adrenergic stimulation of Ca^{2+} current or after endogenous release of lipid metabolites which interfere with Na^+ channel inactivation [19]. Stretch-responsive channels have been described in ventricular myocardium [20,21] and proposed to contribute to EADs in heart failure [11,15] but their physiological significance remains controversial.

The ability to isolate viable human ventricular myocytes enabled the dissection of the changes in membrane current that occur in myocardial failure. The inward Na^+ and Ca^{2+} currents do not appear to be altered, at least under basal conditions. Sakakaibara et al. found no disease-related changes in the time course or amplitude of Na^+ currents in human ventricular cells [22]. Measurements of dihydropyridine binding sites [23] and inward Ca^{2+} current [13,24] in ventricular myocytes from failing hearts reveal no changes relative to nonfailing control cells, despite a modest decrease in steady-state messenger RNA levels.

Human ventricular myocytes contain several distinct classes of voltage-dependent K^+ channels. The inward rectifier K^+ current, I_{K1}, sets the resting membrane potential and contributes to the terminal phase of repolarization. The density of I_{K1} is reduced by nearly 40% in cells from myopathic ventricles compared with controls; this reduction occurs in the absence of changes in the voltage dependence of gating or kinetics [13,25]. Another important K^+ current is the transient outward current, I_{to}. Unlike the inward rectifier, I_{to} is expressed in heart cells in a species- and cell type-specific fashion. This current plays a crucial role in the early phases of repolarization and in determining the voltage of the plateau of the action potential, which in turn influences all currents active during the remainder of the action potential. Ventricular myocytes from the mid-portion of the ventricular wall have a substantial I_{to} that is specifically blocked by 4-aminopyridine (4-AP). Figure 1 (right panels) shows the 4-AP-sensitive I_{to} recorded from normal (top) and failing (bottom) ventricular myocytes. This current is significantly reduced (35-40%) in cells isolated from failing ventricles and, as in the case of I_{K1}, there is no other significant change in the current [25]. Similar changes in I_{to} have been noted in diseased human atria [26], chronically infarcted canine ventricle [27], and hypertrophied rat ventricle [28], all of which are arrhythmogenic substrates.

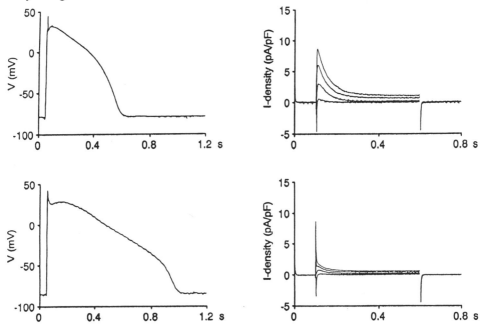

Figure 1. Prolongation of action potentials and reduction in the transient outwardcurrent (I_{to}) in human heart failure. The whole-cell patch clamp data were adapted from the work of Beuckelmann et al. [13]. Action potentials and I_{to} were recorded from human ventricular myocytes isolated from the mid-myocardial wall of the left ventricle. The cells were obtained from normal and myopathic ventricles using identical isolation protocols. The records on the top are from cells isolated from a normal ventricle and on the bottom from a myocyte isolated from a failing heart. The action potentials were recorded in modified Tyrode's solution at $37°C$ and with a stimulus frequency of 0.5 Hz. I_{to} was recorded at room temperature in the same Tyrode's solution with 0.3 mM $CdCl_2$ to block Ca^{2+} currents and a high K^+ solution in the patch pipette [13]. Reproduced from ref. 10 by permission of the American Heart Association.

The heart failure-associated prolongation of the action potential alone would not necessarily suffice to produce ventricular arrhythmias, particularly if the prolongation were homogeneous. Variations in action potential duration would, however, create dispersion of repolarization and refractoriness that could be arrhythmogenic [29]. Regional differences in the density of K^+ currents, particularly I_{to}, have been described in several experimental animal models [30]. Human hearts have recently been reported to exhibit similar gradients of K^+ currents, with I_{to} being much larger in the subepicardium than in the subendocardium [31,32-34]. It is plausible that reduction in repolarizing K^+ current density does not occur uniformly in heart failure. Thus, enhanced regional variability and disease-related changes in K^+ current density may conspire to produce large spatial inhomogeneities of repolarization. Another plausible contributor involves the influence of the autonomic nervous system, which figures prominently in the heart failure phenotype. Heterogeneity of sympathetic innervation is well described in cardiomyopathy patients [33] and has been correlated with heterogeneity of recovery of excitability [34].

The cellular electrophysiologic abnormalties are consistent with the clinical arrhythmias observed in heart failure patients. Abnormalities of action potential duration and afterdepolarizations may produce arrhythmias by triggered mechanisms or may predispose the myocardium to reentry by inhomogeneous changes in excitability and dispersion of refractoriness [35]. Except for patients who present with sustained monomorphic VT [36,37], evidence to support a reentrant mechanism for arrhythmias in nonischemic cardiomyopathy is scarce even in settings where inhomogeneities of action potential duration or refractoriness have been described [38,39]. The failure of programmed stimulation of the ventricle to predict sudden death in either animal models or humans also argues against an excitable-gap reentry mechanism for ventricular arrhythmia production in nonischemic cardiomyopathy.

Prognostic Indicators and Risk Stratification of Heart Failure Patients

Just as the basic mechanisms of sudden cardiac death in heart failure are uncertain, the care of patients is complicated by the limited utility of conventional clinical prognostic indicators of risk for sudden death. Ventricular ectopic activity is commonly observed in patients with left ventricular dysfunction and congestive heart failure, with up to 80% having nonsustained ventricular tachycardia. Unlike patients with a recent myocardial infarction, in whom there is a clear association between ventricular ectopy and the risk of sudden death, the prognostic significance of ventricular ectopy in heart failure patients is unclear. Some studies suggest that the presence of nonsustained VT in patients with cardiomyopathy is predictive of sudden death, while others indicate that its presence is merely a marker for a failing ventricle [8,40].

The controversy regarding the utility of asymptomatic ventricular ectopic activity as an independent predictor of sudden cardiac death may relate to ambiguities regarding the definition and cause of sudden death in heart failure patients. The mechanism of death in the majority of patients with organic heart disease who die suddenly is sustained ventricular tachyarrhythmias, based on studies of heterogeneous populations of patients with out-of-hospital cardiac arrest [41-43]. A recently reported series of unexpected cardiac arrests in hospitalized patients with NYHA class III or IV heart failure found 15 out of 29 cases (52%) of sudden death were due to VT/VF, the others resulting from bradyarrhythmias or electromechanical dissociation [44,45]. However, this group of patients was highly selected, having end-stage heart failure awaiting cardiac transplantation. The authors were careful to acknowledge that the population was not representative of the majority of heart failure patients, most of whom are ambulatory. Irrespective of the mechanism, the lack of specificity of ventricular ectopy in predicting sudden death in heart failure patients is clear. This has motivated a search for other modalities that might provide improved prognostic information regarding sudden death risk in heart failure patients.

Electrophysiological testing also has limited value for predicting the risk of arrhythmic death in patients with dilated nonischemic cardiomyopathy. Induction of sustained monomorphic VT in patients with dilated cardiomyopathy and no clinical history of this arrhythmia is uncommon [36,37,46-49]. Nonspecific electrophysiological endpoints such as polymorphic VT and VF occur commonly but have dubious prognostic significance. Even the absence of an inducible arrhythmia in this patient population does not predict a low risk for sudden death [36,37,48].

Various studies suggest that the signal averaged ECG might be prognostically useful in patients with dilated cardiomyopathy [50,51]. In a prospective study, patients with an abnormal signal averaged ECG were more likely to develop sustained ventricular arrhythmias or sudden death than patients with either a normal signal averaged ECG or bundle branch block [50]. This study supports the importance of an arrhythmic substrate in predicting the survival of patients with dilated cardiomyopathy. The presence of a prolonged high frequency QRS duration was the most common signal averaged ECG abnormality. This finding is suggestive of slowed conduction through the ventricular myocardium but does not permit discrimination among slowed conduction due to abnormal cell-cell coupling, action potential upstroke characteristics, or abnormalities of repolarization.

Other clinical parameters thought to be indicative of hemodynamic derangement in heart failure, such as left ventricular ejection fraction, plasma norepinephrine levels, peak exercise oxygen consumption, and cardiothoracic ratio on chest x-ray are predictors of all-cause mortality [3-6,52], but in general these parameters do not discriminate between sudden deaths and deaths from other causes.

Despite multiple randomized trials of therapy in heart failure, our understanding of sudden cardiac death and how to prevent it remains unclear. The role of antiarrhythmic therapy (particularly with amiodarone) is also uncertain and is the subject of several ongoing multicenter trials. Our inability to identify heart failure patients who will die suddenly may be the result of the empirical approaches utilized to date, none of which applies our understanding of the fundamental mechanisms to the investigation of arrhythmogenesis in this patient population.

Does Evaluation of the Spatial and Temporal Inhomogeneity of Repolarization Have Prognostic Significance?

Alteration of the action potential duration is likely to produce changes in cardiac repolarization. The QT interval on the surface ECG is a readily measurable reflection of cardiac repolarization. It is possible that patients with heart failure and prolonged action potential durations will have abnormalities of the QT interval. The problem with a single measurement of the QT interval is that this is a static, global index of cardiac repolarization, which is a spatially and temporally dynamic process certain to vary on a beat-to-beat basis and when measured from different body surface leads.

The prototypic clinical entities associated with abnormalities of cardiac repolarization, polymorphic ventricular tachycardia and sudden death are the syndromes of congenital and acquired prolongation of the QT interval [53]. Ventricular arrhythmias characteristic of this syndrome may occur in predisposed patients even with normal QT and QTc intervals on a resting ECG. These arrhythmias may be explained by temporal changes in the QT interval, possibly related to changing antiarrhythmic drug regimens and/or serum electrolyte levels [54]. Similar temporal variability may be operative in producing ventricular arrhythmias in patients with heart failure even in the absence of QT prolongation on a resting ECG.

The QT interval may vary regionally in the heart, such spatial variability in the QT interval has been recognized since the 1930s [55], although the biological significance of this variability has only recently been tested. Regional differences in repolarization, assessed by dispersion of endocardial monophasic action potential duration [56,57] or QT [58] intervals, have been documented in conditions associated with torsades des pointes and polymorphic VT. In patients with congenital or acquired long QT syndrome and acute myocardial infarction it has been suggested that it is not the absolute duration of the single-lead QT or QTc that predicts arrhythmia risk, but rather the regional dispersion of the QT (ΔQT) defined as the maximal difference in the QT intervals measured in various leads on a standard 12-lead electrocardiogram [59-61]. Regional dispersion of repolarization may, in and of itself, be arrhythmogenic, creating conditions which support reentry or which permit the propagation of an afterdepolarization-triggered arrhythmia. Regional dispersion of depolarization also exists in patients with dilated cardiomyopathy and is predictive of increased risk for sudden death [62].

In addition to spatial heterogeneity of repolarization there is indirect evidence for temporal heterogeneity in some situations, for example the lability of the QT interval and the occurrence of long QT-associated arrhythmias in patients with normal resting ECGs [58,63]. This lability of the QT interval is probably multifactorial but in part reflects the influence of the autonomic nervous system and may provide prognostic information in patients with heart failure. Variability in the heart rate has proven very useful as an index of autonomic nervous system input to the heart, for example after myocardial infarction, decreased heart rate variability associated with low parasympathetic nervous system tone or high sympathetic activity is a powerful predictor of mortality [64,65]. The effect of heart failure on heart rate variability has also been described. Parameters of variability in both the time- and frequency-domain [66-70] are severely depressed in advanced myocardial failure, consistent with a reduction in vagal input and increased sympathetic input to the heart. A limitation of heart rate variability as an index of autonomic nervous system tone on the ventricle is that it is indirect, reflecting changes in the RR by way of reflex mechanisms mediated by the sinus node. The QT interval is a reflection of ventricular repolarization that is directly influenced by myocardial health and autonomic nervous system activity. It may be that the variability of the QT should more directly and accurately predict cardiac risk than RR variability. A new algorithm for automated quantification of the QT interval has recently been developed and used by Berger et al. [63] to analyze a large cohort of patients with dilated cardiomyopathy. They found that QT variability is markedly increased in heart failure; breakdown by functional class revealed that only patients with symptomatic heart failure (New York Heart Association classes II, III, and IV) exhibited a significant increase in repolarization variability. This study, while provocative, did not follow patients over time to determine whether those with increased QT variability are at greater risk for sudden death. Follow-up will be required to assess of the prognostic importance of increased QT variability.

Summary

Heart failure remains a lethal disease, claiming a substantial number of lives suddenly. Our ability to predict the risk for sudden death is poor; likewise, there is no effective preventive strategy. On the cellular level, human and animal models of myocardial failure are associated with prolongation of action potential duration possibly as a result of decreased density of repolarizing K^+ currents. The consequences of abnormalities of cellular repolarization in the intact failing human heart have not been examined despite the fact that they are potentially arrhythmogenic. Novel indices of abnormal repolarization merit further investigation as potentially useful markers for propensity to sudden death in heart failure patients. Elucidation and recognition of the fundamental pathophysiology of arrhythmias in heart failure may ultimately suggest new therapeutic strategies, including the prospect of somatic gene transfer to correct the presumed abnormalities in ion channel gene expression.

Acknowledgements

Supported by a Specialized Center of Research in Sudden Cardiac Death from the National Heart, Lung and Blood Institute (P50 HL52307). The authors thank their collaborators (notably David Kass, Ronald Berger, Dirk Beuckelmann, and Hugh Calkins) for helpful discussions and access to unpublished data.

References

1.   Packer M. Prolonging life in patients with congestive heart failure: The next frontier. Circulation 1987;75(IV):1-3.
2.   Kannel WB, Plehn JF, Cupples LA. Cardiac failure and sudden death in the Framingham study. Am Heart J 1988;115:869-75.
3.   Cohn J, Archibald D, Ziesche S, et al. Effect of vasodilator therapy on mortality in chronic congestive heart failure: Results of a Veterans Administration cooperative study (V-HeFT). N Engl J Med 1986;314:1547-52.
4.   Cohn J, Johnson G, Ziesche S, et al. A comparison of enalapril with hydralazine-isosorbide dinitrate in treatment of chronic congestive heart failure: V-HeFT II. N Engl J Med 1991;325: 303-10.
5.   CONSENSUS Trial study group. Effects of enalapril on mortality in severe congestive heart failure: Results of the Cooperative North Scandinavian Enalapril Survival Study

(CONSENSUS). N Engl J Med 1987;316:1429-35.

6.   SOLVD Investigators. Effect of enalapril on survival in patients with reduced left ventricular ejection fractions and congestive heart failure. N Engl J Med 1991;325:293-302.

7.   Ho KKL, Anderson KM, Kannel WB, Grossman W, Levy D. Survival after the onset of congestive heart failure in Framingham Heart Study subjects. Circulation 1993;88:107-15.

8.   Packer M. Lack of relation between ventricular arrhythmias and sudden death in patients with chronic heart failure. Circulation 1992;85(I):50-56.

9.   Gradman A, Deedwania P, Cody R, Massie B, Packer M, Pitt B, Goldstein S, for the Captopril-Digoxin Study Group. Predictors of total mortality and sudden death in mild to moderate heart failure. J Am Coll Cardiol 1989;14:564-70.

10.   Tomaselli, GF, Beuckelmann, DJ, Calkins, et al. Sudden death in heart failure. The role of abnormal repolarization. Circulation 1994;90:2534-39.

11.   Aronson RS. Characteristics of action potentials of hypertrophied myocardium from rats with renal hypertension. Circ Res 1980;47:443-54.

12.   Scamps F, Mayoux E, Charlemange D, Vassort G. Calcium current in single cells isolated from normal and hypertrophied rat heart: Effects of β-adrenergic stimulation. Circ Res 1990; 67:199-208.

13.   Beuckelmann DJ, Näbauer M, Erdmann E. Alterations of K^+-currents in isolated human ventricular myocytes from patients with terminal heart failure. Circ Res 1993;73:379-85.

14.   Gwathmey JK, Copelas L, MacKinnon R, et al. Abnormal intracellular calcium handling in myocardium from patients with end-stage heart failure. Circ Res 1987;61:70-76.

15.   Aronson RS, Ming Z. Cellular mechanisms of arrhythmias in hypertrophied and failing myocardium. Circulation 1993;87(VII):76-83.

16.   Leier CV, Dei Cas L, Metra M. Clinical relevance and management of the major electrolyte abnormalities in congestive heart failure: Hyponatremia, hypokalemia, and hypomagnesemia. Am Heart J 1994;128:564-74.

17.   Corabouef E, Deroubaix E, Coulombe A. Acidosis-induced abnormal repolarizations and repetitive activity in isolated dog Purkinje fibers. J Physiol (Paris) 1980;76:97-106.

18.   Furukawa T, Bassett A, Furukawa N, Kimura S, Myerberg RJ. The ionic mechanism of reperfusion-induced early afterdepolarization in feline left ventricular hypertrophy. J Clin Invest 1993;91:1521-31.

19.   Undrovinas AI, Fleidervish IA, Makielski JC. Inward sodium current at resting potentials in single cardiac myocytes induced by the ischemic metabolite lysophosphatidylcholine. Circ Res 1992;71:1231-41.

20.   Hansen DE, Borganelli M, Stacy GP Jr, Taylor K. Dose-dependent inhibition of stretch-induced arrhythmias by gadolinium in isolated canine ventricles: Evidence for a unique mode of antiarrhythmic action. Circ Res 1991;69:820-31.

21.   Morris CE, Sigurdson WJ. Stretch-inactivated channels coexist with stretch-activated ion channels. Science 1989;243:807-9.

22.   Sakakibara Y, Furukawa T, Singer DH, Jia H, Arentzen CE, Wasserstrom JA. Sodium current in isolated human ventricular myocytes. Am J Physiol 1993;265:H1301-H1309.

23.   Rasmussen PR, Minobe W, Bristow MR. Calcium antagonist binding sites in failing and nonfailing human ventricular myocardium. Biochem Pharmacol 1990;39:691-96.

24.   Beuckelmann DJ, Näbauer M, Erdmann E. Characteristics of calcium current in isolated human ventricular myocytes from patients with terminal heart failure. J Mol Cell Cardiol 1991;23:929-37.

25.   Kääb S, Nuss HB, Chiamvimonvat N, O'Rourke B, Kass DA, Marban E, Tomaselli GF. Ionic

mechanism of action potential prolongation in ventricular myocytes from dogs with pacing-induced heart failure. Circ Res 1996;78:262-73.

26.   Mansourati J, Le Grand B. Absence of transient outward current in diseased young human atria. Am J Physiol 1993;265:H1466-H1470.

27.   Lue WM, Boyden P. Abnormal electrical properties of myocytes from chronically infarcted canine heart. Alterations in V_{max} and the transient outward current. Circulation 1992;85:1175-88.

28.   Xu X, Best PM. Decreased transient outward current in ventricular myocytes from acromegalic rats. Am J Physiol 1991;260:H935-42.

29.   Brugada P, Wellens HJJ. Early afterdepolarizations: Role in conduction block, prolonged repolarization-dependent re-excitation, and tachyarrhythmias in the human heart. PACE 1985; 8:889-96.

30.   Anzelevitch C, Sicouri S, Litovsky SH, et al. Heterogeneity within the ventricular wall. Electrophysiology and electropharmacology of epicardial, endocardial and M cells. Circ Res 1991;69:1227-49.

31.   Näbauer M, Beuckelmann DJ, Uberfuhr P, Steinbeck G. Regional differences in current density and rate-dependent properties of the transient outward current in subepicardial and subendocardial myocytes of human left ventricle. Circulation 1996;93:168-77.

32.   Wettwer E, Amos GJ, Posival H, Ravens U. Transient outward current in human ventricular myocytes of subepicardial and subendocardial origin. Circ Res 1994;75:473-82.

33.   Henderson EB, Kahn JK, Corbett JR, et al. Abnormal I-123 metaiodobenzylguanidine myocardial washout and distribution may reflect myocardial adrenergic derangement in patients with congestive cardiomyopathy. Circulation 1988;78:1192-99.

34.   Calkins H, Allman K, Bolling S,Kirsch M, Wieland D, Morady F, Schwaiger M. Correlation between scintigraphic evidence of regional sympathetic neuronal dysfunction and ventricular refractoriness in the human heart. Circulation 1993;88:172-79.

35.   Kuo C-S, Munakata K, Reddy CP, Surawicz B. Characteristics and possible mechanism of ventricular arrhythmia dependent on the dispersion of action potential durations. Circulation 1983;67:1356-67.

36.   Das SK, Morady F, DiCarlo L Jr., et al. Prognostic usefulness of programmed ventricular stimulation in idiopathic dilated cardiomyopathy with symptomatic ventricular arrhythmias. Am J Cardiol 1986;58:998-1000.

37.   Poll DS, Marchlinski FE, Buxton AE, Josephson ME. Usefulness of programmed stimulation in idiopathic dilated cardiomyopathy. Am J Cardiol 1986,58:992-97.

38.   Cameron JS, Myerburg RJ, Wong S, et al. Electrophysiological consequences of chronic experimentally induced left ventricular pressure overload. J Am Coll Cardiol 1983;2:481-87.

39.   Kowey PR, Frichling TD, Sewter J, et al. Electrophysiologic effects of left ventricular hypertrophy: Effects of calcium and potassium channel blockade. Circulation 1991;83:2067-75.

40.   Podrid PJ, Fogel RI, Fuchs TT. Ventricular arrhythmia in congestive heart failure. Am J Cardiol 1992;69:82G-96G.

41.   Roberts WC. Sudden cardiac death: Definitions and causes. Am J Cardiol 1986;57:1410-13.

42.   Wilber D, Garan H, Finkelstein D, et al. Out-of-hospital cardiac arrest: Use of electrophysiologic testing in the prediction of long-term outcome. N Engl J Med 1988;318:19-24.

43.   Liberthson RR, Nagel EL, Hirschman JC, Nussenfeld SR. Prehospital ventricular fibrillation: Prognosis and follow-up course. N Engl J Med 1974;219:317-21.

44. Luu M, Stevenson WG, Stevenson LW, Baron K, Walden J. Diverse mechanisms of unexpected cardiac arrest in advanced heart failure. Circulation 1989;80:1675-80.

45. Stevenson WG, Stevenson LW, Middlekauff HR, Saxon LA. Sudden death prevention in patients with advanced ventricular dysfunction. Circulation 1993;88:2953-61.

46. Meinertz T, Treese N, Kasper W, et al. Determinants of prognosis in idiopathic dilated cardiomyopathy as determined by programmed electrical stimulation. Am J Cardiol 1985; 56:337-41.

47. Stamato NJ, O'Connell JB, Murdock DK, Moran JF, Loeb HS, Scanlon PJ. The response of patients with compex ventricular arrhythmias secondary to dilated cardiomyopathy to programmed electrical stimulation. Am Heart J 1986;112:505-8.

48. Veltri EP, Platia EV, Griffith LSC, Reid PR. Programmed electrical stimulation and long-term follow-up in asymptomatic, nonsustained ventricular tachycardia. Am J Cardiol 1985;56:309-14.

49. Milner PG, DiMarco JP, Lerman BB. Electrophysiological evaluation of sustained ventricular tachyarrhythmia in idiopathic dilated cardiomyopathy. PACE 1988;11:562-68.

50. Mancini DM, Wong KL, Simson MB. Prognostic value of an abnormal signal-averaged electrocardiogram in patients with nonischemic cardiomyopathy. Circulation 1993;87:1083-92.

51. Poll DS, Marchlinski FE, Falcone RA, Simson MB. Abnormal signal averaged ECG in nonischemic congestive cardiomyopathy: Relationship to sustained ventricular tachyarrhythmias. Circulation 1986;72:1308-13.

52. Cohn J, Levine TB, Olivari MT, et al. Plasma norepinephrine as a guide to prognosis in patients with chronic congestive heart failure. N Engl J Med 1984;311:819-23.

53. Keren A, Tzivoni D, Gavish D, et al. Etiology, warning signals and therapy of torsades de pointes: A study of 10 patients. Circulation 1981;64:1167-74.

54. Nguyen PT, Scheinmann MM, Seger J. Polymorphous ventricular tachycardia: Clinical characterization, therapy, and the QT interval. Circulation 1986;74:340-9.

55. Wilson FN. The T deflection of the electrocardiogram. Trans Assoc Am Physicians 1931;46:29.

56. Gavrilescu S, Luca C. Right ventricular monophasic action potentials in patients with long QT syndrome. Br Heart J 1978;40:1014-18.

57. Bonatti V, Rolli A, Botti G. Recording of monophasic action potentials of the right ventricle in long QT syndrome complicated by severe ventricular arrhythmias. Eur Heart J 1983;4:168-79.

58. Zareba W, Badilini F, Moss AS. Automatic detection of spatial and dynamic heterogenity of repolarization. J Electrocardiol 1994;27:566-72.

59. Hii JTY, Wyse DG, Gillis AM, Duff HJ, Solylo MA, Mitchell LB. Precordial QT interval dispersion as a marker of torsade de pointes. Disparate effects of class Ia antiarrhythmic drugs and amiodarone. Circulation 1992;86:1376-82.

60. Day CP, McComb JM, Campbell RWF. QT dispersion: An indication of arrhythmia risk in patients with long QT intervals. Br Heart J 1990;63:342-44.

61. Day CP, McComb JM, Matthews, Campbell RWF. Reduction in QT dispersion by sotalol following myocardial infarction. Eur Heart J 1991;12:423-27.

62. Barr CS, Naas A, Freeman M, Lang CC, Struthers AD. QT dispersion and sudden unexpected death in chronic heart failure. Lancet 1994;343:327-29

63. Berger RD, Kasper EK, Baughman KL, Marban E, Calkins H, Tomaselli GF. Beat-to-beat QT interval variability: Novel evidence for repolarization lability in dilated cardiomyopathy.

Circulation 1997; in press.
64.   Kleiger RE, Miller JP, Bigger JT, Moss AJ and the Multicenter Post-Infarction Research Group. Decreased heart rate variability and its association with increased mortality after acute myocardial infarction. Am J Cardiol 1987;59:256-62.
65.   Bigger JT, Kleiger RE, Fleiss JL, Rolnitzky LM, Steinman RC, Miller JP and the Multicenter Post-Infarction Research Group. Components of heart rate variability measured during healing of acute myocardial infarction. Am J Cardiol 1988;61:208-15.
66.   Saul JP, Arai Y, Berger RD, Lilly LS, Colucci WS, Cohen RJ. Assessment of autonomic regulation in chronic congestive heart failure by heart rate spectral analysis. Am J Cardiol 1988;61:1292-99.
67.   Casolo G, Bali E, Taddei T, Amuhasi J, Gori C. Decreased spontaneous heart rate variability in congestive heart failure. Am J Cardiol 1989;64:1162-67.
68.   Coumel P, Hermida J-S, Wennerblöm, Leenhardt A, Maison-Blanche P, Cauchemez B. Heart rate variability in left ventricular hypertrophy and heart failure, and the effects of beta-blockade. Eur Heart J 1991;12:412-22.
69.   Woo MA, Stevenson WG, Moser DK, Trelease RB, Harper RM. Patterns of beat-to-beat heart rate variability in advanced heart failure. Am Heart J 1992;123:704-10.
70.   Kienzle MG, Ferguson DW, Birkett CL, Myers GA, Berg WJ, Mariano J. Clinical hemodynamic and sympathetic neural correlates of heart rate variability in congestive heart failure. Am J Cardiol 1992;69:761-67.

Subject index

Medical Science Symposia Series

1. A.M. Gotto, C. Lenfant, R. Paoletti (eds.) and M. Soma (ass.ed.): *Multiple Risk Factors in Cardiovascular Disease.* 1992   ISBN 0-7923-1938-9
2. A.L. Catapano, A.M. Gotto, Jr., L.C. Smith and R. Paoletti (eds.): *Drugs Affecting Lipid Metabolism.* 1993   ISBN 0-7923-2232-0
3. T. Godfraind, S. Govoni, R. Paoletti and P.M. Vanhoutte (eds.): *Calcium Antagonists. Pharmacology and Clinical Research.* 1993   ISBN 0-7923-2259-2
4. D. Galmarini, L.R. Fassati, R. Paoletti and S. Sherlock (eds.): *Drugs and the Liver: High Risk Patients and Transplantation.* 1993   ISBN 0-7923-2307-6
5. P.M. Vanhoutte, P.R. Saxena, R. Paoletti, N. Brunello (eds.) and A.S. Jackson (ass.ed.): *Serotonin. From Cell Biology to Pharmacology and Therapeutics.* 1993   ISBN 0-7923-2518-4
6. A.G. Dalgleish, A. Albertini and R. Paoletti (eds.): *The Impact of Biotechnology on Autoimmunity.* 1994   ISBN 0-7923-2724-1
7. P.G. Crosignani, R. Paoletti, P.M. Sarrel, N.K. Wenger (eds.), M. Meschia and M. Soma (ass.eds.): *Women's Health in Menopause. Behaviour, Cancer, Cardiovascular Disease, Hormone Replacement Therapy.* 1994   ISBN 0-7923-3068-4
8. A.M. Gotto Jr., C. Lenfant, A.L. Catapano and R. Paoletti (eds.): *Multiple Risk Factors in Cardiovascular Disease.* 1995   ISBN 0-7923-3503-1
9. T. Godfraind, G. Mancia, M.P. Abbracchio, L. Aguilar-Bryan and S. Govoni (eds.): *Pharmacological Control of Calcium and Potassium Homeostasis. Biological, Therapeutical, and Clinical Aspects.* 1995   ISBN 0-7923-3604-6
10. A.M. Gotto Jr., R. Paoletti, L.C. Smith, A.L. Catapano and A.S. Jackson (eds.): *Drugs Affecting Lipid Metabolism. Risk Factors and Future Directions.* 1996   ISBN 0-7923-4167-8
11. R. Paoletti, P.G. Crosignani, P. Kenemans, G. Samsioe, M. Soma and A.S. Jackson (eds.): *Women's Health and Menopause.* Risk Reduction Strategies. 1997   ISBN 0-7923-4697-1
12. A.M. Gotto Jr., C. Lenfant, R. Paoletti, A.L. Catapano and A.S. Jackson (eds.): *Multiple Risk Factors in Cardiovascular Disease.* Strategies of Prevention of Coronary Heart Disease, Cardiac Failure, and Stroke. 1998   ISBN 0-7923-5023-5

KLUWER ACADEMIC PUBLISHERS – DORDRECHT / BOSTON / LONDON